Regulatory Policies and Technical Guidances on Traditional Chinese Medicines in China

中国中药监管政策与技术指引

BILINGUAL EDITION　　VOLUME 1

英中双语版　第一辑

Edited by　Editorial Board

本书编委会　编

中国健康传媒集团　China Health Media Group

中国医药科技出版社　China Medical Science Press

图书在版编目（CIP）数据

中国中药监管政策与技术指引. 第一辑 : 英、汉 /
《中国中药监管政策与技术指引》英中双语版编辑委员会
编 . -- 北京 : 中国医药科技出版社，2024. 8. -- ISBN
978-7-5214-4773-6

Ⅰ. R288

中国国家版本馆 CIP 数据核字第 2024FW4938 号

出版　**中国健康传媒集团**｜中国医药科技出版社
地址　北京市海淀区文慧园北路甲 22 号
邮编　100082
电话　发行：010-62227427　邮购：010-62236938
网址　www.cmstp.com
规格　710×1000mm $\frac{1}{16}$
印张　$33\frac{1}{4}$
字数　595 千字
版次　2024 年 8 月第 1 版
印次　2024 年 8 月第 1 次印刷
印刷　北京盛通印刷股份有限公司
经销　全国各地新华书店
书号　ISBN 978-7-5214-4773-6
定价　**136.00 元**

Regulatory Policies and Technical Guidances on Traditional Chinese Medicines in China

Editorial Board

《中国中药监管政策与技术指引》

编辑委员会

名誉主编 赵军宁

主　　编 董江萍　　王海南　　周思源

副 主 编 曹莉莉　　王翔宇　　于江泳

顾问委员 叶祖光

编　　委（按姓氏拼音顺序排列）

艾　华　蔡　毅　曹　晖　曹　宜　陈文星

程　龙　程翼宇　郭　青　果德安　韩　玲

黄芳华　季　申　赖　寒　梁　纯　马秀璟

聂黎行　彭　健　石上梅　舒　融　唐健元

唐民科　吴啟南　许文杰　阳长明　杨　渝

张体灯　张永文　赵　明　周　恒

执行编委 史赤天　洪　耕

执行编辑 王　珂

Introduction

With the acceleration of the modernization and globalization of traditional Chinese medicines (TCMs), their spread and influence have been increasingly enlarged in the world, attracting a mounting number of attention and recognition from people all over the world. A pattern of all-round, multi-angle, wide-range, and high-level cooperation in the field of international cooperation in TCMs is taking shape. However, the globalization of TCMs is not always smooth, and one of the biggest challenges is the harmonization of regulation. The TCMs are characterized by their complex composition, unique preparation and treatment concepts that are different from those of western medicine, which make the safety, efficacy, and quality control of TCMs a difficult regulatory issue. As TCMs go global, how to establish a regulatory system that can safeguard the characteristics of TCMs and at the same time comply with international standards has become an urgent issue.

At present, the National Medical Products Administration is developing a world-leading excellent regulatory system for TCMs with Chinese characteristics, in line with the characteristics of traditional Chinese medicines, and establishing a transformation mechanism for the research fruits of TCMs regulation science. We also actively promote to develop a regulatory coordination mechanism for the globalization of TCMs. In 2023, the Measures on Further Strengthening the Scientific Regulation of Traditional Chinese Medicines to Promote Its Preservation and Innovative Development was issued as Document No. 1, taking "promoting cooperation in the globalization of the regulation of TCMs" as an important initiative to comprehensively implement the "promoting the preservation and innovative development of TCMs". The CCFDIE actively promotes the translation of relevant documents, regulations, and technical guidelines for TCMs regulation, invites experts to translate important documents and relevant technical guidelines for the review and approval of TCMs, and contributes to the Chinese experience in the international rules and standards for the regulation of TCMs.

This collection of technical guidelines covers the registration classification of TCMs and the requirements for application dossiers, standard format and writing guidelines, manufacturing process, specifications, pharmacological and toxicological studies, clinical studies, etc. Chinese version has been officially released by the National Medical Product Administration. The corresponding English version is a supporting translation version, aiming at provide reference and guidance for TCMs industry, regulatory authorities, academic institutions, as well as readers from domestic and abroad who interested in the globalization of TCMs.

In the days ahead, the path to globalization of TCMs may be full of challenges, but also full of opportunities. This series of technical guidelines aspires to be a driving force in introducing TCMs to the world, contributing a modest effort to the international exchange and collaboration of TCMs. We believe that with the promotion of scientific, standardized and transparent regulation of TCMs, the global interest on TCMs will continue to improve, the regulatory system will be further improved, the path to the globalization of TCMs will broaden, and ultimately achieve the global development of TCMs.

Here, I would like to thank all the experts, scholars, colleagues from industry and everyone who thrives to the compilation, translation and revision of this series of books. The publication of this series of books is inseparable from their hard work and valuable opinions. At the same time, I would also like to express my gratitude to the TCMs review & approval team from the CDE of NMPA for your long-term commitment to research and your contribution to a technical system for evaluation that not only follows the general rules of international drug development and evaluation but also conforms to the characteristics of TCMs, laying solid technical support for the international coordination of TCMs regulation.

Then, I would also like to thank the readers for your reading and support. I hope this series of books can provide you with valuable information and inspiration. Through this series of books, your witness on the globalization process of TCMs and exploration for its unique value and far-reaching significance in global health are highly appreciated.

Hope that the TCMs go further on the global stage and make even greater contributions to the health industry for humanity!

ZHAO Junning

July 2024

序 言

随着中药现代化、全球化进程加速，中药在世界范围的传播与影响日益扩大，越来越多地受到世界各地人民的关注和认可。中药对外合作全方位、多角度、宽领域、高层次合作格局正在形成。然而，中药"走出去"进程并非一帆风顺，其中最大的挑战之一便是监管的国际化。中药的特色在于其复杂的成份、独特的制备过程以及与西方医学不同的治疗理念，这些特点使得中药的安全性、有效性和质量控制成为监管的难点。随着中药走向世界，如何建立一个既能够保障中药特性又能够符合国际标准的监管体系，成为一个亟待解决的问题。

目前，国家药监局正加快打造具有中国特色、符合中药特点、全球领先的中药卓越监管体系，建立中药监管科学研究转化机制，积极推动构建全球化中药（传统药）监管政策协调机制。2023 年以 1 号文件印发《关于进一步加强中药科学监管促进中药传承创新发展的若干措施》，将"推进中药监管全球化合作"作为全面贯彻"促进中医药传承创新发展"重大战略部署的重要举措。中国食品药品国际交流中心积极推进中药监管相关政策规定和技术指导原则翻译工作，组织专家分批次对中药审评审批重要文件和相关技术指导原则进行翻译，为国际传统草药监管规则和标准制修订贡献"中国经验"。

本系列技术指导原则涵盖中药注册分类及申报资料要求、通用格式和撰写指南、生产工艺、质量标准、药理毒理研究、临床研究等方面内容，其中文版业已由国家药监局正式发布。英文版为配套翻译版本，旨在为国内外中药企业、监管机构、研究人员以及对中药"走出去"感兴趣的读者提供参考和指导。

在未来的日子里，中药"走出去"的道路或许充满挑战，但也充满机遇。本书期望成为推动中药走向世界的一份力量，为中药的国际交流与合作贡献一份绵薄之力。我们相信，随着对中药监管科学化、标准化和透明化的推动，全球对中药认知将得到不断提升、监管体系将更加完善，中药"走出去"之路将越走越宽广，最终实现中药的全球化发展。

在此，我要感谢所有为本系列丛书的编纂、翻译、审校提供帮助的专家学者、业界同仁和工作人员，本系列丛书的出版离不开他们的辛勤工作和宝贵意见。同时，也感谢国家药监局药品审评中心的中药审评技术团队，你们长期致力于研究构建既遵循国际药物研发和评价一般规律又符合中医药特点的技术评价体系，为中药监管国际协调打下扎实的技术支撑。

还要感谢广大读者的阅读和支持，希望本系列丛书能够为您提供有价值的信息和启发。欢迎各位读者通过本系列丛书，一同见证中药"走出去"进程，探寻其在全球健康事业中的独特价值与深远意义。

祝愿中药在全球的传播之路越走越远，为人类的健康事业作出更大贡献！

赵军宁

2024 年 7 月

Contents
目 录

Regulatory Policies
监 管 政 策

Technical Guidances
技 术 指 引

Regulatory Policies
监管政策

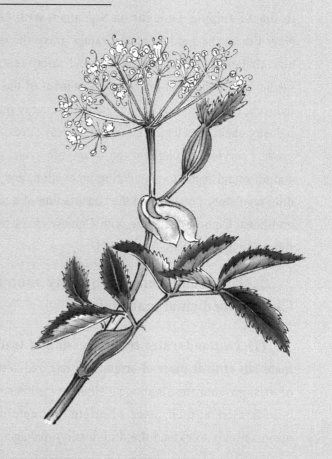

Several Measures to Further Strengthen the Scientific Regulation of Traditional Chinese Medicine and Promote the Inheritance, Innovation and Development of Traditional Chinese Medicine

In order to thoroughly implement the spirit of the 20th Party Congress, fully implement the 20th Party Congress Report on the major strategic deployment of "strengthening food and drug safety regulation" and "promoting the inheritance, innovation and development of traditional Chinese medicine (TCM)", adhere to the Xi Jinping Thought on Socialism with Chinese Characteristics for a New Era as the guidance, accurately grasp the new situation, new tasks and new challenges facing the quality and safety regulation of traditional Chinese medicine and the high-quality development of the traditional Chinese medicine industry, comprehensively strengthen the quality management of the whole TCM industry chain, accelerate the whole process of review and approval, and enhance product services throughout the whole life cycle, global regulatory cooperation and all-round regulatory scientific innovation, and promote the Chinese modern drug regulatory practice and the construction of a scientific regulatory system for traditional Chinese medicine with Chinese characteristics to a deeper extent, the following measures are formulated.

I. To strengthen the quality management of traditional Chinese medicinal materials

(I) To standardize the processing of traditional Chinese medicinal materials at their place of origin. It is required to further mobilize the enthusiasm of local governments, traditional Chinese medicinal materials manufacturers and base farmers at their place of origin, promote traditional Chinese medicine manufacturers to extend the drug quality management system to the cultivation and processing of traditional Chinese medicinal materials, and promote the combination of traditional Chinese medicinal materials production and processing with the construction of ecological civilization and rural revitalization. The provincial medical products regulatory authorities shall strengthen the regulation over manufacturers of TCM prepared slices to purchase and process (cut while fresh) traditional Chinese medicinal materials at the place of origin, standardize the processing and purchase of traditional Chinese medicinal materials at the place of origin, and strengthen the quality management of fresh cut traditional Chinese medicinal materials on the basis of conforming to the *Good Agricultural Practice* (GAP).

(II) To promote the implementation of the *Good Agricultural Practice* (GAP). It is required to give full play to the important role of GAP in the regulation of the production quality of traditional Chinese medicinal materials, establish a national GAP expert working group, study and improve the implementation promotion plan and supporting technical requirements, and promote the standardization, industrialization and large-scale cultivation of traditional Chinese medicinal materials. Through GAP extended inspection, compliance inspection and daily supervision and inspection, traditional Chinese medicine manufacturers are encouraged to adopt self-construction, co-construction, joint construction or sharing of traditional Chinese medicine planting and breeding bases, stabilize the supply of traditional Chinese medicinal materials, and use traditional Chinese medicinal materials that meet GAP requirements. Through variety-by-variety and step-by-step studies, the traditional Chinese medicinal materials used in the production of some key or high-risk traditional Chinese medicines should meet the requirements of GAP. In principle, the traditional Chinese medicinal materials used in the production of traditional Chinese medicine injections should meet the requirements of GAP.

(III) To improve the registration regulation of traditional Chinese medicinal materials. Jointly with the National Administration of Traditional Chinese Medicine, the *Catalogue of Traditional Chinese Medicinal Materials Subject to Approval Management* has to be formulated to carry out the approval and management of traditional Chinese medicinal materials that meet the requirements in accordance with the law. It is required to strengthen the management of local folk medicinal materials, revise the *Provision for Local Common Medicinal Materials*, guide the provincial medical products regulatory authorities to formulate and revise the local folk medicinal materials standards, and ensure the coordination and consistence of local standards and national standards of drug.

(IV) To establish the quality monitoring mechanism of traditional Chinese medicinal materials. It is required to organize comprehensive analysis of the quality monitoring data of traditional Chinese medicinal materials, pay attention to quality differences of traditional Chinese medicinal materials in different places of origin, and study to issue the quality monitoring report of traditional Chinese medicinal materials. It is also required to build a national basic database for the quality of traditional Chinese medicinal materials that covers the information of the variety, place of origin, quality and safety of traditional Chinese medicinal materials, and promote the sharing of data and information of traditional Chinese medicinal materials.

(V) To improve the import management of traditional Chinese medicinal materials. It is required to continue to strengthen the inspection capacity building for imported medicinal materials and improve the quality traceability level thereof. According to the requirements of the national strategic regional planning, it is required to carry out the on-site assessment and evaluation of the application for adding ports for drug import or border ports for medicinal materials import in an orderly manner, and approve such application in a reasonable manner.

II. To strengthen the regulation of TCM prepared slices and traditional Chinese medicine formula granules

(VI) To strengthen the review and approval management of TCM prepared slices. It is required to follow the theories and laws of traditional Chinese medicine, focus on the quality and safety risks, promote the research on the processing mechanism of TCM prepared slices, and establish and improve the relevant quality evaluation system. Jointly with the National Administration of Traditional Chinese Medicine, the *Catalogue of TCM prepared slices Subject to Approval Management* and supporting documents have to be formulated to carry out the review and approval management of TCM prepared slices that meet the requirements in accordance with the law.

(VII) To improve the processing standards of TCM prepared slices. It is required to release, implement and continuously improve the *National Standards for the Processing of TCM prepared slices* in batches, strengthen the filing management of the provincial standards for the processing of TCM prepared slices, and guide the formulation and revision of the provincial standards for the processing of TCM prepared slices. It is also required to strengthen the regulation over the implementation of the provincial standards for the processing of TCM prepared slices, and improve the production, circulation, and use management of TCM prepared slices produced in accordance with the provincial standards for the processing of TCM prepared slices.

(VIII) To standardize the production and quality traceability of TCM prepared slices. It is required to follow the processing characteristics of TCM prepared slices, combine traditional processing methods and modern production techniques, study to improve the good manufacturing practice of TCM prepared slices, explore to establish a tracing system for the production and circulation of TCM prepared slices, so as to gradually realize the mutual sharing of information on the source, destination and traceability of key varieties. It is also required to issue and implement the *Regulations on the Management of Packaging Labels of TCM prepared slices (Trial)* and related supporting technical documents to standardize the labeling contents of TCM prepared slices.

(IX) To promote the improvement of the production and distribution modes of TCM prepared slices. It is required to guide and urge the manufacturers of TCM prepared slices to optimize and adjust the production structure of varieties in combination with industrial planning, resource advantages, technical capabilities and other production practices, to gradually promote the intensive, high-quality and large-scale production mode of TCM prepared slices.

(X) To strengthen the production process management of traditional Chinese medicine formula granules. It is required to regulate and urge the manufacturers of traditional Chinese medicine formula granules to produce in strict accordance with the filed manufacturing process, strictly inspect the suppliers, strengthen the quality management of the whole process of identification of traditional Chinese medicinal materials, processing of TCM prepared slices, granules production, inspection and release, to ensure that the whole production process conforms to the corresponding drug standards and the *Good Manufacturing Practice.*

III. To optimize the management of traditional Chinese medicine preparations in medical institutions

(XI) **To give full play to the role of traditional Chinese medicine preparations in medical institutions.** It is required to promote medical institutions to adapt big data, AI, real-world research and other technical means, and carry out research on traditional Chinese medicine preparations in medical institutions based on clinical orientation, suitable population, usage and dosage, course of treatment and evaluation indicators reflecting the characteristics and advantages of traditional Chinese medicine. It is also required to give full play to the role of human use experience in supporting the safety and effectiveness of traditional Chinese medicine preparations in medical institutions, and support the transformation of traditional Chinese medicine preparations in medical institutions with definite curative effect, obvious characteristic advantages and less adverse reactions into new drugs.

(XII) **To strictly file and regulate the use of traditional Chinese medicine preparations in medical institutions.** It is required to carry out the filing management of traditional Chinese medicine preparations prepared by medical institutions in strict accordance with the regulations, timely check the data and on-site inspection of the filed medical institutions' preparations, and carry out sampling inspection in accordance with relevant regulations when necessary. It is also required to standardize the use of traditional Chinese medicine preparations in medical institutions, and support the implementation of multi-center clinical research in different medical institutions through adjustment. The provincial medical products regulatory authorities shall standardize and strengthen the supervision of the regional preparation workshop of traditional Chinese medicine preparations in medical institutions, and strictly supervise the quality of traditional Chinese medicine preparations in accordance with the relevant provisions of the *Good Manufacturing Practice*.

(XIII) To strengthen the monitoring of adverse reactions of traditional Chinese medicine preparations in medical institutions. It is required to promote medical institutions to establish and improve the pharmacovigilance system, take the initiative to monitor, identify, evaluate and control the suspected adverse reactions of traditional Chinese medicine preparations in medical institutions, conduct research and comprehensive evaluation on the effectiveness and safety of traditional Chinese medicine preparations in medical institutions when necessary, and take the initiative to apply to the local provincial medical products regulatory authority for cancellation of relevant approval documents or cancellation for filing if the effect is uncertain, adverse reactions are serious, or there are other reasons endangering human health.

IV. To improve the review and approval mechanism of traditional Chinese medicine

(XIV) To continue to promote the research and innovation of the evaluation system of traditional Chinese medicine. It is required to optimize the review and approval system and mechanism of traditional Chinese medicine, promote the change of registration acceleration "at the final stage" to the whole process of acceleration with "frontward" extension, formulate and implement the *Special Provisions on the Administration of Registration of Traditional Chinese Medicine*, accelerate the construction of the "three-in-one" review evidence system of traditional Chinese medicine theory, human use experience, and clinical trials, and establish and improve the clinical value-oriented diversified technical standards and clinical efficacy evaluation methods of traditional Chinese medicine.

(XV) To improve the emergency review and approval mechanism of traditional Chinese medicine. It is required to respond to public health emergencies quickly and effectively, and implement special review and approval procedures for traditional Chinese medicines that are urgently needed according to the health administration or traditional Chinese medicine administration under the State Council. It is also required to encourage and support the research and development of new traditional Chinese medicine for major diseases, rare diseases or children, and give priority to the review and approval of relevant registration applications that meet the prescribed circumstances.

(XVI) To improve the classification management of prescription and OTC drugs of traditional Chinese medicine. It is required to optimize the technical guidance system and requirements related to OTC drug registration and post-marketing conversion, standardize the technical evaluation of the conversion of prescription drugs into OTC drugs, study to formulate technical requirements for the evaluation of OTC drugs, and further give full play to the role of traditional Chinese patent medicines in self-medication.

V. To pay attention to the post–marketing regulation of traditional Chinese medicine

(XVII) To improve the post-marketing management mechanism of traditional Chinese medicine. It is required to strengthen the whole life cycle services of drugs, urge drug marketing authorization holders to fulfill their primary responsibilities and obligations, develop the post-marketing risk management plan according to product characteristics, proactively carry out post-marketing study and post-marketing evaluation, and conduct comprehensive analysis and evaluation on the benefits and risks of drugs. According to the evaluation results, it is required to take measures such as revising package inserts, suspending production and sales, recalling drugs, and actively applying for cancellation of drug approval documents according to law. In addition, it is also required to urge drug marketing authorization holders to proactively carry out post-marketing study and evaluation of traditional Chinese medicine injections and continuously improve their pharmacovigilance level and ability for traditional Chinese medicine injections.

(XVIII) To strengthen the regulation of post-marketing changes of traditional Chinese medicine. It is required to improve the management of post-marketing changes based on risk control, further clarify the criteria for risk level classification of different changes, and strengthen the review and approval of high-risk change varieties. It is also required to strengthen the sense of primary responsibility of drug marketing authorization holders to proactively improve the quality of traditional Chinese medicine, give full play to the advantages of terminal policy effect, and improve the whole life cycle management ability of marketing authorization holders for drugs.

(XIX) To strengthen the monitoring of adverse reactions of traditional Chinese medicine. It is required to research and develop monitoring tools for adverse drug reaction signals of traditional Chinese medicine that conform to the characteristics of traditional Chinese medicine, conduct comprehensive analysis and judgment on the identified safety risk signals in time, take corresponding risk control measures, strengthen the monitoring and disposal of adverse drug reaction aggregation events, and timely prevent and control risks in drug use.

VI. To improve the standard management level of traditional Chinese medicine

(XX) To optimize the standard management of traditional Chinese medicine. It is required to study to formulate special regulations for the standard management of traditional Chinese medicine. Taking the revision of Chinese Pharmacopoeia (Volume I) as an opportunity, it is required to explore the implementation of national standards for traditional Chinese medicine to formulate quality management specifications, and timely transform scientific, mature and applicable registration standards for traditional Chinese medicine, international standards, group standards or enterprise internal control standards into national standards. In addition, it is also required to establish the rapid revision mechanism and procedures for national standards of traditional Chinese medicine, strengthen the construction of the special committee on traditional Chinese medicine of Pharmacopoeia Committee, and improve the selection and determination mechanism of committee members.

(XXI) To scientifically improve the standards for traditional Chinese medicine. It is required to continue to promote the formulation and revision of standards for traditional Chinese medicine, and accelerate the release and implementation of national standards for the processing of TCM prepared slices and standards for the traditional Chinese medicine formula granules. It is also required to reasonably set the limit requirements and test methods for pesticide residues, heavy metals and harmful elements, mycotoxins and other harmful substances in traditional Chinese medicine as well as for plant growth regulators. In addition, it is required to strengthen the research on testing technology and risk assessment system of endogenous toxic components of traditional Chinese medicine, formulate the limit standard of endogenous toxic components in line with the characteristics of traditional Chinese medicine, and improve the usage and dosage.

(XXII) **To strengthen the research & development and supply of standard substances for traditional Chinese medicine.** It is required to improve the mechanism for the research & development and continuous supply of standard substances for traditional Chinese medicine , strengthen the mechanism for dynamic early warning and information feedback, carry out demand analysis and develop the research & development plan, and strengthen quality monitoring. In addition, it is required to classify and improve the technical requirements for the research & development and calibration of standard substances for traditional Chinese medicine such as chemical reference substances, reference medicinal materials and reference extracts.

(XXIII) **To improve the digital management level of traditional Chinese medicine standards.** It is required to establish and improve the dynamic database of national drug standards and drug registration standards of traditional Chinese medicine, accelerate the construction of digital standards, timely update the data, to realize the informatization of the release, query, analysis, research and maintenance of drug standards.

VII. To strengthen the safety regulation of traditional Chinese medicine

(XXIV) **To innovate the quality regulation mode of traditional Chinese medicine.** It is required to gradually build a "grid" regulation mode, improve the construction of the regulation system for the production of traditional Chinese medicine, and study, formulate and supervise the implementation of the *Good Manufacturing Practice for Traditional Chinese Medicine*. It is also required to gradually establish and improve the risk analysis and judgment mechanism for the regionalization of traditional Chinese medicine production, continue to strengthen the regulation and inspection of TCM prepared slices, traditional Chinese medicine formula granules and traditional Chinese patent medicine for key enterprises, key varieties and key links, and carry out the extended inspection of traditional Chinese medicine in an orderly manner. In addition, it is required to further standardize the circulation and distribution order of TCM prepared slices, traditional Chinese medicine formula granules and traditional Chinese patent medicines, and strengthen the quality regulation in the use.

(XXV) To strengthen the quality sampling inspection and monitoring of traditional Chinese medicine. It is required to continue to promote and improve the quality sampling inspection of TCM prepared slices, traditional Chinese medicine formula granules and traditional Chinese patent medicines, scientifically carry out exploratory research based on regulatory needs and the actual development of the industry, comprehensively analyze and judge the sampling inspection and monitoring data, take corresponding risk prevention and control or quality improvement measures according to the risk, optimize the working mechanism for the release of traditional Chinese medicine quality announcements, publish the sampling inspection and monitoring results according to law, and objectively and accurately transmit the quality and safety information of traditional Chinese medicine to the public.

(XXVI) To severely crack down on violations of laws and regulations. It is required to strictly investigate and punish drug marketing authorization holders, manufacturers and/or distributors suspected of falsification in registration and filing, as well as adulteration, fabrication of records, illegal sales and other violations of laws and regulations in accordance with the law. It is also required to strictly crack down on illegal and criminal activities such as the manufacture and sales of counterfeit traditional Chinese medicines in "dens", make full use of clues such as online monitoring, complaints and reports, and work jointly with public security organs, judicial and other departments to resolutely investigate the source and pursue it to the end, prosecute the criminal responsibility of criminals in accordance with the law, and stick to the bottom line for traditional Chinese medicine safety.

VIII. To promote global cooperation in the regulation of traditional Chinese medicine

(XXVII) To give full play to the role of international cooperation platform. It is required to further deepen the international cooperation among the World Health Organization (WHO), the International Regulatory Cooperation for Herbal Medicines (IRCH) and the Forum for the Harmonization of Herbal Medicines (FHH), give full play to platforms such as "The Belt and Road Initiative" international cooperation framework, the "China-ASEAN Drug Cooperation and Development Summit Forum" and the WHO Collaborating Centre for Traditional Medicine, and actively promote the further formation of international consensus on traditional herbal medicine regulation and cooperation, and standard coordination.

(XXVIII) To support the international registration of traditional Chinese medicine. It is required to actively promote and exchange international registration policies for traditional Chinese medicines, support the international registration of domestic traditional Chinese medicines with clinical advantages, and encourage the implementation of international multi-center clinical trials of traditional Chinese medicines. In addition, it is required to organize the inspection of the place of origin of imported medicinal materials, production fields such as the initial processing field, etc., and the research & development and production of traditional Chinese medicines (natural medicines) abroad according to the plan.

(XXIX) To share "Chinese experience" in the regulation of traditional Chinese medicine. It is required to accelerate the translation of policies and regulations related to the regulation of traditional Chinese medicine and technical guidelines, release English version of technical guidelines related to traditional Chinese medicine, promote international publicity, and share "Chinese experience" to the revision of international regulatory rules and standards for traditional herbal medicines.

IX. Supporting measures

(XXX) To strengthen inter-departmental collaboration. It is required to strengthen the coordination and linkage with the National Health Commission, the National Healthcare Security Administration, the National Administration of Traditional Chinese Medicine and other departments, strengthen communication and exchange in the process of formulating major policies related to traditional Chinese medicine, and form a good situation for all departments to jointly promote the inheritance, innovation and development of traditional Chinese medicine.

(XXXI) To vigorously develop the regulatory science of traditional Chinese medicine. It is required to research and formulate scientific development strategies and key paths for traditional Chinese medicine regulation, and promote the development of the scientific action plan for drug regulation of the National Medical Products Administration. It is also required to actively prepare for the establishment of a national key laboratory for drug regulatory science, rely on the National Medical Products Administration's drug regulatory science base, key laboratories and key project implementation, promote the research of new tools, methods and standards for the evaluation of traditional Chinese medicine, and establish a transformation recognition process to promote their use in the regulation of traditional Chinese medicine, establish and improve a scientific system for the regulation of traditional Chinese medicine with Chinese characteristics, and solve basic, critical, frontier and strategic technical problems in the regulation of traditional Chinese medicine.

(XXXII) To strengthen the construction of high-end think tanks. It is required to give full play to the role of high-end think tanks, establish an expert advisory committee on strategic decision-making of traditional Chinese medicine management composed of academicians, traditional Chinese medicine masters and senior experts in the field of traditional Chinese medicine and other related disciplines, establish an expert panel on scientific work of traditional Chinese medicine regulation, provide relevant policy and legal advice for the National

Medical Products Administration, put forward decision-making references and work suggestions, to ensure the scientific and authoritative nature of major decisions on traditional Chinese medicine regulation.

(XXXIII) To pay attention to the training of regulatory science talents. It is required to strengthen the cooperation with high-level research institutions, colleges and universities, industry associations, and research associations, etc., build a curriculum system for the training of traditional Chinese medicine regulation talents, carry out regulation ability and practical training by category, and cultivate a regulation team compatible with the high-quality development of traditional Chinese medicine.

(XXXIV) To consolidate the infrastructure of traditional Chinese medicine regulation. It is required to strengthen the construction of basic data of traditional Chinese medicine regulation, carry out data science research, and promote the construction of intelligent regulation mode of traditional Chinese medicine with data as the core from the aspects of technical standards, quality traceability, process monitoring and risk monitoring, etc.

(XXXV) To fully implement the national regional strategy. It is required to implement national regional development strategies such as the "Beijing-Tianjin-Hebei Coordinated Development", "Yangtze River Delta Regional Integration" and "Guangdong-Hong Kong-Macao Greater Bay Area Construction", and build a demonstration zone for the comprehensive reform of traditional Chinese medicine, and encourage the medical products regulatory authorities in well-developed areas to take the lead in strengthening quality and safety regulation of traditional Chinese medicine and promoting the higher quality development of the traditional Chinese medicine industry.

关于进一步加强中药科学监管
促进中药传承创新发展的若干措施

为深入贯彻党的二十大精神，全面落实二十大报告关于"强化食品药品安全监管""促进中医药传承创新发展"的重大战略部署，坚持以习近平新时代中国特色社会主义思想为指导，准确把握当前中药质量安全监管和中药产业高质量发展面临的新形势、新任务和新挑战，全面加强中药全产业链质量管理、全过程审评审批加速、全生命周期产品服务、全球化监管合作、全方位监管科学创新，向纵深推进中国式现代化药品监管实践和具有中国特色的中药科学监管体系建设，特制定以下若干措施。

一、加强中药材质量管理

（一）**规范中药材产地加工**。进一步调动中药材产地地方政府、中药材生产企业、基地农户积极性，推动中药生产企业将药品质量管理体系向中药材种植加工环节延伸，促进中药材生产加工与生态文明建设和乡村振兴结合。省级药品监督管理部门要加强中药饮片生产企业采购产地加工（趁鲜切制）中药材监管，在符合《中药材生产质量管理规范》（GAP）的基础上，规范中药材产地加工及采购行为，加强趁鲜切制中药材质量管理。

（二）**推进实施《中药材生产质量管理规范》（GAP）**。充分发挥GAP在中药材生产质量监管的重要作用，组建国家GAP专家工作组，研究完善实施工作推进方案和配套技术要求，促进中药材规范化、产业化、规模化种植养殖。通过GAP延伸检查、符合性检查和日常监督检查，推动中药生产企业采取自建、共建、联建或共享中药材种植养殖基地，稳定中药材供给，使用符合GAP要求的中药材。分品种、分步骤研究明确部分重点或高风险中药品种生产使用的中药材应当符合GAP要求。中药注射剂生产所用的中药材，原则上应当符合GAP要求。

（三）**完善中药材注册管理**。会同国家中医药管理局制定《实施审批管理的中药材品种目录》，依法对符合规定情形的中药材品种实施审批管理。加强对地区性民间习用药材管理，修订《地区性民间习用药材管理办法》，指导省级药品监督管理部门制修订地区性民间习用药材标准，确保地方药材标准与国家药品标准协调统一。

（四）**建立中药材质量监测工作机制**。组织综合分析中药材质量监测数据，关注不同产地中药材质量的差异，研究发布中药材质量监测报告。构建涵盖药材品种考证、产地、质量、安全等信息的国家中药材质量基本数据库，促进中药材数据信息的共享和共用。

（五）**改进中药材进口管理**。持续强化进口药材检验能力建设，提升进口药材质量追溯水平。根据国家战略区域规划要求，有序开展对申请增设允许药品进口的口岸或允许药材进口的边境口岸现场考核评估工作，合理增设允许药品进口的口岸或允许药材进口的边境口岸。

二、强化中药饮片、中药配方颗粒监管

（六）**加强中药饮片审批管理**。遵循中医药理论和用药规律，围绕质量安全风险，推动中药饮片炮制机理研究，建立健全中药饮片质量评价体系。会同国家中医药管理局制定《实施审批管理的中药饮片目录》及配套文件，依法对符合规定情形的中药饮片实施审批管理。

（七）**完善中药饮片炮制规范**。分批发布实施并不断提高完善《国家中药饮片炮制规范》，加强对省级中药饮片炮制规范的备案管理，指导省级中药饮片炮制规范的制定和修订。强化省级中药饮片炮制规范监督实施，完善按照省级中药饮片炮制规范生产中药饮片的生产、流通、使用管理等规定。

（八）**规范中药饮片生产和质量追溯**。遵循中药饮片炮制特点，结合传统炮制方法和现代生产技术手段，研究完善中药饮片生产质量管理规范，探索建立中药饮片生产流通追溯体系，逐步实现重点品种来源可查、去向可追和追溯信息互通互享。发布实施《中药饮片包装标签管理规定（试行）》及相关配套技术文件，规范中药饮片标签的标识内容。

（九）**推动改进中药饮片生产经营模式**。引导和督促中药饮片生产企业结合产业规划、资源优势、技术能力等生产实际，优化调整品种生产结构，逐步推进实现中药饮片集约化、精品化、规模化的生产模式。

（十）**强化中药配方颗粒生产过程管理**。督促中药配方颗粒生产企业严格按照备案的生产工艺生产，严格供应商审核，加强中药材鉴别、中药饮片炮制、颗粒生产、检验放行等全环节质量管理，确保生产全过程符合相应的药品标准和药品生产质量管理规范。

三、优化医疗机构中药制剂管理

（十一）积极发挥医疗机构中药制剂作用。 推动医疗机构采用大数据、人工智能、真实世界研究等技术手段，围绕临床定位、适用人群、用法用量、疗程以及体现中药作用特点和优势的评价指标等对医疗机构中药制剂开展研究。发挥人用经验对医疗机构中药制剂的安全性、有效性的支持作用，支持将疗效确切、特色优势明显，不良反应少的医疗机构中药制剂品种向新药转化。

（十二）严格备案和调剂使用医疗机构中药制剂。 严格按照规定开展医疗机构应用传统工艺配制中药制剂的备案管理工作，及时对已备案的医疗机构制剂进行资料核查和现场检查，必要时按照相关规定开展抽样检验。规范调剂使用医疗机构中药制剂，支持通过调剂在不同医疗机构内开展多中心临床研究。省级药品监督管理部门参照《药品生产质量管理规范》等相关规定，规范和加强医疗机构中药制剂区域配制车间监管，严格监管其配制中药制剂的质量。

（十三）加强医疗机构中药制剂不良反应监测。 推动医疗机构建立和完善药物警戒体系，主动开展对医疗机构中药制剂疑似不良反应的监测、识别、评估和控制，必要时对医疗机构中药制剂的有效性、安全性开展研究和综合评价，对疗效不确切、不良反应大或者其他原因危害人体健康的，主动向所在地省级药品监督管理部门申请注销有关批准证明文件或注销备案。

四、完善中药审评审批机制

（十四）持续推动中药评价体系的研究和创新。 优化中药审评审批体系和机制，推进注册"末端"加速变为向"前端"延伸的全程加速，制定发布实施《中药注册管理专门规定》，加快推进中医药理论、人用经验、临床试验"三结合"审评证据体系建设，建立完善以临床价值为导向的多元化中药评价技术标准和临床疗效评价方法。

（十五）完善中药应急审评审批机制。 快速有效应对公共突发卫生事件，对国务院卫生健康或者中医药管理部门认定急需中药实施特别审批程序。鼓励并扶持用于重大疾病、罕见病，或者儿童用中药新药的研制，对符合规定情形的相关注册申请实行优先审评审批。

（十六）完善中药处方药与非处方药分类管理。 优化非处方药上市注册与上市后转换相关技术指导原则体系和要求，规范开展中药处方药转换为非处方药技术评价，研究制定中药非处方药审评技术要求，进一步发挥中成药在自我药疗中的作用。

五、重视中药上市后管理

（十七）**完善中药上市后管理工作机制**。加强药品全生命周期服务，督促药品上市许可持有人履行主体责任和义务，根据产品特点制定上市后风险管理计划，主动开展上市后研究和上市后评价，对药品的获益和风险进行综合分析评估。根据评估结果，依法采取修订药品说明书、暂停生产销售、召回药品、主动申请注销药品批准证明文件等措施。督促药品上市许可持有人主动开展中药注射剂上市后研究和评价，持续提升对中药注射剂的药物警戒水平和能力。

（十八）**强化中药上市后变更管理**。完善基于风险控制的上市后变更管理，进一步明确不同变更风险等级划分的标准，加强对高风险变更品种的审评审批。强化药品上市许可持有人主动提升中药质量的主体责任意识，发挥末端政策发力优势，提升药品上市许可持有人对产品的全生命周期管理能力。

（十九）**加强中药不良反应监测**。组织研究开发符合中药特点的中药不良反应信号监测工具，对发现的安全性风险信号及时开展综合分析研判，采取相应的风险控制措施，加强对不良反应聚集性事件的监测和处置力度，及时防控用药风险。

六、提升中药标准管理水平

（二十）**优化中药标准管理**。研究制定中药标准管理专门规定。以《中国药典》（一部）修订为契机，探索实施中药国家标准制定质量管理规范，及时将科学、成熟、适用的中药相关注册标准、国际标准、团体标准或企业内控标准等转化为国家标准。建立中药国家标准快速修订机制和修订程序。加强药典委员会中药相关专委会建设，完善委员遴选和产生机制。

（二十一）**科学完善中药标准**。持续推进中药标准制定、修订，加快国家中药饮片炮制规范、中药配方颗粒标准发布实施。合理设置中药中农药残留、重金属与有害元素、真菌毒素等有害物质以及植物生长调节剂等的限量要求和检测方法。加强中药内源性有毒成份检测技术研究和风险评估体系建设，制订符合中药特点的内源性有毒成份限度标准和完善用法用量。

（二十二）**加强中药标准物质研制和供应保障**。完善中药标准物质研制和持续保障供应机制，强化动态预警和信息反馈机制，开展需求分析并制订研制计划，加强质量监测。分类完善中药化学对照品、对照药材和对照提取物等中药标准物质的研制和标定技术要求。

（二十三）**提升中药标准数字化管理水平**。建立完善中药国家药品标准、药品注册标准动态数据库，加快推进数字化标准建设，及时更新数据，实现药品标准的发布、查询、分析、研究、维护信息化。

七、加大中药安全监管力度

（二十四）创新中药质量监管模式。逐步构建"网格化"监管模式，完善中药生产监管制度建设，研究制定并监督实施《中药生产质量管理规范》。逐步建立并完善中药生产区域化风险研判机制，针对重点企业、重点品种、重点环节，持续加强中药饮片、中药配方颗粒和中成药监督检查，有序开展中药材延伸检查。进一步规范中药饮片、中药配方颗粒和中成药流通经营秩序，强化使用环节质量监管。

（二十五）加强中药质量抽检监测。持续推进和完善中药饮片、中药配方颗粒、中成药质量抽检，结合监管需求和行业发展实际科学开展探索性研究，对抽检监测数据进行综合分析研判，依风险采取相应的风险防控或质量提升措施，优化中药质量公告发布工作机制，依法发布抽检监测结果，向公众客观准确传递中药质量安全信息。

（二十六）严厉打击违法违规行为。依法严查重处药品上市许可持有人、生产和/或经营企业涉嫌注册、备案造假，以及掺杂掺假、编造记录、违规销售等违法违规行为。严厉打击"窝点"制售中药假药等违法犯罪活动，充分利用网络监测、投诉举报等线索，联合公安、司法等部门，坚决查清源头、一追到底，依法追究犯罪人员刑事责任，坚守中药安全底线。

八、推进中药监管全球化合作

（二十七）充分发挥国际合作平台作用。进一步深化世界卫生组织（WHO）、国际草药监管合作组织（IRCH）、西太区草药监管协调论坛（FHH）国际合作，充分发挥"一带一路"国际合作框架、"中国–东盟药品合作发展高峰论坛"、世界卫生组织传统医药合作中心等平台作用，积极推动在传统草药监管合作、标准协调等方面进一步形成国际共识。

（二十八）支持中药开展国际注册。积极开展中药国际注册政策宣贯和交流，支持国内具有临床优势的中药开展国际注册，鼓励开展中药国际多中心临床试验。按计划组织对进口药材的产地、初加工等生产现场以及境外中药（天然药物）的研制、生产实施检查。

（二十九）传播中药监管"中国经验"。加快推进中药监管相关政策规定和技术指导原则翻译工作，分批次印制中药相关技术指导原则外文版本，加快国际推广，为国际传统草药监管规则和标准制修订贡献"中国经验"。

九、保障措施

（三十）**强化部门联动、协同推进**。强化与卫生健康委、医保局、中医药局等部门协同联动，在中药相关重大政策制定过程中加强沟通交流，形成各部门共同推进中药传承创新发展良好局面。

（三十一）**大力发展中药监管科学**。研究制定中药监管科学发展战略和关键路径，推进开展国家药监局药品监管科学行动计划。积极筹建药品监管科学全国重点实验室，依托国家药监局药品监管科学基地、重点实验室和重点项目实施，推动研究用于中药评价的新工具、新方法和新标准，并建立促进其用于中药监管的转化认定程序，建立完善具有中国特色的中药监管科学体系，解决中药监管基础性、关键性、前沿性和战略性技术问题。

（三十二）**加强高端智库建设**。充分发挥高端智库作用，组建由中医药领域和其他相关学科领域的院士、国医大师以及资深专家组成的中药管理战略决策专家咨询委员会，建立中药监管科学工作专家组，为国家药监局提供相关政策、法律咨询，提出决策参考、工作建议，确保中药监管工作重大决策的科学性、权威性。

（三十三）**重视监管科学人才队伍培养**。加强与高水平研究机构、高等院校以及行业学会、研究会等合作，构建中药监管人才培养课程体系，分类别开展监管能力和实务培训，培养一支适应中药高质量发展的监管队伍。

（三十四）**夯实中药监管基础建设**。加强中药监管基础数据建设，开展数据科学研究，从技术标准、质量追溯、过程监控、风险监测等方面，推动构建以数据为核心的中药智慧监管模式。

（三十五）**全面落实国家区域战略**。落实推进"京津冀协同发展""长江三角洲区域一体化""粤港澳大湾区建设"等国家区域发展战略和中医药综合改革示范区建设，鼓励条件成熟地区药品监督管理部门在加强中药质量安全监管，促进中药产业更高质量发展等方面先行先试。

Special Regulations on Registration and Management of Traditional Chinese Medicines

Chapter 1   General Provisions

Article 1   In order to promote the inheritance, innovation, and development of traditional Chinese medicine, follow the patterns of TCM research, and strengthen the development and registration management of new TCMs, the regulations are hereby formulated in accordance with "the Drug Administration Law of the People's Republic of China" "the Law of the People's Republic of China on Traditional Chinese Medicine" "Implementation Regulations of the Drug Administration Law of the People's Republic of China" "Measures for the Drug Registration Management" and other laws, regulations, and rules.

Article 2   The research and development of new TCMs should focus on reflecting the original thinking and holistic view of TCM, and it should be encouraged to research and develop TCMs by using TCM theory-oriented research methods and modern science and technology. It is supported to develop the new TCMs with rich clinical practice experience in TCM based on ancient classic formulas, empirical formulas prescribed by prestigious veteran TCM practitioners, and TCM preparations prepared by medical institutions (hereinafter referred to as medical institution TCM preparations); it is supported to develop the new TCMs with systemic regulatory intervention functions on the human body, etc., and it is encouraged to study and explain the mechanism of TCMs' actions by applying emerging science and technology.

Article 3   The development of new TCMs should adhere to being oriented by clinical value, pay attention to clinical benefit and risk assessment, give full play to the unique advantages and functions of TCMs in disease prevention and treatment, and focus on meeting unmet clinical needs.

Article 4   The development of new TCMs should be in line with the theory of TCM. Under the guidance of TCM theory, formulas should be reasonably formulated, and functions, main syndromes to be treated, applicable population, dosage, duration of treatment, efficacy characteristics, and contraindications should be drawn up. It is encouraged to observe patterns of disease progression, syndrome transformation, symptom changes, drug reactions, etc. in TCM clinical practice to provide supportive evidence under TCM theory for the development of new TCMs.

Article 5   The new TCMs derived from TCM clinical practice should be developed on the basis of summarizing individual medication experience; they should gradually clarify the main functions, applicable population, dosage regimens, and clinical benefits and formulate a fixed formula through clinical practice to develop a new TCM suitable for group medication. It is encouraged to carry out research with high quality based on application experience in human in TCM clinical practice, clarify the clinical positioning and clinical value of TCMs, and continuously analyze and summarize based on scientific methods to obtain sufficient evidence to support registration.

Article 6   The registration review of TCMs should adopt an evidence system for review that combines TCM theory, application experience in human, and clinical trials to comprehensively evaluate the safety, effectiveness, and quality controllability of TCMs.

Article 7   The evaluation of the efficacy of TCMs should be based on the clinical treatment characteristics of TCMs, and the indicators in terms of the efficacy outcome should be determined to be compatible with the clinical positioning of TCMs and reflect their functional characteristics and advantages. The efficacy of TCMs can be evaluated by using indicators including the recovery from disease or delayed progress of disease, the improvement of the condition or symptoms, the improvement of the patient's disease-related body functions or quality of life, increasing efficacy and reducing toxicity of TCMs through use in combination with chemical pharmaceuticals, or reducing the dosage of chemical pharmaceuticals with obvious side effects.

It is encouraged to evaluate the efficacy of TCMs by using real-world research, new biomarkers, surrogate endpoint decision-making, patient-centered drug development, adaptive design, enrichment design, etc.

Article 8   The safety and benefit-risk ratio of TCMs should be comprehensively evaluated, and the full life cycle management of TCMs should be strengthened based on the composition and characteristics of formulas, TCM theory, application experience in human, clinical trials, and results from necessary research on non-clinical safety.

Article 9   The registration applicant (hereinafter referred to as the applicant) who develops TCMs should strengthen the quality control on the source of raw TCM material and prepared TCM pieces, conduct an assessment on the available resources of raw materials, ensure the source traceability of raw materials, and clarify their origins, provenances, collecting periods, etc. It should strengthen quality control throughout the entire production process to maintain stable and controllable quality between batches. TCM ingredients in a formula can be fed after their respective quality uniformities are fulfilled.

Article 10   Applicants should ensure the sustainable availability of resources for raw TCM materials and pay attention to the impact on the ecological environment. Those involving endangered wild animals and plants must comply with relevant national regulations.

Chapter 2   Registration Classification and Marketing Approval for TCMs

Article 11   The registration classification of TCMs includes innovative TCMs, modified new TCMs, complex-formulated TCM preparations derived from ancient classical formulas and from formulas prescribed by prestigious veteran practitioners, TCMs with identical names and identical formulas, etc. The TCMs registration classification with specific conditions and the required corresponding application dossier should be implemented in accordance with the requirements set in the relevant regulations with regard to the registration classification and application dossier for TCMs.

Article 12   The research and development of new TCMs should be based on the registration classification of TCMs, and the path and model should be selected for research and development in line with the characteristics of TCMs. The TCMs with efficacy characteristics should be discovered and explored based on TCM theory and application experience in human; their efficacy should be confirmed mainly through application experience in human and/or necessary clinical trials; TCMs to be developed based on pharmacological screening studies should undergo necessary Phase I clinical trials; and Phase II and III clinical trials should be carried out in a sequential manner.

Article 13   Simplified registration and approval will be implemented for marketing applications of complex-formulated TCM preparations derived from ancient classical formulas and formulas prescribed by prestigious veteran practitioners, and specific requirements should be implemented in accordance with relevant regulations.

Article 14   Review and approval with priority will be implemented for registration applications of new TCMs with clear clinical positioning and obvious clinical value in the following cases:

(1) medicine for the prevention and treatment of major diseases, emerging and unexpected contagious diseases, and rare diseases;

(2) medication with an urgent clinical need and a shortage in the market;

(3) medication for children;

(4) newly discovered raw TCM materials and their preparations, or new officinal parts in raw TCM materials and their preparations;

(5) TCMs with a clear profile of medicinal substances and a basically clear mechanism of action.

Article 15   In the case that TCMs are used for the treatment of serious life-threatening diseases for which there is no effective treatment method, and TCMs are urgently needed as determined by the State Council's health department or competent department of TCM, if the existing data from clinical trials and empirical evidence based on application experience in human with high quality can show efficacy and predict clinical value, it can be approved with additional conditions, and the relevant matters should be stated in the drug registration certificate.

Article 16   In the event of a public health emergency, if TCMs are deemed urgently needed by the State Council's health department or competent department of TCM, the TCMs may be directly applied for clinical trials, marketing licenses, or adding functions and indications in accordance with special approval procedures by using empirical evidence based on application experience in human.

Chapter 3   The Rational Application of Empirical Evidence Based on Application Experience in Human

Article 17   Application experience in human for TCMs is usually accumulated in clinical practice and has certain regularity, repeatability and clinical value, including the understanding and summary of TCM formulas and preparations in terms of clinical positioning, applicable population, dosage, efficacy characteristics and clinical benefits, etc., which are accumulated in the process of clinical use.

Article 18   Applicants may collect and collate application experience in human through multiple channels and should be responsible for the authenticity and traceability of the data. The standardized collection, collation, and evaluation of application experience in human should meet relevant requirements. As the data on application experience in human is regarded as the key evidence to support the registration application, the drug regulatory administration should organize and carry out the corresponding drug registration verification in accordance with relevant procedures.

Article 19   Application experience in human for which there is reasonable and sufficient analysis conducted on data and the correct interpretation given to the result can be used as evidence to support the registration application. Applicants can determine follow-up research strategies and provide corresponding application dossiers according to the degree to which the evidence supports based on application experience in human in terms of the safety and effectiveness of TCM.

Article 20   The ingredients in a formula (including origin, officinal parts, preparation, etc.) and dosage of TCMs should be fixed in application experience in human that are regarded as key evidence to support registration applications. The key pharmaceutical information and quality of the applied preparation should be basically consistent with the TCMs in application experience in human. If the preparation process, excipients, etc. are changed, an evaluation should be conducted, and data on research and evaluation that supports the relevant changes should be provided.

Article 21   In the case that the formulas of innovative TCMs are derived from ancient classic formulas and formulas described by prestigious veteran practitioners or from TCM clinically experienced formulas, if their formulas' composition, clinical positioning, usage, dosage, etc. are basically consistent with those in previous clinical applications, their traditional processes are basically consistent with those used in clinics, and their functions and indications, applicable population, dosage regimen, clinical benefits, etc. can be preliminary determined through application experience in human, the research on non-clinical effectiveness may not be conducted.

Article 22   For the complex-formulated TCM preparations composed of prepared TCM pieces, the data should be generally provided in terms of single-dose and repeated-dose toxicity trials on rodent, and other data on toxicological trials should be provided when necessary.

In the case that the prepared TCM pieces in a formula of complex-formulated TCM preparation have national drug standards or drug registration standards, and the formula does not contain toxic ingredients or does not contain prepared TCM pieces that have been proven to be toxic by modern toxicology and likely cause serious adverse reactions, and if the preparation uses traditional techniques, and is not used for special groups such as pregnant women and children, and if no obvious toxicity is found in the preparation by single-dose and the repeated-dose toxicity trials on one animal, generally, there is no need to provide the repeated-dose toxicity trials on another animal, nor trial data on pharmacological safety, genotoxicity, carcinogenicity, reproductive toxicity and other.

The term "toxic ingredients" mentioned in this regulation refers to the toxic TCM species included in the "Measures for the Administration of Toxic Drugs for Medical Use."

Article 23   In the case that the new TCMs are derived from clinical practice, if application experience in human can provide research and supportive evidence in terms of clinical positioning, screening of the applicable population, exploration of treatment courses, dosage exploration, etc., phase II clinical trials may not be conducted.

Article 24   If there are application experience in human for the clinical research and development of TCMs and the data exists in an applicable real-world setting with high quality on the basis of fixed formulas and production processes, and if the real-world evidence being formed through well-designed clinical studies is scientific and sufficient, the applicant can apply to use real-world evidence as one of the bases to support product marketing after communicating and reaching an agreement with the national agency of drug evaluation on the real-world research proposal.

Article 25   Medical institutions are responsible for the safety, effectiveness, and quality controllability of TCM preparations administered in the institutions. They should continue to collect and collate the data on the application experience in human of TCM preparations used in medical institutions in a standardized manner and report them to the local provincial drug regulatory administrations on an annual basis. Submit a report on the collection, collation, and evaluation of application experience in human in TCM preparations used in medical institutions.

Article 26   For the new TCMs developed by medical institutions, if formula composition, process route, clinical positioning, usage and dosage, etc. are basically consistent with previous clinical applications, if their functions and indications, applicable population, usage and dosage are consistent with those in previous clinical applications, and if applicable populations, dosage regimens, and clinical benefits can be preliminary determined through application experience in human, studies on non-clinical effectiveness may not be carried out. If the formula composition, extraction process, dosage form, immediate packaging, etc. of the TCM preparation to be developed are consistent with that used in medical institutions, research information may not be provided, such as dosage form selection, process route screening, and research on immediate packaging, based on pharmaceutical research information on the preparation provided by the medical institution.

Article 27　According to specific product conditions, applicants may communicate with the national agency of drug evaluation about TCM theory, research proposals, and data on application experience in human during the critical stage of research and development.

Chapter 4　Innovative TCMs

Article 28　Innovative TCMs should have sufficient evidence of effectiveness and safety, and randomized controlled clinical trials should principally be conducted before marketing.

Article 29　It is encouraged, as per TCM clinical practice, to explore the use of sequential combination medication on the basis of clinical treatment plans to carry out clinical trials and efficacy evaluations of innovative TCMs.

Article 30　It is encouraged for clinical trials of innovative TCMs to give priority to the use of placebo controls, or placebo controls loaded with basic treatment, if they meet ethical requirements.

Article 31　Prepared TCM pieces, extracts, etc. can be used as formula components of complex-formulated TCM preparations. If the prepared TCM pieces or extracts contained in a formula do not have national drug standards or drug registration standards, their quality standards should be appended to the standard of the TCM preparation.

Article 32　Extracts and their preparations should have sufficient basis for establishing research subjects to conduct research on effectiveness, safety, and quality control. A reasonable preparation process should be studied and fixed. The structural type of a large class of homologous compounds and the structures of major components should be studied and clarified, and the quality of the extracts and preparations should be fully characterized to ensure uniformity and stability in quality between different batches of extracts and preparations by establishing quality control items in quality standards in terms of assays and fingerprints or characteristic chromatography for the main components and large class of homologous compounds.

Article 33   In the case that new extracts and their preparations are applied for registration, if preparations made by a single ingredient or extract from a single ingredient are already on the market and the functions and indications between applying one and marketed one are basically the same, comparative studies of such preparations between non-clinic and clinic preparations should be conducted to illustrate their advantages and characteristics.

Article 34   In the case that new raw TCM materials and their preparations are applied for registration, it should provide research information on the nature and flavor, channel tropism, efficacy, etc. for the raw TCM materials, and relevant research should provide supportive evidence for the proposed nature and flavor, channel tropism, efficacy, etc. for the new raw TCM materials.

Article 35   The complex-formulated TCM preparations can be divided into different cases according to different indications:

(1) The complex-formulated TCM preparations whose indications are described with syndromes refer to the preparations used to treat TCM syndromes under the guidance of TCM theory, including those to treat TCM diseases or TCM symptoms. The functions and indications should be expressed in the professional terminology of TCM;

(2) The complex-formulated TCM preparations whose indications are described with diseases in combination with syndromes. The "diseases" involved refer to the diseases under modern medical science, while the "syndromes" involved refer to the syndromes under TCM theory. The functions should be expressed in professional terms of TCM, and the indications should be expressed with diseases under modern medical science in combination with syndromes under TCM theory;

(3) The complex-formulated TCM preparations whose indications are described with diseases refer to the preparations specially used to treat special diseases for which the formulas are formulated under the guidance of TCM theory. The "diseases" involved refer to diseases under modern medical science; the functions should be expressed in professional terms of TCM, and indications should be expressed in terms of modern medical diseases.

Article 36　In the case that applicants apply for registration of innovative TCMs, phased research may be conducted according to the characteristics of TCMs and the general patterns of new drug research and development, it should focus on the main purpose of each phase, such as applying for clinical trials, pre-phase Ⅲ clinical trials, and applying for marketing authorization. Phased research on TCMs should reflect the concept of quality coming from design and focus on the integrity and systematicity of the research.

Article 37　Dosage form and administration route should be reasonably selected for innovative TCMs according to the formula composition, flavor and nature of the ingredient, drawing on medication experience in order to meet clinical needs based on comprehensive analysis such as production process, physical and chemical properties, traditional medication methods, biological characteristics, dosage form characteristics, clinical medication safety, patient medication compliance, etc. Injection administration is not encouraged if oral administration is allowed.

Article 38　It should conduct corresponding non-clinical safety trials for the development of innovative TCMs based on the safety information obtained from the TCM characteristics, clinical application, etc. Corresponding non-clinical safety trials can be carried out according to different registration classifications, risk assessment situations, and development processes.

Article 39　The samples used in non-clinical safety trials should be samples of pilot scale or above. When it is applied for clinical trials, information should be provided to describe the preparation samples used for non-clinical safety trials. TCM preparations for clinical trials should generally use production-scale samples. When it is applied for marketing authorization, information should be provided to describe the preparation of samples for clinical trials, including experimental samples and placebos.

Article 40　Phase I clinical trials should necessarily be carried out under the following circumstances:

(1) The formula contains a toxic ingredient;

(2) The formulas contain prepared TCM pieces and extracts that do not have national drug standards or drug registration standards, in addition to those containing prepared TCM pieces that have a history of customary use and are included in the provincial standards for processing TCM pieces;

(3) Results from non-clinical safety trials show obvious toxic reactions and indicate that there may be certain safety risks to the human body;

(4) TCM registration applications that require data on human pharmacokinetics to guide clinical medication.

Chapter 5　Modified New TCMs

Article 41　It is to support holders of drug marketing authorization (hereinafter referred to as holders) to carry out research on modified new TCMs. The research and development of modified TCMs should follow the principles of necessity, scientificity, and rationality, and the purpose of modification should be clear. Research should be conducted on the existing TCMs on the market and based on an objective, scientific, and comprehensive understanding of the modified TCMs, focusing on the defects of the modified TCMs or the newly discovered therapeutic characteristics and potentialities during clinical application. When modified new TCMs are developed for children, the development should be consistent with the children's growth and development characteristics and medication habits.

Article 42　The modified new TCMs applying for changing the dosage form or administration route of the existing marketed TCMs should have advantages and characteristics in clinical application, such as increased effectiveness, improved safety, enhanced compliance, etc., or should promote environmental protection and upgrade safety levels of production, etc. under the prerequisite that the modified TCMs' effectiveness and safety are not reduced.

Article 43 The rationality and necessity for changing the administration route should be explained when a marketed TCM is applied for registration to change the administration route, corresponding non-clinical research should be conducted, and clinical trials should be carried out by focusing on the purpose of modification to prove the advantages and characteristics in clinical application for changing the administration route.

Article 44 In the case that a marketed TCM is applied for registration to change the dosage form, sufficient evidence should be provided to demonstrate its scientific rationality based on the clinical treatment needs, the medicine's physical and chemical properties, and its biological properties. Applicants should carry out corresponding pharmaceutical research based on the specific situations of the new dosage form and conduct non-clinical research on effectiveness and safety, as well as clinical trials when necessary.

In the case that medication is for children and special groups (such as those with dysphagia, etc.), or some marketed TCMs aim to be improved in terms of clinical use compliance through changing dosage forms due to inconvenient use caused by special usage, clinical trials may not be conducted if comparative studies show that there is no significant change in the substance profile and absorption and the utilization of medicinal components exiting in the TCM with the changed dosage form, and if the TCM with the original dosage form has sufficient evidence on the clinical value.

Article 45 In the case that a TCM is applied for registration to add functions and indications, in addition to the cases specified in Articles 23 and 46, the data on non-clinical effectiveness research should be provided, and phase II and phase III clinical trials should be carried out sequentially.

In the case that a TCM is applied for registration to extend the medication cycle or increase the dose, data on non-clinical safety research should be provided. New tests on non-clinical safety do not need to be conducted if relevant studies on non-clinical safety have been conducted before marketing that can support extending the cycle or increasing the dose.

If the applicant who is not a holder of a marketed TCM applies for registration to add functions and indications to the marketed TCM, a registration application for the new TCM with the identical name and identical formula should be submitted.

Article 46   In the case that a marketed TCM is applied for registration to add functions and indications, the data on the non-clinical effectiveness test does not need to be provided if empirical evidence in human application supports the corresponding clinical positioning. The data on non-clinical safety tests does not need to be provided if the dosage and treatment duration do not increase and the applicable population remains unchanged.

Article 47   It is encouraged to apply new technologies and new processes suitable for products' characteristics to improve marketed TCMs. If modified production processes or modified excipients of a marketed TCM cause significant changes in the component profile or the absorption and utilization of the medicinal components existing in the modified TCM, relevant trials on non-clinical effectiveness and safety should be carried out by taking an objective at a study on improving effectiveness or safety, and phase II and phase III clinical trials should be submitted according to the registration application for the modified new drug.

Chapter 6   The TCM Complex–Formulated Preparations Derived from Ancient Classic Formulas or Formulas Prescribed by Prestigious Veteran Practitioners

Article 48   In the case that the TCM complex-formulated preparations derived from ancient classic formulas or the formulas prescribed by prestigious veteran practitioners do not contain incompatible ingredients, virulent toxic and highly toxic ingredients labeled in TCM standards, or toxic ingredients proven by modern toxicology, traditional process techniques and traditional administration routes should be applied, and functions and indications should be expressed in TCM terms. The development of this category of TCM complex-formulated preparations does not require research on non-clinical effectiveness or clinical trials. A special format should be given to the TCM approval number.

Article 49 The TCM complex-formulated preparations derived from ancient classic formulas or the formulas prescribed by prestigious veteran practitioners are reviewed by a model based on expert opinions. The Expert Review Committee for the TCM complex-formulated preparations derived from ancient classic formulas or the formulas prescribed by prestigious veteran practitioners, which primarily consists of TCM masters, academicians, and nationally renowned TCM practitioners, conducts technical reviews on this category of preparations and issues technical review opinions on whether to agree with marketing the preparation.

Article 50 In the case that TCM complex-formulated preparations are applied for marketing in light of the catalog of ancient classic formulas or the formulas prescribed by prestigious veteran practitioners, the applicant should conduct corresponding pharmaceutical research and research on non-clinical safety. In principle, preparations' formula composition, origins and officinal parts of raw TCM materials as ingredients, processing specifications, converted dosage, usage and dosage, functions, and indications should be consistent with the key information of ancient classic formulas or formulas prescribed by prestigious veteran practitioners issued by the country.

Article 51 In the case that other TCM complex-formulated preparations derived from ancient classic formulas or the formulas prescribed by prestigious veteran practitioners are applied for registration, corresponding pharmaceutical research and data on non-clinical safety trials should be provided; additionally, the key information and basis of ancient classic formulas should be provided; and a systematic summary of the TCM clinical practice should be provided as well to illustrate its clinical value. The addition, subtraction, and modification of ancient classic formulas or the formulas prescribed by prestigious veteran practitioners should be carried out under the guidance of TCM theory.

Article 52 Applicants are encouraged to communicate with the national drug evaluation agency on major issues such as research on benchmark samples and non-clinical safety, standardized collection and collation of application experience in human , and a summary of TCM clinical practice at the critical stage of research and development based on the characteristics of ancient classic formulas and the formulas prescribed by prestigious veteran practitioners.

Article 53   After marketing a TCM complex-formulated preparation derived from ancient classic formulas or the formulas prescribed by prestigious veteran practitioners, the holder should carry out post-market clinical research on the preparation and continuously enrich and improve the evidence of clinical effectiveness and safety. The holder should continue to collect information on adverse reactions, timely revise and improve the package insert, and timely conduct studies on non-clinical safety when unexpected adverse reactions are discovered during clinical use.

Chapter 7   TCMs with the Identical Name and Identical Formula

Article 54   Low-level duplication should be avoided in the development of TCMs with identical names and identical formulas. Applicants should evaluate the clinical value of marketed TCMs with identical names and identical formulas that are used as controls (hereinafter referred to as the control TCM with the identical name and identical formula). Regarding the registration of applications for the TCMs to be developed with the identical name and formula of the marketed TCM, the safety, effectiveness, and quality controllability should be no less than those of the marketed TCM.

Article 55   The TCMs to be developed with the identical name and identical formula should be compared with the control TCM with the identical name and identical formula in terms of quality control of the entire process of TCM, including prepared TCM pieces, intermediates, preparations, etc. The applicant should evaluate whether to conduct research on non-clinical safety and clinical trials based on the evidence of the effectiveness and safety of the control TCM with identical name and identical formula, as well as the comparison results of the process techniques, excipients, etc. between the TCM to be developed and the control TCM with identical name and identical formula.

Article 56   Applicants should select a control TCM with an identical name and identical formula as per the results of the clinical value evaluation.

Control TCM with an identical name and identical formula should have sufficient evidence of effectiveness and safety. The evidence of effectiveness and safety can generally be regarded as sufficient, such as TCMs that have been approved for marketing after clinical trials that have been carried out in accordance with the requirements with reference to drug registration and management, the marketed TCMs listed in the current version of the Pharmacopoeia of the People's Republic of China, and marketed TCMs that have ever obtained TCM protection certificates.

The term "marketed TCM that have ever obtained TCM protection certificates," as mentioned in the preceding paragraph, refers to protected TCMs that are over the validity period and other protected TCMs that comply with the relevant provisions in the TCM protection system.

Article 57　In the case that TCMs with identical names and identical formulas are applied for registration and need to be compared through clinical trials with control TCMs with identical names and identical formulas, at least Phase III clinical trials must be conducted. The TCM made from an extracted single component can be proven to be consistent with the control TCM with an identical name and identical formula through bioequivalence testing.

Article 58　For TCMs with national drug standards but without a drug approval number, registration applications should be submitted in line with the TCMs with identical names and identical formulas. Applicants should conduct necessary clinical trials based on the TCM theory and application experience in human.

Article 59　In the case that the control TCM with identical name and identical formula has sufficient evidence of effectiveness and safety and the TCM to be developed has the same process techniques and excipients as the control TCM with identical name and identical formula, or if the changes in the process techniques and excipients of the TCM to be developed with identical name and identical formula do not cause obvious changes in the medicinal substance profile or the absorption and utilization of medicinal components after research and evaluation, there is generally no need to conduct research on non-clinical safety and clinical trials.

Chapter 8   Post–Marketing Changes

Article 60   Changes to the marketed TCM should follow the characteristics and patterns of TCMs and meet the relevant requirements on necessity, scientificity, and rationality. The holder should perform the main responsibilities of research, evaluation, and management on changes and comprehensively evaluate and verify the impact of changes on TCM's safety, effectiveness, and quality controllability. The categories of change management for marketed TCMs should be determined based on the results of research, evaluation, and related verification. The implementation of changes should be carried out or reported after approval and filing in accordance with regulations. The holder can timely communicate with the corresponding drug regulatory administrations during the research process of post-marketing changes.

Article 61   Changes in pharmaceutical strength should follow the principle of being consistent with the corresponding ingredients in formula and the principle of being compatible with the applicable population, usage and dosage, and filling specifications.

If a product has the same TCM on the market, the applied pharmaceutical strength should generally be consistent with the one with the same TCM on the market.

Article 62   Changes in production processes and excipients should not cause obvious changes in the absorption and utilization of medicinal substances or the medicine. The selection of production equipment should meet the requirements of production processes and quality assurance.

Article 63   In the case that a TCM applies for changes in usage and dosage or expending the scope of the applicable population without changing the administration route, research data on non-clinical safety that can support the changes should be provided, and clinical trials should be conducted when necessary. In addition to the cases stipulated in Article 64, If clinical trials are required when the usage and dosage is changed, or scope of the applicable population is expended, phase Ⅱ and phase Ⅲ clinical trials should be conducted in sequence.

If the medication [usage and dosage] of marketed TCMs for children is unclear, necessary clinical trials should be carried out based on the characteristics of children's medication and application experience in human to clarify the dosage and treatment course for children of different ages.

Article 64   In the case that a marketed TCM applies for changes in the usage and dosage or expending the scope of the applicable population, if the functions and indications, and the administration route remain unchanged, and the empirical evidence in application experience in human supports the new usage and dosage or the usage and dosage of the new applicable population after the changes, only phase Ⅲ clinical trials are needed while phase Ⅱ clinical trials are allowed to be exempted.

Article 65   In the case that a TCM is applied for substituting or subtracting toxic ingredients or endangered ingredients in the formulas listed in a national TCM standard, studies on pharmacy and non-clinical effectiveness and/or non-clinical safety should be carried out in contrast with the original TCM based on the formula composition and efficacy in accordance with relevant technical requirements. If toxic ingredients are clarified in the formula as substituted or subtracted ones, phase Ⅲ clinical trials should be carried out in contrast with placebo. If ingredients are clarified in the formula as endangered species, at least the studies on the phase Ⅲ clinical trials should be carried out in contrast with the original TCM. The generic name of the TCM should be changed simultaneously when needed.

Article 66   In the case that the extracts approved as new TCMs and contained in a formula of TCM complex-formulated preparation are applied for changes from outsource to self-extracted source, the applicant should provide accordingly the research data, including but not limited to the pharmacy research on the extract obtained through self-development and on its TCM preparation, as well as the data on studies on the phase Ⅲ clinical in contrast with the original TCM preparation. The quality standard of the extract should be appended to the preparation standard.

Article 67　In the case that the TCM is applied for deletion of functions and indications or deletion of the scope of the applicable population, the rationale for deletion should be explained. Generally, clinical trials are exempted.

Chapter 9　Registration Standards for TCMs

Article 68　The research and formulation of registration standards for TCMs should aim at achieving a stable and controllable quality of TCMs and establish control indicators that reflect the overall quality of TCMs based on products' characteristics. Reflect on the quality status of products as much as possible, and pay attention to the relationship between the effectiveness and safety of TCMs.

Article 69　It is to support the use of new technologies and new methods to explore and establish fingerprints or characteristic chromatographs, biological effect detection, etc. for quality control of intermediates and preparations of new complex-formulated TCM. The testing items in the registration standards for TCMs, including assays, should have a reasonable limit range.

Article 70　The holder should formulate internal control standards in enterprise that are no lower than the registration standards of the TCM based on products' characteristics and the real case, and improve the quality of TCM preparations by continuously revising and improving its testing items, methods, limits, etc.

Article 71　After a TCM is put on the market, data on production should be accumulated, and a holistic quality standard system including raw TCM materials, prepared TCM pieces, intermediates, and preparations should be continuously revised and improved to ensure the stability and controllability of the TCM quality based on the development of science and technology.

Chapter 10　TCM Name and Package Insert

Article 72　The naming of Chinese proprietary medicines should comply with the requirements with regard to the "Technical Guidelines for Naming Generic Names of Chinese Proprietary Medicines" and relevant national regulations.

Article 73   If a TCM formula contains toxic ingredients or contains other prepared TCM pieces that have been proven to be toxic by modern toxicology and can easily cause serious adverse reactions, the name of the toxic ingredient contained in the formula should be indicated under the [ingredients] item in the package insert of the TCM and should be indicated in warning that the preparation contains the toxic TCM pieces.

Article 74   [Precautions] in the package inserts for new TCMs involving use under syndrome differentiation should include, but are not limited to, the following:

(1) Situations that require use with caution due to factors such as TCM syndrome, pathogenesis, physical constitution, etc., as well as drug-related precautions in terms of diet, compatibility, etc.

(2) If there is post-medication care, it should be clarified.

Article 75   The holder should strengthen the management of the entire life cycle of TCMs, strengthen the monitoring, evaluation, and analysis of safety risks, and refer to relevant technical guidelines to timely improve [contraindications], [adverse reactions], and [precautions] in the package insert of TCMs.

When a TCM is applied for re-registration, re-registration will not be granted in accordance with the law if any of the [Contraindications], [Adverse Reactions], and [Precautions] in the package insert of the TCM are still "unclear" after three years from the date of implementation of these regulations.

Article 76   The package insert for TCMs derived from ancient classic formulas or formulas prescribed by prestigious veteran practitioners should list the [source of formula], [theoretical basis for functions and indications], etc.

For new TCMs that use application experience in humans as evidence for approval for marketing or for adding functions and indications, [TCM Clinical Practice] should be included as an item in the package insert.

Chapter 11   Supplementary Provisions

Article 77   Pharmaceutical quality control of natural medicines may be implemented by consulting these regulations. In order to confirm the therapeutic effect of innovative natural medicines, data on at least one Phase III clinical trial should be used to demonstrate their effectiveness. The rest should comply with the relevant requirements with regard to research on new natural medicines.

Article 78   In the case that TCMs and natural medicines are applied for import, the application should comply with the requirements on drug management in the exported countries or regions and should also meet the requirements on safety, effectiveness, and quality controllability of domestic TCMs and natural medicines. Registration application dossiers should be provided in accordance with the requirements for innovative TCMs. It should prevail if the country has other regulations.

Article 79   The development of injections derived from TCMs and natural medicines should comply with the general technical requirements for injection research. The necessity and rationality for choosing an administration route should be demonstrated through sufficient non-clinical studies based on the availability of existing treatment methods. The active components and mechanisms of TCMs' functions should be clarified, comprehensive studies on non-clinical effectiveness and safety should be carried out, and phase I, phase II, and phase III clinical trials should be carried out sequentially.

After the injections of TCMs and natural medicine are launched on the market, holders should carry out post-marketing clinical studies on the medicines, continuously enrich and improve the evidence of clinical effectiveness and safety, continue to collect information on adverse reactions, and timely revise and improve the package inserts. Studies on non-clinical safety should be carried out in a timely manner if any unexpected adverse reactions are discovered during clinical use. Holders should strengthen quality control on injections.

Article 80   The provincial drug regulatory administrations should submit annual reports to the national drug regulatory administration about the approval and filing status of TCM preparations used in medical institutions. The national drug regulatory administration will include information about the approval and filing status of TCM preparations used in medical institutions in the annual national drug review report based on the reports from provincial drug regulatory administrations.

Article 81　The general requirements for drug registration management that are not covered by these regulations should be implemented in accordance with the "Measures for Drug Registration Management." Regulations on the registration and management of raw TCM materials and prepared TCM pieces that need to be implemented upon approval will be formulated separately.

Article 82　These regulations came into effect on July 1, 2023. The "Notice on Issuing Supplementary Regulations on Registration and Management of Traditional Chinese Medicines" issued by the former National Food and Drug Administration's (National Food and Drug Administration Note〔2008〕No.3) was abolished simultaneously.

中药注册管理专门规定

第一章 总 则

第一条 为促进中医药传承创新发展，遵循中医药研究规律，加强中药新药研制与注册管理，根据《中华人民共和国药品管理法》《中华人民共和国中医药法》《中华人民共和国药品管理法实施条例》《药品注册管理办法》等法律、法规和规章，制定本规定。

第二条 中药新药研制应当注重体现中医药原创思维及整体观，鼓励运用传统中药研究方法和现代科学技术研究、开发中药。支持研制基于古代经典名方、名老中医经验方、医疗机构配制的中药制剂（以下简称医疗机构中药制剂）等具有丰富中医临床实践经验的中药新药；支持研制对人体具有系统性调节干预功能等的中药新药，鼓励应用新兴科学和技术研究阐释中药的作用机理。

第三条 中药新药研制应当坚持以临床价值为导向，重视临床获益与风险评估，发挥中医药防病治病的独特优势和作用，注重满足尚未满足的临床需求。

第四条 中药新药研制应当符合中医药理论，在中医药理论指导下合理组方，拟定功能、主治病证、适用人群、剂量、疗程、疗效特点和服药宜忌。鼓励在中医临床实践中观察疾病进展、证候转化、症状变化、药后反应等规律，为中药新药研制提供中医药理论的支持证据。

第五条 来源于中医临床实践的中药新药，应当在总结个体用药经验的基础上，经临床实践逐步明确功能主治、适用人群、给药方案和临床获益，形成固定处方，在此基础上研制成适合群体用药的中药新药。鼓励在中医临床实践过程中开展高质量的人用经验研究，明确中药临床定位和临床价值，基于科学方法不断分析总结，获得支持注册的充分证据。

第六条 中药注册审评，采用中医药理论、人用经验和临床试验相结合的审评证据体系，综合评价中药的安全性、有效性和质量可控性。

第七条 中药的疗效评价应当结合中医药临床治疗特点，确定与中药临床定位相适应、体现其作用特点和优势的疗效结局指标。对疾病痊愈或者延缓发展、病情或者症状改善、患者与疾病相关的机体功能或者生存质量改善、与化学药品等合用增效减毒或者减少毒副作用明显的化学药品使用剂量等情形的评价，均可用于中药的疗效评价。

鼓励将真实世界研究、新型生物标志物、替代终点决策、以患者为中心的药物研发、适应性设计、富集设计等用于中药疗效评价。

第八条 应当根据处方组成及特点、中医药理论、人用经验、临床试验及必要的非临床安全性研究结果，综合评判中药的安全性和获益风险比，加强中药全生命周期管理。

第九条 注册申请人（以下简称申请人）研制中药应当加强中药材、中药饮片的源头质量控制，开展药材资源评估，保证中药材来源可追溯，明确药材基原、产地、采收期等。加强生产全过程的质量控制，保持批间质量的稳定可控。中药处方药味可经质量均一化处理后投料。

第十条 申请人应当保障中药材资源的可持续利用，并应当关注对生态环境的影响。涉及濒危野生动植物的，应当符合国家有关规定。

第二章 中药注册分类与上市审批

第十一条 中药注册分类包括中药创新药、中药改良型新药、古代经典名方中药复方制剂、同名同方药等。中药注册分类的具体情形和相应的申报资料要求按照中药注册分类及申报资料要求有关规定执行。

第十二条 中药新药的研发应当结合中药注册分类，根据品种情况选择符合其特点的研发路径或者模式。基于中医药理论和人用经验发现、探索疗效特点的中药，主要通过人用经验和／或者必要的临床试验确认其疗效；基于药理学筛选研究确定拟研发的中药，应当进行必要的Ⅰ期临床试验，并循序开展Ⅱ期临床试验和Ⅲ期临床试验。

第十三条 对古代经典名方中药复方制剂的上市申请实施简化注册审批，具体要求按照相关规定执行。

第十四条 对临床定位清晰且具有明显临床价值的以下情形中药新药等的注册申请实行优先审评审批：

（一）用于重大疾病、新发突发传染病、罕见病防治；

（二）临床急需而市场短缺；

（三）儿童用药；

（四）新发现的药材及其制剂，或者药材新的药用部位及其制剂；

（五）药用物质基础清楚、作用机理基本明确。

第十五条 对治疗严重危及生命且尚无有效治疗手段的疾病以及国务院卫

生健康或者中医药主管部门认定急需的中药，药物临床试验已有数据或者高质量中药人用经验证据显示疗效并能预测其临床价值的，可以附条件批准，并在药品注册证书中载明有关事项。

第十六条　在突发公共卫生事件时，国务院卫生健康或者中医药主管部门认定急需的中药，可应用人用经验证据直接按照特别审批程序申请开展临床试验或者上市许可或者增加功能主治。

第三章　人用经验证据的合理应用

第十七条　中药人用经验通常在临床实践中积累，具有一定的规律性、可重复性和临床价值，包含了在临床用药过程中积累的对中药处方或者制剂临床定位、适用人群、用药剂量、疗效特点和临床获益等的认识和总结。

第十八条　申请人可以多途径收集整理人用经验，应当对资料的真实性、可溯源性负责，人用经验的规范收集整理与评估应当符合有关要求。作为支持注册申请关键证据的人用经验数据，由药品监督管理部门按照相关程序组织开展相应的药品注册核查。

第十九条　对数据进行合理、充分的分析并给予正确结果解释的人用经验，可作为支持注册申请的证据。申请人可根据已有人用经验证据对药物安全性、有效性的支持程度，确定后续研究策略，提供相应的申报资料。

第二十条　作为支持注册申请关键证据的人用经验所用药物的处方药味（包括基原、药用部位、炮制等）及其剂量应当固定。申报制剂的药学关键信息及质量应当与人用经验所用药物基本一致，若制备工艺、辅料等发生改变，应当进行评估，并提供支持相关改变的研究评估资料。

第二十一条　中药创新药处方来源于古代经典名方或者中医临床经验方，如处方组成、临床定位、用法用量等与既往临床应用基本一致，采用与临床使用药物基本一致的传统工艺，且可通过人用经验初步确定功能主治、适用人群、给药方案和临床获益等的，可不开展非临床有效性研究。

第二十二条　由中药饮片组成的中药复方制剂一般提供啮齿类动物单次给药毒性试验和重复给药毒性试验资料，必要时提供其他毒理学试验资料。

如中药复方制剂的处方组成中的中药饮片均具有国家药品标准或者具有药品注册标准，处方不含毒性药味或者不含有经现代毒理学证明有毒性、易导致严重不良反应的中药饮片，采用传统工艺，不用于孕妇、儿童等特殊人群，且单次给药毒性试验和一种动物的重复给药毒性试验未发现明显毒性的，一般不需提供另一种动物的重复给药毒性试验，以及安全药理学、遗传毒性、致癌性、生殖毒性等试验资料。

本规定所称毒性药味，是指《医疗用毒性药品管理办法》中收载的毒性中药品种。

第二十三条 来源于临床实践的中药新药，人用经验能在临床定位、适用人群筛选、疗程探索、剂量探索等方面提供研究、支持证据的，可不开展Ⅱ期临床试验。

第二十四条 已有人用经验中药的临床研发，在处方、生产工艺固定的基础上，存在适用的高质量真实世界数据，且通过设计良好的临床研究形成的真实世界证据科学充分的，申请人就真实世界研究方案与国家药品审评机构沟通并达成一致后，可申请将真实世界证据作为支持产品上市的依据之一。

第二十五条 医疗机构对医疗机构中药制剂的安全性、有效性及质量可控性负责，应当持续规范收集整理医疗机构中药制剂人用经验资料，并按年度向所在地省级药品监督管理部门提交医疗机构中药制剂人用经验收集整理与评估的报告。

第二十六条 来源于医疗机构制剂的中药新药，如处方组成、工艺路线、临床定位、用法用量等与既往临床应用基本一致，且可通过人用经验初步确定功能主治、适用人群、给药方案和临床获益等的，可不开展非临床有效性研究。如处方组成、提取工艺、剂型、直接接触药品的包装等与该医疗机构中药制剂一致的，在提供该医疗机构中药制剂的药学研究资料基础上，可不提供剂型选择、工艺路线筛选、直接接触药品的包装材料研究等研究资料。

第二十七条 申请人可根据具体品种情况，在关键研发阶段针对中医药理论、人用经验研究方案和人用经验数据等，与国家药品审评机构进行沟通交流。

第四章　中药创新药

第二十八条 中药创新药应当有充分的有效性、安全性证据，上市前原则上应当开展随机对照的临床试验。

第二十九条 鼓励根据中医临床实践，探索采用基于临床治疗方案进行序贯联合用药的方式开展中药创新药临床试验及疗效评价。

第三十条 鼓励中药创新药临床试验在符合伦理学要求的情况下优先使用安慰剂对照，或者基础治疗加载的安慰剂对照。

第三十一条 中药饮片、提取物等均可作为中药复方制剂的处方组成。如含有无国家药品标准且不具有药品注册标准的中药饮片、提取物，应当在制剂药品标准中附设其药品标准。

第三十二条 提取物及其制剂应当具有充分的立题依据，开展有效性、安全性和质量可控性研究。应当研究确定合理的制备工艺。应当研究明确所含大类成份的结构类型及主要成份的结构，通过建立主要成份、大类成份的含量测定及指纹或者特征图谱等质控项目，充分表征提取物及制剂质量，保证不同批次提取物及制剂质量均一稳定。

第三十三条 新的提取物及其制剂的注册申请，如已有单味制剂或者单味提取物制剂上市且功能主治（适应症）基本一致，应当与该类制剂进行非临床及临床对比研究，以说明其优势与特点。

第三十四条 新药材及其制剂的注册申请，应当提供该药材性味、归经、功效等的研究资料，相关研究应当为新药材拟定的性味、归经、功效等提供支持证据。

第三十五条 中药复方制剂根据主治的不同，可以分为不同情形：

（一）主治为证候的中药复方制剂，是指在中医药理论指导下，用于治疗中医证候的中药复方制剂，包括治疗中医学的病或者症状的中药复方制剂，功能主治应当以中医专业术语表述；

（二）主治为病证结合的中药复方制剂，所涉及的"病"是指现代医学的疾病，"证"是指中医的证候，其功能用中医专业术语表述、主治以现代医学疾病与中医证候相结合的方式表述；

（三）主治为病的中药复方制剂，属于专病专药，在中医药理论指导下组方。所涉及的"病"是现代医学疾病，其功能用中医专业术语表述，主治以现代医学疾病表述。

第三十六条 中药创新药的注册申请人可根据中药特点、新药研发的一般规律，针对申请临床试验、Ⅲ期临床试验前、申请上市许可等不同研究阶段的主要目的进行分阶段研究。中药药学分阶段研究应当体现质量源于设计理念，注重研究的整体性和系统性。

第三十七条 中药创新药应当根据处方药味组成、药味药性，借鉴用药经验，以满足临床需求为宗旨，在对药物生产工艺、理化性质、传统用药方式、生物学特性、剂型特点、临床用药的安全性、患者用药依从性等方面综合分析的基础上合理选择剂型和给药途径。能选择口服给药的不选择注射给药。

第三十八条 中药创新药的研制，应当根据药物特点、临床应用情况等获取的安全性信息，开展相应的非临床安全性试验。可根据不同注册分类、风险评估情况、开发进程开展相应的非临床安全性试验。

第三十九条 非临床安全性试验所用样品，应当采用中试或者中试以上规模的样品。申报临床试验时，应当提供资料说明非临床安全性试验用样品制备情况。临床试验用药品一般应当采用生产规模的样品。申报上市时，应当提供资料说明临床试验用药品的制备情况，包括试验药物和安慰剂。

第四十条 以下情形，应当开展必要的I期临床试验：

（一）处方含毒性药味；

（二）除处方含确有习用历史且被省级中药饮片炮制规范收载的中药饮片外，处方含无国家药品标准且不具有药品注册标准的中药饮片、提取物；

（三）非临床安全性试验结果出现明显毒性反应且提示对人体可能具有一定的安全风险；

（四）需获得人体药代数据以指导临床用药等的中药注册申请。

第五章　中药改良型新药

第四十一条 支持药品上市许可持有人（以下简称持有人）开展改良型新药的研究。改良型新药的研发应当遵循必要性、科学性、合理性的原则，明确改良目的。应当在已上市药品的基础上，基于对被改良药品的客观、科学、全面的认识，针对被改良中药存在的缺陷或者在临床应用过程中新发现的治疗特点和潜力进行研究。研制开发儿童用改良型新药时，应当符合儿童生长发育特征及用药习惯。

第四十二条 改变已上市中药剂型或者给药途径的改良型新药，应当具有临床应用优势和特点，如提高有效性、改善安全性、提高依从性等，或者在有效性、安全性不降低的前提下，促进环境保护、提升生产安全水平等。

第四十三条 改变已上市药品给药途径的注册申请，应当说明改变给药途径的合理性和必要性，开展相应的非临床研究，并围绕改良目的开展临床试验，证明改变给药途径的临床应用优势和特点。

第四十四条 改变已上市中药剂型的注册申请，应当结合临床治疗需求、药物理化性质及生物学性质等提供充分依据说明其科学合理性。申请人应当根据新剂型的具体情形开展相应的药学研究，必要时开展非临床有效性、安全性研究和临床试验。

对儿童用药、特殊人群（如吞咽困难者等）用药、某些因用法特殊而使用不便的已上市中药，通过改变剂型提高药物临床使用依从性，若对比研究显示改剂型后药用物质基础和药物吸收、利用无明显改变，且原剂型临床价值依据充分的，可不开展临床试验。

第四十五条 中药增加功能主治，除第二十三条和第四十六条规定的情形外，应当提供非临床有效性研究资料，循序开展Ⅱ期临床试验及Ⅲ期临床试验。

延长用药周期或者增加剂量者，应当提供非临床安全性研究资料。上市前已进行相关的非临床安全性研究且可支持其延长周期或者增加剂量的，可不进行新的非临床安全性试验。

申请人不持有已上市中药申请增加功能主治的，应当同时提出同名同方药的注册申请。

第四十六条 已上市中药申请增加功能主治，其人用经验证据支持相应临床定位的，可不提供非临床有效性试验资料。使用剂量和疗程不增加，且适用人群不变的，可不提供非临床安全性试验资料。

第四十七条 鼓励运用适合产品特点的新技术、新工艺改进已上市中药。已上市中药生产工艺或者辅料等的改变引起药用物质基础或者药物的吸收、利用明显改变的，应当以提高有效性或者改善安全性等为研究目的，开展相关的非临床有效性、安全性试验及Ⅱ期临床试验、Ⅲ期临床试验，按照改良型新药注册申报。

第六章　古代经典名方中药复方制剂

第四十八条 古代经典名方中药复方制剂处方中不含配伍禁忌或者药品标准中标有剧毒、大毒及经现代毒理学证明有毒性的药味，均应当采用传统工艺制备，采用传统给药途径，功能主治以中医术语表述。该类中药复方制剂的研制不需要开展非临床有效性研究和临床试验。药品批准文号给予专门格式。

第四十九条 古代经典名方中药复方制剂采用以专家意见为主的审评模式。由国医大师、院士、全国名中医为主的古代经典名方中药复方制剂专家审评委员会对该类制剂进行技术审评，并出具是否同意上市的技术审评意见。

第五十条 按古代经典名方目录管理的中药复方制剂申请上市，申请人应当开展相应的药学研究和非临床安全性研究。其处方组成、药材基原、药用部位、炮制规格、折算剂量、用法用量、功能主治等内容原则上应当与国家发布的古代经典名方关键信息一致。

第五十一条 其他来源于古代经典名方的中药复方制剂的注册申请，除提供相应的药学研究和非临床安全性试验资料外，还应当提供古代经典名方关键信息及其依据，并应当提供对中医临床实践进行的系统总结，说明其临床价值。对古代经典名方的加减化裁应当在中医药理论指导下进行。

第五十二条 鼓励申请人基于古代经典名方中药复方制剂的特点，在研发的关键阶段，就基准样品研究、非临床安全性研究、人用经验的规范收集整理及中医临床实践总结等重大问题与国家药品审评机构进行沟通交流。

第五十三条 古代经典名方中药复方制剂上市后，持有人应当开展药品上市后临床研究，不断充实完善临床有效性、安全性证据。持有人应当持续收集不良反应信息，及时修改完善说明书，对临床使用过程中发现的非预期不良反应及时开展非临床安全性研究。

第七章　同名同方药

第五十四条 同名同方药的研制应当避免低水平重复。申请人应当对用于对照且与研制药物同名同方的已上市中药（以下简称对照同名同方药）的临床价值进行评估。申请注册的同名同方药的安全性、有效性及质量可控性应当不低于对照同名同方药。

第五十五条 同名同方药的研制，应当与对照同名同方药在中药材、中药饮片、中间体、制剂等全过程质量控制方面进行比较研究。申请人根据对照同名同方药的有效性、安全性证据，以及同名同方药与对照同名同方药的工艺、辅料等比较结果，评估是否开展非临床安全性研究及临床试验。

第五十六条 申请人应当基于临床价值评估结果选择对照同名同方药。对照同名同方药应当具有有效性、安全性方面充分的证据，按照药品注册管理要求开展临床试验后批准上市的中药、现行版《中华人民共和国药典》收载的已上市中药以及获得过中药保护品种证书的已上市中药，一般可视作具有充分的有效性、安全性证据。

前款所称获得过中药保护证书的已上市中药，是指结束保护期的中药保护品种以及符合中药品种保护制度有关规定的其他中药保护品种。

第五十七条 申请注册的同名同方药与对照同名同方药需要通过临床试验进行比较的，至少需进行Ⅲ期临床试验。提取的单一成份中药可通过生物等效性试验证明其与对照同名同方药的一致性。

第五十八条 有国家药品标准而无药品批准文号的品种，应当按照同名同方药提出注册申请。申请人应当根据其中医药理论和人用经验情况，开展必要的临床试验。

第五十九条 对照同名同方药有充分的有效性和安全性证据，同名同方药的工艺、辅料与对照同名同方药相同的，或者同名同方药的工艺、辅料变化经研究评估不引起药用物质基础或者药物吸收、利用明显改变的，一般无需开展非临床安全性研究和临床试验。

第八章　上市后变更

第六十条　已上市中药的变更应当遵循中药自身特点和规律，符合必要性、科学性、合理性的有关要求。持有人应当履行变更研究及其评估、变更管理的主体责任，全面评估、验证变更事项对药品安全性、有效性和质量可控性的影响。根据研究、评估和相关验证结果，确定已上市中药的变更管理类别，变更的实施应当按照规定经批准、备案后进行或者报告。持有人在上市后变更研究过程中可与相应药品监督管理部门及时开展沟通交流。

第六十一条　变更药品规格应当遵循与处方药味相对应的原则以及与适用人群、用法用量、装量规格相协调的原则。

对于已有同品种上市的，所申请的规格一般应当与同品种上市规格一致。

第六十二条　生产工艺及辅料等的变更不应当引起药用物质或者药物吸收、利用的明显改变。生产设备的选择应当符合生产工艺及品质保障的要求。

第六十三条　变更用法用量或者增加适用人群范围但不改变给药途径的，应当提供支持该项改变的非临床安全性研究资料，必要时应当进行临床试验。除符合第六十四条规定之情形外，变更用法用量或者增加适用人群范围需开展临床试验的，应当循序开展Ⅱ期临床试验和Ⅲ期临床试验。

已上市儿童用药【用法用量】中剂量不明确的，可根据儿童用药特点和人用经验情况，开展必要的临床试验，明确不同年龄段儿童用药的剂量和疗程。

第六十四条　已上市中药申请变更用法用量或者增加适用人群范围，功能主治不变且不改变给药途径，人用经验证据支持变更后的新用法用量或者新适用人群的用法用量的，可不开展Ⅱ期临床试验，仅开展Ⅲ期临床试验。

第六十五条　替代或者减去国家药品标准处方中的毒性药味或者处于濒危状态的药味，应当基于处方中药味组成及其功效，按照相关技术要求开展与原药品进行药学、非临床有效性和 / 或者非临床安全性的对比研究。替代或者减去处方中已明确毒性药味的，可与安慰剂对照开展Ⅲ期临床试验。替代或者减去处方中处于濒危状态药味的，至少开展Ⅲ期临床试验的比较研究。必要时，需同时变更药品通用名称。

第六十六条　中药复方制剂处方中所含按照新药批准的提取物由外购变更为自行提取的，申请人应当提供相应研究资料，包括但不限于自行研究获得的该提取物及该中药复方制剂的药学研究资料，提取物的非临床有效性和安全性对比研究资料，以及该中药复方制剂Ⅲ期临床试验的对比研究资料。该提取物的质量标准应当附设于制剂标准后。

第六十七条 对主治或者适用人群范围进行删除的，应当说明删除该主治或者适用人群范围的合理性，一般不需开展临床试验。

第九章 中药注册标准

第六十八条 中药注册标准的研究、制定应当以实现中药质量的稳定可控为目标，根据产品特点建立反映中药整体质量的控制指标。尽可能反映产品的质量状况，并关注与中药有效性、安全性的关联。

第六十九条 支持运用新技术、新方法探索建立用于中药复方新药的中间体、制剂质量控制的指纹图谱或者特征图谱、生物效应检测等。中药注册标准中的含量测定等检测项目应当有合理的范围。

第七十条 根据产品特点及实际情况，持有人应当制定不低于中药注册标准的企业内控标准，并通过不断修订和完善其检验项目、方法、限度范围等，提高中药制剂质量。

第七十一条 药品上市后，应当积累生产数据，结合科学技术的发展，持续修订完善包括中药材、中药饮片、中间体和制剂等在内的完整的质量标准体系，以保证中药制剂质量稳定可控。

第十章 药品名称和说明书

第七十二条 中成药命名应当符合《中成药通用名称命名技术指导原则》的要求及国家有关规定。

第七十三条 中药处方中含毒性药味，或者含有其他已经现代毒理学证明具有毒性、易导致严重不良反应的中药饮片的，应当在该中药说明书【成份】项下标明处方中所含的毒性中药饮片名称，并在警示语中标明制剂中含有该中药饮片。

第七十四条 涉及辨证使用的中药新药说明书的【注意事项】应当包含，但不限于以下内容：

（一）因中医的证、病机、体质等因素需要慎用的情形，以及饮食、配伍等方面与药物有关的注意事项；

（二）如有药后调护，应当予以明确。

第七十五条 持有人应当加强对药品全生命周期的管理，加强对安全性风险的监测、评价和分析，应当参照相关技术指导原则及时对中药说明书【禁忌】、【不良反应】、【注意事项】进行完善。

中药说明书【禁忌】、【不良反应】、【注意事项】中任何一项在本规定施行之日起满 3 年后申请药品再注册时仍为"尚不明确"的，依法不予再注册。

第七十六条 古代经典名方中药复方制剂说明书中应当列明【处方来源】、【功能主治的理论依据】等项。

人用经验作为批准上市或者增加功能主治证据的中药新药，说明书中应当列入【中医临床实践】项。

第十一章 附 则

第七十七条 天然药物的药学质量控制可参照本规定执行。天然药物创新药在治疗作用确证阶段，应当至少采用一个 III 期临床试验的数据说明其有效性。其余均应当符合天然药物新药研究的有关要求。

第七十八条 申请进口的中药、天然药物，应当符合所在国或者地区按照药品管理的要求，同时应当符合境内中药、天然药物的安全性、有效性和质量可控性要求。注册申报资料按照创新药的要求提供。国家另有规定的，从其规定。

第七十九条 中药、天然药物注射剂的研制应当符合注射剂研究的通用技术要求。应当根据现有治疗手段的可及性，通过充分的非临床研究说明给药途径选择的必要性和合理性。药物活性成份及作用机理应当明确，并应当开展全面的非临床有效性、安全性研究，循序开展 I 期临床试验、II 期临床试验和 III 期临床试验。

中药、天然药物注射剂上市后，持有人应当开展药品上市后临床研究，不断充实完善临床有效性、安全性证据，应当持续收集不良反应信息，及时修改完善说明书，对临床使用过程中发现的非预期不良反应及时开展非临床安全性研究。持有人应当加强质量控制。

第八十条 省级药品监督管理部门应当按年度向国家药品监督管理部门提交医疗机构中药制剂审批、备案情况的报告。国家药品监督管理部门根据省级药品监督管理部门提交的报告，将医疗机构中药制剂的审批、备案情况纳入药品审评年度报告。

第八十一条 本规定未涉及的药品注册管理的一般性要求按照《药品注册管理办法》执行。实施审批管理的中药材、中药饮片注册管理规定另行制定。

第八十二条 本规定自 2023 年 7 月 1 日起施行。原国家食品药品监督管理局《关于印发中药注册管理补充规定的通知》（国食药监注〔2008〕3 号）同时废止。

Technical Guidances
技术指引

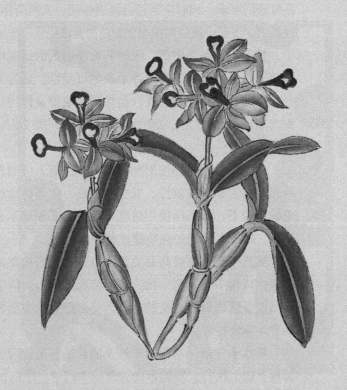

Registration Classifications and Requirements for Application Dossiers of Traditional Chinese Medicines (TCMs)

—————— Table of Contents ——————

Ⅰ. Registration Classifications of TCMs

TCMs refer to medicinal substances and their preparations used based on the TCM theories.

1. Innovative TCMs, which refer to the new TCM formula preparations that have clinical value and have not been marketed overseas, and whose formulas are not included in the national drug standards, national drug registration standards, or *Directory of Ancient Classic Formulas of Traditional Chinese Medicines* issued by the National Administration of Traditional Chinese Medicine. This includes the following circumstances in general:

1.1 Compound preparations of TCMs, which refer to preparations made with multiple prepared slices/decoction pieces and extracts, etc. based on TCM theories.

1.2 Extracts obtained from single plant, animal or mineral materials and their preparations.

1.3 New TCM crude drugs and their preparations, which refer to TCM crude drugs not included in the national drug standards, national drug registration standards or provincial standards, and their preparations, as well as new medicinal parts of TCM crude drugs included by the above standards, and their preparations.

2. Improved new TCMs, which refer to the preparations that change the administration routes and/or dosage forms to marketed TCMs, with clinical application advantages and characteristics, or add functions and indications, etc. This includes the following circumstances in general:

2.1 Preparations with a changed administration route and/or drug-absorbing sites to the marketed TCMs.

2.2 Preparations with a changed dosage form to the marketed TCMs, without changing the administration route.

2.3 TCMs with added functions and indications.

2.4 TCMs with changes in manufacturing process or excipients to marketed TCMs, causing substantial changes in medicinal substances or their absorption and utilization.

3. Compound preparations of TCMs originated from ancient classic formulas, which refer to the prescriptions recorded in ancient TCM classics that conform to the regulations of the *Law of the People's Republic of China on Traditional Chinese Medicines* and are still used currently in practice, with confirmed efficacy and significant characteristics and advantages. This includes the following circumstances:

3.1 Compound preparations of TCMs managed in accordance with the *Directory of Ancient Classic Formulas of Traditional Chinese Medicines*.

3.2 Other compound preparations of TCMs originated from ancient classic formulas, including compound preparations of TCMs originated from ancient classic formulas not listed in the *Directory of Ancient Classic Formulas of Traditional Chinese Medicines* and those with addition or subtraction of ingredients, based on ancient classic formulas.

4. TCMs with identical name and formula (to marketed TCMs), which refer to the preparations that have safety, efficacy and quality control not inferior to those of marketed TCMs, and whose generic name, formula, dosage form, functions and indications, usage and daily dose of decoction pieces are the same as those of marketed TCMs.

Natural medicines refer to natural medicinal substances and their preparations used based on modern medicine theories. The registration and classification of natural medicines should be in accordance with those of TCMs.

Others, mainly include preparations of TCMs and natural medicines marketed overseas but not marketed in China.

II. Requirements for Registration Application Dossiers of TCMs

The following items of and requirements for application dossiers are applicable to innovative TCMs, improved new TCMs, compound preparations of TCMs originated from ancient classic formulas, and TCMs with identical name and formula to marketed TCMs. The applicants should provide corresponding data based on registration classifications, application stages and requirements in the *Guidelines for Registration Application Acceptance Review of Traditional Chinese Medicines*. The dossiers provided by applicants should follow the item number, and if the documents are not should be offered according to cases of different classifications or different application phases, the item number and name should still be kept, and "No relevant study contents" or "N/A" can be indicated under the item. The applicants should provide explanation in the cases of exemption of documents. The applicants should also refer to relevant regulations, technical requirements and relevant stipulations in technical guidelines when drafting dossiers. Certificates issued by overseas drug administrations and all technical data for drugs produced overseas should be translated into Chinese, with the original text attached.

Application dossiers for preparations of natural medicines should be subject to requirements in this document, while the technical requirements should be subject to those for the study of natural medicines. The intended use of natural medicines should be expressed by indications.

Relevant study data on preparations of TCMs and natural medicines that are marketed overseas but not in China should be provided in reference to innovative TCMs.

(I) Administrative documents and drug information

1.0 Cover letter (details in the Attachment: Cover Letter)

It mainly includes a summary and description of key information of the application.

1.1 Directory

The directory of application dossiers should be submitted by chapters.

1.2 Application form

It mainly includes basic product information such as the name, dosage form, specification, registration classification, and application items, etc.

1.3 Product information related materials

1.3.1 Package insert

1.3.1.1 Package insert for investigational drugs and revision instructions (applicable to application for clinical trials)

1.3.1.2 Package insert for marketed drugs and revision instructions (applicable to application for marketing authorization)

A draft of drug package insert should be prepared, and instructions for all the items in the draft should be written in accordance with relevant regulations, and the latest literature references related to the drug's safety and efficacy should be provided.

For drugs marketed overseas, original package inserts approved by the overseas drug administration in the marketing country or region should be provided, and Chinese translation should be attached.

1.3.2 Packaging label

1.3.2.1 Packaging label of investigational drugs (applicable to application for clinical trials)

1.3.2.2 Packaging label of marketed drugs (applicable to application for marketing authorization)

For drugs marketed overseas, samples of packaging labels used in the overseas marketing country or region also should be provided.

1.3.3 Product quality standards and manufacturing processes

Product quality standards should be written according to the format and contents of *Chinese Pharmacopoeia.*

Manufacturing process data (applicable to application for marketing authorization) should be written according to the relevant requirements for format and contents.

1.3.4 Key information of ancient classic formulas

For compound preparations of TCMs originated from ancient classic formulas, the key information including the formula, origin of TCM crude drugs, medicinal parts, processing method, dose, usage and dosage, and functions and indications, etc. should be provided. Compound preparations of TCMs managed in accordance with the *Directory of Ancient Classic Formulas of Traditional Chinese Medicines* should be consistent with relevant information released by the State.

1.3.5 Application dossiers for approval of generic names of drugs

For drugs not listed in the national drug standards or national drug registration standards, application dossiers for approval of generic names of drugs should be provided when applying for marketing authorization.

1.3.6 Inspection related information (applicable to application for marketing authorization)

Including a drug development information sheet, a drug production information sheet, a list of site master documents, an information sheet of clinical trial for drug registration, a clinical trial information sheet and a test report.

1.3.7 Product-related certificates

1.3.7.1 Certificates for TCM crude drugs and prepared slices/decoction pieces, extracts and other ingredients, pharmaceutical excipients and pharmaceutical packaging materials.

Certificates for the source of TCM crude drugs and prepared slices/decoction pieces, extracts and other ingredients.

Certificates for a legal source of pharmaceutical excipients and pharmaceutical packaging materials, including supply agreement and invoices, etc. (applicable to TCM preparations whose medicinal substances, excipients and/or packaging materials have not been registered).

Usage Authorization Letter for pharmaceutical excipients and pharmaceutical packaging materials (applicable to TCM preparations whose medicinal substances, excipients and packaging materials have been registered).

1.3.7.2 Patent information and certificates

A description on the status of any existing patents and its proprietorship for the drug, its formula, manufacturing process and intended use, a declaration of non-infringement on the drug, and relevant supporting documents.

1.3.7.3 Project approval documents for special drugs

Copies of project approval documents for narcotic drugs and psychotropic drugs should be provided.

1.3.7.4 Certificates for the source of control drugs

1.3.7.5 Drug clinical trial related certificates (applicable to application for marketing authorization)

Approval Document for Drug Clinical Trials/Notice of Clinical Trials, Quality Standards of Investigational Drugs and Registration Number of Clinical Trials (internal audit).

1.3.7.6 Qualification certificates of institutions

Non-clinical safety evaluation institutions should provide approval certificates or inspection reports and other certificates conforming to the *Good*

Laboratory Practice (GLP), issued by medical products regulatory authorities. The clinical institutions should provide filing certificates.

1.3.7.7 Certificates for market authorization of drugs (applicable to drugs marketed overseas)

Certificates issued by overseas drug administrations for marketing authorization of drugs, notarial certificates and Chinese translations should be provided. The certificate of approval for export by the species control authority of the exporting country or region should be provided.

1.3.8 Other documents related to the product.

1.4 Application status (if applicable)

1.4.1 Previous approval

Provide descriptions of previous applications related to the current application and approval/rejection certificates (internal audit).

1.4.2 Application for adjusting the clinical trial protocol, suspending or terminating clinical trials

1.4.3 Application for restoring clinical trials after suspension

1.4.4 Re-application for clinical trials after termination

1.4.5 Application for withdrawing the drug clinical trial application and marketing authorization application that have not been approved

1.4.6 Application for changes during the review period of marketing authorization application, which include only changes in the applicant' name, registered address and name, and other changes that do not involve technical review contents

1.4.7 Application for revoking the drug registration certificate

1.5 Application for expedited marketing authorization procedure (if applicable)

1.5.1 Application for expedited marketing authorization procedure

Including the breakthrough therapeutic drug procedure, conditional approval procedure, priority review and approval procedure, and special approval procedure

1.5.2 Application for terminating the expedited marketing authorization procedure

1.5.3 Other applications for expedited registration procedure

1.6 Communication and exchange meeting (if applicable)

1.6.1 Meeting application

1.6.2 Meeting background information

1.6.3 Meeting related letters, minutes and replies

1.7 Clinical trial process management information (if applicable)

1.7.1 Added functions and indications during clinical trials

1.7.2 Changes in the clinical trial protocol, non-clinical or PCMC changes or new findings, etc., that may increase safety risk of the subjects

1.7.3 Requests for adjusting the clinical trial protocol, and suspending or terminating drug clinical trials by the sponsor

1.8 Pharmacovigilance and risk management (if applicable)

1.8.1 Development Safety Update Report (DSUR) and appendixes

1.8.1.1 Development Safety Update Report (DSUR)

1.8.1.2 Cumulative summary table of serious adverse reactions

1.8.1.3 List of domestic dead subjects during the reporting period

1.8.1.4 List of subjects dropped out of clinical trials due to any adverse events during the reporting period

1.8.1.5 Summary table of changes in the drug clinical trial protocol or new clinical findings, and non-clinical or PCMC changes or findings during the reporting period

1.8.1.6 Outline of the overall study plan for the next reporting period

1.8.2 Other potential serious safety risk information

1.8.3 Risk management plan

Including the pharmacovigilance activity plan and risk minimization measures, etc.

1.9 Post-market studies (if applicable)

Including Phase IV studies and studies with specific purposes, etc.

1.10 Certificates of the applicant/manufacturer

1.10.1 Qualification certificates of the applicant/manufacturer of domestically produced drug

Legal registration certificate of the applicant/manufacturer (Business License, etc.). When applying for marketing authorization, the applicant and the manufacturer should have acquired corresponding *Drug Manufacturing Certificate* and changing records (internal audit).

If applying for clinical trials, the applicant should provide descriptions of the preparation of the investigational drug under the condition of following the *Good Manufacturing Practice*.

1.10.2 Qualification certificates of the applicant/manufacturer of drugs produced overseas

Certificates demonstrating that the manufacturing plant and the packaging plant conform to the *Good Manufacturing Practice*, notarial certificates and Chinese translations.

If applying for clinical trials, the applicant should provide descriptions of the preparation of the investigational drug under the condition of following the *Good Manufacturing Practice*.

1.10.3 Certificates of registration agency

When an overseas applicant designates an enterprise legal representative in China to handle relevant drug registration matters, copies of the entrustment document, notarial certificate and their Chinese translations as well as the Business License of the registration agency should be provided.

1.11 Certificates of small and micro enterprises (if applicable)

Notes: 1. Documents marked "if applicable" refer to the applicable documents that should be submitted by the applicant in accordance with the characteristics of the drug under application and application items in connection with the whole life cycle management requirements of the drug. 2. Documents marked "internal audit" refer to documents to be reviewed by the medical products regulatory authorities, while the applicant is not forced to submit such documents. 3. If certificates (including certificates of marketing authorization of drugs, GMP certificates and certificates allowing changes in drugs) issued by overseas drug administrations or regions and submitted for drugs produced overseas conform to the unified format recommended by the World Health Organization (WHO), they may not be notarized by notarial organizations of the country or certified by the Chinese Embassies and Consulates stationed in the country where they were issued.

Attachment: Covering Letter

Application of XX Company for XX of XX Product

1. Brief description

Including but not limited to: product name (proposed), functions and indications, usage and dosage, dosage form and specification.

2. Background information

Briefly describe the product's registration classification and basis, application items and relevant supporting studies.

Application for expedited marketing authorization procedure (including breakthrough therapeutic drug procedure, conditional approval procedure, priority review and approval procedure, and special approval procedure, etc.) and their bases (if applicable).

Additional application items, such as clinical exemption, OTC drugs or pediatric drugs, etc. (if applicable).

3. Other important relevant information that needs special explanation

(II) Overview

2.1 Overview of the submitted TCMs

Briefly describe the drug's name, registration classification and application stage.

Briefly describe the formula, excipients, total produced amount, specification, functions and indications under application, proposed usage and dosage (including dose and duration of administration), and daily human dosage (the dosage of preparation and dosage of TCM crude drugs should be specified).

Briefly describe the project basis, source of formula, and application experience in humans, etc. For improved new TCMs, provide relevant information of the original preparation (e.g., marketing authorization holder, drug approval document No., and current standards, etc.), and briefly describe their similarities and differences in terms of the formulas, manufacturing processes, and quality standards, etc. For TCMs with identical name and formula, provide relevant information of those marketed TCMs with identical name and formula (e.g., marketing authorization holder, drug approval document No., and current standards, etc.) and the selection basis, briefly describe their comparison in terms of the formula, manufacturing processes, and quality control, etc., and explain whether they are consistent or not.

When applying for clinical trials, the applicant should briefly describe the communications and exchanges with the Center for Drug Evaluation, National Medical Products Administration, before the application.

When applying for marketing authorization, the applicant should briefly describe the communications and exchanges with the Center for Drug Evaluation, National Medical Products Administration; describe the conditions of the clinical trial approval document/clinical trial notice, and briefly describe the performance of the study contents and relevant work required to be completed as stated in the clinical trial approval document/clinical trial notice; in case of changes during the clinical trial period, the applicant should describe the changes, whether an application for such changes has been made as required by relevant regulations, and the approval status.

When applying for compound preparations of TCMs originated from ancient classic formulas, the applicant should briefly describe key information such as formula, origin of TCM crude drugs, medicinal parts, processing methods of decoction pieces, dose, usage and dosage, and functions and indications, etc. For compound preparations of TCMs managed in accordance with the *Directory of Ancient Classic Formulas of Traditional Chinese Medicines*, the consistency with information released by the State should be described.

2.2 Summary report of PCMC studies

The summary report of PCMC studies is the summary, analysis and evaluation of the PCMC study results. Their contents and data should be consistent with the relevant PCMC studies, and should be drafted based on different stages.

2.2.1 Summary of main PCMC study results

(1) Supplementary PCMC studies during the clinical trial period (applicable to application for marketing authorization)

Briefly describe the situation and results of supplementary PCMC studies during the clinical trial period.

(2) Ingredients and evaluation of TCM crude drug resources

The applicant should describe the sources of the quality standards for ingredients, and new quality control methods and limits for ingredients. For ingredients that have not been included in the national drug standards, national drug registration standards or provincial standards, the applicant should describe whether studies or applications have been done according to relevant technical requirements, and should briefly describe the results.

The applicant should briefly describe the results of evaluation of TCM crude drug resources.

(3) Processing of decoction pieces

The applicant should briefly describe processing methods of the decoction pieces. When applying for marketing authorization, consistency of processing methods of the decoction pieces in various R&D stages should be specified. In case of any change, relevant reasons and information should be described.

(4) Manufacturing process

The applicant should briefly describe the formula and manufacturing method. Besides, the applicant should also describe changes in the manufacturing process in case of applying for improved new TCMs or TCMs with identical name and formula.

The applicant should briefly describe reasons for the selection of dosage form and the confirmation of specification.

The applicant should briefly describe manufacturing routes, process parameters and the reasons for process verification. If relevant quality control methods for intermediates being established, the applicant should describe the information and report test results.

When applying for clinical trials, the applicant should briefly describe the pilot-scale study results and quality test results, evaluate the rationality of the process, and analyze the feasibility of the process. When applying for marketing authorization, the applicant should briefly describe batches, scales and quality test results, etc. of the scale-up samples and commercial process samples, and should estimate whether the process is stable and feasible.

The applicant should describe standards of excipients. When applying for marketing authorization, the applicant should also describe the information of the pharmaceutical excipient joint review.

(5) Quality standards

The applicant should describe the main contents of the quality standard and their bases, the source of reference substances and the self- test results of the samples.

When applying for marketing authorization, the applicant should briefly describe the changes in quality standards during the phase of clinical trials.

(6) Stability study

The applicant should briefly describe the stability study conditions and results, evaluate the stability of the samples, and propose shelf life and storage conditions.

The applicant should specify primary pharmaceutical packaging materials and containers of the drugs and their standards. When applying for marketing authorization, the applicant should also describe the information of pharmaceutical packaging materials joint review

2.2.2 Analysis and evaluation of PCMC study results

Summarize the results of the ingredient study, evaluation of TCM crude drug resource, selection of dosage form, process studies, quality control studies and stability studies, and comprehensively analyze and evaluate the product quality control results. When applying for clinical trials, the applicant should, in connection with the clinical application backgrounds, pharmacology and toxicology study results and relevant literatures, etc., analyze the correlation between PCMC study results and drug safety and efficacy, evaluate the rationality of the process and quality control, and make a preliminary judgment on stability. When applying for marketing authorization, the applicant should, in connection with the clinical trial results, etc., analyze the correlation between the PCMC study results and the drug safety and efficacy, and evaluate the feasibility of the process, quality control and stability of the drugs.

For compound preparations of TCMs managed in accordance with the *Directory of Ancient Classic Formulas of Traditional Chinese Medicines*, the applicant should describe the correlation of quality among TCM crude drugs, decoction pieces, the samples prepared in accordance with relevant key information of the ancient classic formulas released by the State and records in ancient books, intermediates and preparations.

2.2.3 References

Relevant references should be provided, and full texts should be provided when necessary.

2.3 Summary report of pharmacology and toxicology study data

The summary report of pharmacology and toxicology study data should include comprehensive and critical evaluation of the pharmacology, pharmacokinetics and toxicology studies. The pharmacology and toxicology study strategies should be discussed, and the reasons should be described. GLP compliance of the studies submitted should be described.

For drugs applying for clinical trials, whether the clinical trials under application are supported by the existing pharmacology and toxicology study data should be analyzed and described. During the clinical trial process, if pharmacology and toxicology studies have been performed to support the corresponding clinical trial stage or development progress, the pharmacology and toxicology study data should be updated timely, and relevant study reports should be provided. In case of changes (e.g., changes in process) during the clinical trial period, the pharmacology and toxicology studies should be performed according to such changes, and relevant study reports should be provided. For drugs applying for marketing authorization, pharmacology and toxicology studies performed during the clinical trial period should be described, and comprehensive analysis should be performed to determine whether the existing pharmacology and toxicology study data support the marketing authorization application of the product.

Draft in the following sequence: Overview of Pharmacology and Toxicology Study Strategies, Summary of Pharmacology Studies, Summary of Pharmacokinetics Studies, Summary of Toxicology Studies, Comprehensive Evaluation and Conclusions, and References.

For drugs applying for marketing authorization, the [Pharmacology and Toxicology] item in the package insert should be drafted in accordance with the data of the pharmacology and toxicology studies performed, and descriptions and supporting basis for the package insert should be provided.

2.3.1 Overview of pharmacology and toxicology study strategies

Introduce the thinking and strategies of pharmacology and toxicology studies in connection with the application classification, formula source or data of application experience in humans, and the functions and indications under application, etc.

2.3.2 Summary of pharmacology studies

Briefly summarize the contents of the pharmacology studies. Draft in the following sequence: Overview, Primary Pharmacodynamics, Secondary Pharmacodynamics, Safety Pharmacology, Pharmacodynamic Drug-drug Interactions (DDI), Discussions and Conclusions, and a tabulated Summary.

The primary pharmacodynamic studies should be summarized and evaluated. If secondary pharmacodynamics studies are performed, they should be summarized and evaluated by the organ system/study type. The safety pharmacology studies should be summarized and evaluated. If pharmacodynamic DDI studies are performed, they should be briefly summarized in this section.

2.3.3 Summary of pharmacokinetics studies

Provide a brief outline of the contents of pharmacokinetics studies. Draft in the following sequence: Overview, Analysis Methods, Absorption, Distribution, Metabolism, Excretion, Pharmacokinetic Drug-drug Interactions (DDI), Other Pharmacokinetics Studies, Discussions and Conclusions, and a tabulated Summary.

2.3.4 Summary of toxicology studies

Briefly summarize the toxicology study results, and describe the GLP compliance of the studies and the test substances in the toxicology studies.

Draft in the follow sequence: Overview, Single-dose Toxicity Study, Repeated-dose Toxicity Study, Genotoxicity Study, Carcinogenicity Study, Reproductive Toxicity Study, Preparation Safety Study (irritation, hemolysis and allergy studies, etc.), Other Toxicity Studies, Discussions and Conclusions, and a tabulated Summary.

2.3.5 Comprehensive analysis and evaluation

Comprehensively analyze and evaluate the pharmacology, pharmacokinetics and toxicology studies.

Analyze the dose-effect relationship (e.g., the effective dose, the range of effective dose, etc.) and time-effect relationship (e.g., the effective time, duration of effect, or time of best effect, etc.) of the primary pharmacodynamics studies, and comprehensively evaluate the characteristics of pharmacological effects and their correlation with, and the degree of support for the proposed functions and indications.

Safety pharmacology studies are a part of non-clinical safety evaluation, which can be comprehensively evaluated in connection with toxicology study results.

Analyze the characteristics of absorption, distribution, metabolism, excretion, and drug-drug interactions (DDI) in connection with various pharmacokinetics studies, including pharmacokinetic characteristics of the test substance and/or its active metabolites, such as absorption degree and rate, dynamic parameters, main tissues of distribution, bonding degree with plasma proteins, metabolite and possible metabolic pathways, excretion pathways and degree, etc. It is necessary to pay attention to whether the pharmacokinetics study results support the selection of the animal species for the toxicology studies. Analyze various toxicology study results, and comprehensively analyze and evaluate the correlation among the results of various studies, and the differences among species and genders, etc.

Analyze the correlation among the results of pharmacology, pharmacokinetics and toxicology studies.

Comprehensively analyze and evaluate the study results in connection with the PCMC and clinical study data.

2.3.6 References

Relevant references should be provided, and full texts should be provided when necessary.

2.4 Summary report of clinical study data

2.4.1 TCM theories or study background

Provide brief descriptions of the corresponding TCM theories or study background according to the registration classification. For compound preparations of TCMs originated from ancient classic formulas, the formula source, functions and indications, usage and dosage and other key information and their bases, etc. should be described briefly.

2.4.2 Application experience in humans

If there is application experience in humans, a brief summary of the application experience in humans should be provided, and the support of the application experience in humans for the proposed functions and indications or clinical trials to be carried out subsequently should be analyzed and described.

2.4.3 Summary of clinical trial data

It can be drafted in accordance with the relevant requirements in the

Guidelines for the Formats and Contents of the Overview of Traditional Chinese Medicines and Natural Medicines: Overview of Clinical Trial Data.

2.4.4 Clinical value evaluation

Briefly evaluate the clinical value based on benefit-risk evaluation and in connection with the registration classification.

2.4.5 References

Relevant references should be provided, and full texts should be provided when necessary.

2.5 Comprehensive analysis and evaluation

Comprehensively analyze and evaluate the safety, efficacy and quality control of the drug, and the scientificity, normalization and integrity of the studies based on the study results and in connection with the project basis.

When applying for clinical trials, the applicant should evaluate the efficacy for the proposed indications and the safety of clinical application of the product under application based on the study results, comprehensively analyze the correlation among the study results, and weigh risks-benefits of the clinical trials, so as to provide support and basis for determining whether or how to carry out clinical trials.

When applying for marketing authorization, on the basis of having a complete understanding of the drug study results, the applicant should comprehensively evaluate the benefits for the selected target population and potential problems or risks in clinical application.

(III) PCMC study data

The applicant should provide corresponding PCMC study data based on the requirements of application stages. For the corresponding technical requirements, see the relevant technical guidelines for PCMC studies of TCMs.

3.1 Ingredients and evaluation of TCM crude drug resources

3.1.1 Ingredients

TCM ingredients include decoction pieces and extracts, etc.

3.1.1.1 Relevant information of ingredients

Provide the sources of various ingredients in the formula (including the manufacturers/suppliers, etc.), current standards and related supporting information.

Decoction pieces: Provide the origins of TCM crude drugs (including family names, Chinese names and Latin names), medicinal parts (for mineral medicines, the category, family, ore name or rock name, and main ingredients should be indicated), places of origins of TCM crude drugs, harvesting period, processing methods of decoction pieces, and information on whether the TCM crude drugs are planted and cultivated (man-made products) or derived from wild resources. For TCM crude drugs whose origins are easily confused, the origin identification report of the TCM crude drugs needs to be provided. For TCM crude drugs of multiple origins, in addition to conforming to requirements of the quality standards, the origin must be fixed, and the basis for selection of the origin should be provided. The place of origin of TCM crude drugs should be fixed. For TCM crude drugs involving endangered species, they should conform to the relevant regulations of the State and have guaranteed sustainable availability, and special attention must be paid to the legality of their sources.

For decoction pieces used for compound preparations of TCMs managed in accordance with the *Directory of Ancient Classic Formulas of Traditional Chinese Medicines*, the origins of TCM crude drugs, medicinal parts and processing methods, etc. should be consistent with key information of ancient classic formulas released by the State. The basis for selection of the place of origin should be provided, and Daodi (geo-authentic) TCM crude drugs and/or TCM crude drugs from main places of origin should be selected as much as possible.

Extracts: For outsourced extracts, their relevant approval (filing) status, preparation methods and manufacturers/suppliers and other information should be provided. For self-prepared extracts, relevant information of the decoction pieces used and the detailed preparation process and process study data should be provided (the specific requirements are the same as those in "3.3 Preparation process").

3.1.1.2 Quality studies of ingredients

Provide the test reports of ingredients.

For self-formulated quality standards or those improved from the original versions, relevant study data (refer to the relevant requirements in "3.4 Studies of preparation quality and quality standards"), the draft of quality standards and drafting instructions, drug standard substances and relevant data, etc. should be provided.

For compound preparations of TCMs managed in accordance with the *Directory of Ancient Classic Formulas of Traditional Chinese Medicines*, quality study data of multiple batches of TCM crude drugs and prepared slices/decoction pieces should also be provided.

3.1.1.3 Ecological environment, morphological descriptions, growth characteristics, and planting and cultivation (artificial production) technology, etc. of TCM crude drugs

These should be provided for the application of new TCM crude drugs.

3.1.1.4 Plant, animal and mineral specimens. Plant specimens should include all organs such as flower, fruit, and seed, etc.

These should be provided for the application of new TCM crude drugs.

3.1.2 Evaluation of TCM crude drug resources

See relevant technical guidelines for the requirements of evaluation contents and conclusions of TCM crude drug resources.

3.1.3 References

Relevant references should be provided, and full texts should be provided when necessary.

3.2 Processing of decoction pieces

3.2.1 Processing methods of decoction pieces

Specify processing methods of the decoction pieces, and provide processing basis and detailed process parameters of decoction pieces. For decoction pieces used in compound preparations of TCMs managed in accordance with the

Directory of Ancient Classic Formulas of Traditional Chinese Medicines, their processing methods should be consistent with the key information of ancient classic formulas released by the State.

When applying for marketing authorization, consistency of the processing methods of decoction pieces in various R&D stages should be described, and relevant study data should be provided when necessary.

3.2.2 References

Relevant references should be provided, and full texts should be provided when necessary.

3.3 Preparation process

3.3.1 Formula

Provide the formula composition of 1000 preparation units.

3.3.2 Procedure

3.3.2.1 Preparation process flowchart

Provide a complete, intuitive and concise process flowchart in accordance with the preparation process steps, which should cover all process steps, and the main process parameters and extraction solvents used, etc. should be indicated.

3.3.2.2 Detailed descriptions of preparation methods

Provide normative descriptions of the manufacturing process (including the packaging steps), and specify the operation process, process parameters and their ranges.

3.3.3 Dosage form and medicinal substances and excipients

Ingredients and excipients	Dosage	Functions	Current standards
Solvents used but finally removed in the preparation process			

(1) Describe the specific dosage form and specification. List the formula composition of the unit-dose product, in which the functions and current standards of various ingredients (e.g., decoction pieces, extracts) and excipients in the formula should be listed. The solvents used but finally removed in the preparation process should also be listed.

(2) Describe the packaging materials and containers of the product.

3.3.4 Preparation process study data

3.3.4.1 Screening of preparation process route

Provide study data on the screening of preparation process route, and describe the basis for selection of the preparation process route. If the formula comes from hospital preparations, well-proved clinical formulas or has application experience in humans, its specific use conditions in clinical application should be described in detail (e.g., manufacturing process, dosage form, dosage and specification, etc.).

For improved new TCMs, their similarities and differences in the manufacturing process compared with the original preparations and the changes in parameters should also be described.

For compound preparations of TCMs managed in accordance with the *Directory of Ancient Classic Formulas of Traditional Chinese Medicines*, the manufacturing process data from a study carried out in accordance with key information of ancient classic formulas released by the State and records in ancient books should be provided.

For TCMs with identical name and formula, their comparison in manufacturing process with marketed TCMs with identical name and formula should be described, and whether they are consistent or not should also be described.

3.3.4.2 Selection of dosage form

Provide the basis for selection of dosage form.

For compound preparations of TCMs managed in accordance with the *Directory of Ancient Classic Formulas of Traditional Chinese Medicines*, descriptions on the consistency between their dosage form (decoctions can be made into granules) and records in ancient books should be provided.

3.3.4.3 Pre-treatment process of ingredients in prescription

Provide pre-treatment process and specific process parameters of ingredients in prescription. When applying for marketing authorization, key process parameter control points should also be specified.

3.3.4.4 Extraction and purification process study

Describe the extraction and purification process, main process parameters and their ranges, etc.

Provide the basis for determination of the extraction and purification method and main process parameters. Determination of the ranges of manufacturing process parameters should be supported by relevant study data. When applying for marketing authorization, key process parameter control points should also be specified.

3.3.4.5 Concentration process

Describe the concentration method, main process parameters and their ranges, and manufacturing equipment, etc.

Provide the basis for determination of concentration method and main process parameters. Determination of the ranges of manufacturing process parameters should be supported by relevant study data. When applying for marketing authorization, key process parameter control points should also be specified.

3.3.4.6 Drying process

Describe the drying method, main process parameters and their ranges, and manufacturing equipment, etc.

Provide the basis for determination of drying method and main process parameters. Determination of the ranges of manufacturing process parameters should be supported by relevant study data. When applying for marketing authorization, key process parameter control points should also be specified.

3.3.4.7 Molding process of preparation

Describe the molding process of preparation, main process parameters and range, etc.

Provide study data on intermediates, excipients and screening of preparation formulas, and specify the category, grade and dosage, etc. of the excipients.

Provide the basis for determination of molding method and main process parameters. Determination of the ranges of manufacturing process parameters should be supported by relevant study data. Make analysis of physical and chemical properties related to preparation properties. When applying for marketing authorization, key process parameter control points should also be specified.

3.3.5 Pilot-scale and manufacturing process validation

3.3.5.1 Information about sample manufacturer

This should be filled in according to practical situation when applying for clinical trials, and may not be filled in if not applicable.

When applying for marketing authorization, the manufacturer's name and address of the manufacturing site, etc. should be provided. Copies of legal registration certificate and *Drug Manufacturing Certificate* of the sample manufacturer should be provided.

3.3.5.2 Batch formulations

List the batch formulation composition of the product (when applying for clinical trials, take the pilot scale; when applying for marketing authorization, take commercial scale), and list current standards of various ingredients (e.g., decoction pieces, extracts) and excipients. The solvents used but finally removed in the preparation process should also be listed.

Ingredients and excipients	Dosage	Current standards
Solvents used but finally removed in the preparation process		

3.3.5.3 Description of manufacturing process

Describe the manufacturing process (including packaging steps) of the samples according to unit operation process (when applying for clinical trials, take pilot-scale test batch; when applying for marketing authorization, take commercial-scale manufacturing process validation batch), and specify the operation process, process parameters and ranges.

3.3.5.4 Excipients and materials used during manufacturing

Provide the grade, manufacturer/supplier, current standards and relevant certificates, etc. of the excipients and materials used during manufacturing. In case internal control standards have been established for excipients, such standards should be provided. Provide the test report of the excipients and materials used during manufacturing.

If the excipients used need to be refined, the refining process study data, internal control standards and its drafting instructions should be provided.

When applying for marketing authorization, the applicant should describe the information of pharmaceutical excipient joint review.

3.3.5.5 Main manufacturing equipment

Provide information on the main manufacturing equipment used during the pilot-scale (applicable to application for clinical trials) or process validation (applicable to application for marketing authorization) process. For TCMs applying for marketing authorization, it is necessary to pay attention to that selections of the manufacturing equipment should conform to requirements for manufacturing process.

3.3.5.6 Control of key steps and intermediates

List all key steps and control ranges of process parameters. Provide study results to support the basis for determination of key steps and the basis of the control ranges of process parameters. When applying for marketing authorization, key process parameter control points should also be specified.

List quality control standards of intermediates, including the items, methods and limits, and methodological validation data should be provided when necessary.

Specify yield ranges of the intermediates (e.g., extracts).

3.3.5.7 Manufacturing data and process validation data

Provide summary data of samples from representative batches during the R&D process (when applying for clinical trials, including but not limited to pilot scale-up batches; when applying for marketing authorization, including but not limited to pilot scale-up batches, clinical trial batches, and commercial-scale manufacturing process validation batches, etc.), including: batch number, manufacturing time and site, manufacturing data, batch size, intended use (such as for stability study), and quality test results (e.g., content and other main quality indicators). When applying for marketing authorization, the applicant should provide commercial-scale manufacturing process validation data, including the process validation protocol and report, and the manufacturing process must be performed within the predetermined parameter range.

For the manufacturing process study, it is necessary to pay attention to the cohesion between the laboratory conditions and the pilot scale and manufacturing, and consider the feasibility and adaptability of large scale manufacturing equipment. In case of optimization of the manufacturing process, main changes in the manufacturing process study (including changes in batch size, equipment, and process parameters, etc.), and relevant supporting validation study should be described in detail.

For compound preparations of TCMs managed in accordance with the *Directory of Ancient Classic Formulas of Traditional Chinese Medicines*, relevant study data of samples prepared in accordance with key information of ancient classic formulas released by the State and records in ancient books, pilot scale samples and commercial scale samples should be provided.

During the clinical trial period, in case of changes in drug specification and preparation process, etc., study should be carried out based on changes and in reference to relevant technical guidelines, and for significant changes and changes causing obvious changes in absorption and utilization of medicinal substances or preparations, supplementary application should be filed. When applying for marketing authorization, the changes (including changes in equipment and process parameters, etc.), causes for changes, change time and whether relevant changes have obtained approval from the National Medical Products Administration, etc. should be described in detail, and relevant study data should be provided.

3.3.6 Preparation conditions of the samples for studies

3.3.6.1 Samples for toxicology studies

Information on preparation of samples for toxicology studies should be provided, which should generally include:

(1) Summary of manufacturing data of the samples for toxicology studies, including batch number, feeding amount, yield amount and intended use, etc. Samples for toxicology studies should be those at pilot scale and above,

(2) Sources, batch numbers and self-test reports, etc. of the ingredients used for preparing samples for toxicology studies,

(3) Information on main manufacturing equipment used for preparing samples for toxicology studies, and

(4) Quality standards, self-test reports and relevant chromatograms, etc. of the samples for toxicology studies.

3.3.6.2 Investigational drugs (applicable to application for marketing authorization)

When applying for marketing authorization, the applicant should provide preparation information on investigational drugs and placebos for clinical trials (if applicable).

(1) Investigational drugs

Provide copies of batch production records of the investigational drugs. The manufacturing plant/workshop and production line should be specified in the batch production records.

Provide information on origin and place of origin and self-test reports of the ingredients used in the investigational drugs.

Provide the main equipment used during manufacturing and other information.

Provide self-test reports and relevant chromatograms of the investigational drugs.

(2) Placebos

Provide copies of batch production records of the placebos for clinical trials.

Provide information on the formulation, source of formulation ingredients and current standards, etc. of the placebos for clinical trials.

Provide comparative study data on the property and flavor of the placebo and trial sample, and describe consistency of the placebo and trial sample in aspects including appearance, size, color, weight, taste and flavor, etc.

3.3.7 "Manufacturing Process" document (applicable to application for marketing authorization)

For drugs applying for marketing authorization, "Manufacturing Process" document should be provided in reference to common format and guidelines on writing of manufacturing processes for TCMs.

3.3.8 References

Relevant references should be provided, and full texts should be provided when necessary.

3.4 Study on preparation quality and quality standards

3.4.1 Study on chemical components

Provide literature data or trial data of study on chemical components.

3.4.2 Quality study

Provide trial data of the quality study and relevant literatures.

For compound preparations of TCMs managed in accordance with the *Directory of Ancient Classic Formulas of Traditional Chinese Medicines*, study data on the correlation of quality of the TCM crude drugs, decoction pieces, the samples prepared in accordance with key information of ancient classic formulas released by the State and records in ancient books, intermediates and preparations should be provided.

For TCMs with identical name and formula, the quality comparison study results with marketed TCMs with identical name and formula should be provided.

3.4.3 Quality standards

A draft of drug quality standard and the instructions, reference standards and relevant information should be provided. For the reference substances used during the drug development process, the sources, package inserts and batch numbers should be provided. For the reference substances without being standardized by the legal department, when applying for clinical trials, it is necessary to describe whether the study has been carried out in accordance with relevant technical requirements or not, and provide relevant study data; when applying for marketing authorization, it is necessary to describe whether the reference substances has been standardized by the legal department or not, and provide relevant certificates.

The Chinese versions of quality standards provided for drugs produced overseas must be sorted out and submitted in accordance with the format of national drug standards or national drug registration standards in China.

3.4.4 Test report of samples

When applying for clinical trials, the self-test report of at least one batch of samples should be provided. When applying for marketing authorization, the self-test report, as well as the verification of quality standard and following quality control test of 3 continuous batches of samples should be provided.

3.4.5 References

Relevant references should be provided, and full texts should be provided when necessary.

3.5 Stability

3.5.1 Stability summary

Summarize samples, conditions, indicators and results of the stability study, and formulate the storage conditions and shelf life.

3.5.2 Stability study data

Provide stability study data and chromatograms.

3.5.3 Selection of primary packaging materials and containers of the drugs

Illustrate the basis for selection. Provide current standards, test reports, manufacturers/suppliers and relevant certificates, etc. of the packaging materials and containers. Provide data on compatibility study and other studies performed regarding the packaging materials and containers selected (if applicable).

When applying for marketing authorization, the applicant should describe the information of pharmaceutical packaging materials joint review.

3.5.4 Post-market stability study protocol and commitments (applicable to application for marketing authorization)

When applying for drug marketing authorization, the applicant should commit to perform long-term stability study of the first three batches of products manufactured after marketing, and perform long-term stability study of at least one batch of products manufactured every year, and should inform medical products regulatory authorities timely in case of abnormal conditions.

Provide subsequent stability study protocol.

3.5.5 References

Relevant references should be provided, and full texts should be provided when necessary.

(IV) Pharmacology and toxicology study data

The applicant should provide corresponding pharmacology and toxicology study data based on requirements of different application stages. See corresponding detailed requirements in relevant technical guidelines.

The non-clinical safety evaluation study should be carried out in an institution with GLP Certificate.

Pharmacology and toxicology studies of natural medicines should be carried out in reference to technical requirements for corresponding studies.

4.1 Pharmacology study data

The pharmacology study refers to obtaining information on non-clinical efficacy via animal or in vitro or ex vivo studies, including pharmacodynamic effect and characteristics, and mechanism of drug action, etc. The design thought, implementation process, results and evaluation of the study should be listed in the pharmacology application dossiers.

For innovative TCMs, main pharmacodynamic study data should be provided, to provide evidence for entering clinical trials. Evidences for efficacy of the drug entering clinical trials include TCM theories, clinical application experience in humans and pharmacodynamic study. In accordance with differences in formula source and preparation process, etc., the above evidences account for different weights, which should be taken into comprehensive consideration when carrying out studies.

Design of pharmacodynamic trial should take TCM characteristics into consideration, and select appropriate study items in accordance with proposed functions and indications of the test substance.

For extracts and their preparations, the purification degree of extracts should be determined upon screening study. The screening study should be correlated with the proposed functions and indications, and the pharmacology and toxicology studies carried out during the screening process should be embodied in the pharmacology and toxicology application dossiers. In case of marketing of extracts and their preparations with same ingredients, comparison should be made with such extracts and preparations in pharmacodynamics and other aspects, to prove their advantages and characteristics.

For compound preparations of TCMs, the pharmacodynamic study may be appropriately exempted in accordance with the formula source and composition, clinical application experience in humans and preparation process conditions, etc.

For compound preparations of TCMs with application experience in humans, the pharmacodynamic study may be approximately exempted in accordance with support degree of application experience in humans for drug efficacy; if application experience in humans has a certain support effect on drug efficacy, then when the formula composition, process route, clinical positioning, usage and dosage, etc. are basically consistent with previous clinical applications, the pharmacodynamic study data may not be provided.

For compound preparations of TCMs based on modern pharmacology study components, basis of the components should be described by means of study, and information on non-clinical efficacy should be provided via the pharmacodynamic study.

For improved new TCMs, the requirements for pharmacodynamic data should be determined in accordance with the modification purpose and specific changes. If the modification purpose lies in or includes improvement of efficacy, then corresponding comparative pharmacodynamic study data should be provided, to describe advantages of the modification. For added functions and indications of TCMs, pharmacodynamic study data supporting the new functions and indications should be provided, and the pharmacodynamic study may be appropriately exempted in accordance with support degree of application experience in humans for drug efficacy.

The safety pharmacology study belongs to a part of non-clinical safety evaluation, and its requirements are as shown in "4.3 Toxicology study data".

Pharmacology study reports should be submitted in the following sequence:

4.1.1 Primary pharmacodynamics

4.1.2 Secondary pharmacodynamics

4.1.3 Safety pharmacology

4.1.4 Pharmacodynamic drug-drug interactions (DDI)

4.2 Pharmacokinetics study data

The non-clinical pharmacokinetics study is to reveal the rule of dynamic changes of the drug in animal body by in vitro and in vivo studies, obtain basic pharmacokinetic parameters of the drug, and illustrate the absorption, distribution, metabolism and excretion process and characteristics of the drug.

For single-ingredient preparation extracted, reference should be made to non-clinical pharmacokinetics study requirements for chemical drugs.

For other preparations, the pharmacokinetics study or exploratory pharmacokinetics study should be carried out as the case may be (e.g., safety risk degree).

For sustained and controlled release preparations, non-clinical pharmacokinetics study should be performed before the clinical trial, to describe their sustained and controlled release characteristics; for the preparation with a changed dosage form to the marketed TCMs, the pharmacokinetic comparison study should also be performed with the original dosage form; for sustained and controlled release preparations of TCMs with identical name and formula, non-clinical pharmacokinetic comparison study should be performed.

When carrying out non-clinical pharmacokinetics study of TCMs, the complexity of their ingredients should be taken into full consideration, and an appropriate method should be selected in connection with their characteristics to carry out study on in vivo process or active metabolites, so as to provide a reference for subsequent R&D stages.

If combined use with other drugs (especially chemical drugs) is involved in the clinical trial to be performed, in vitro or in vivo study may be performed to evaluate the potential drug-drug interactions.

Pharmacokinetics study reports should be submitted in the following sequence:

4.2.1 Analysis method and verification report

4.2.2 Absorption

4.2.3 Distribution (plasma protein binding rate, tissue distribution, etc.)

4.2.4 Metabolism (in vitro metabolism, in vivo metabolism, possible metabolism pathway, induction or inhibition of drug-metabolizing enzymes, etc.)

4.2.5 Excretion

4.2.6 Pharmacokinetic drug-drug interactions (non-clinical)

4.2.7 Other pharmacokinetics studies

4.3 Toxicology study data

The toxicology study includes: single-dose toxicity study, repeated-dose toxicity study, genotoxicity study, reproductive toxicity study, carcinogenicity study, dependence study, irritation, allergy and hemolysis studies and other preparation safety studies related to local or systemic administration, and other toxicity studies, etc.

For innovative TCMs, more safety information should be obtained as much as possible, to facilitate the evaluation of safety risks. The requirements for toxicology study may differ in accordance with the drug characteristics and differences in the cognition of safety.

For new TCM crude drugs and their preparations, comprehensive toxicology study should be carried out, including safety pharmacology study, single-dose toxicity study, repeated-dose toxicity study, genotoxicity study and reproductive toxicity study, etc., and corresponding preparation safety studies should be carried out in accordance with the administration route and preparation conditions, while the remaining studies should be determined in accordance with specific situations.

For extracts and their preparations, requirements for toxicology study should be determined in accordance with their clinical application status and safety information that can be acquired. If the project of extracts comes from a study, and there is a lack of recognition on their safety, then comprehensive toxicology study should be carried out. If the project of extracts comes from traditional application, and their manufacturing processes are basically consistent with traditional application, then safety pharmacology study, single-dose toxicity study, and repeated-dose toxicity study should be carried out in general, and other studies may need to be carried out when necessary.

For compound preparations of TCMs, in accordance with differences in their formula source and composition, safety application experience in humans and safety risk degree, corresponding toxicology study data should be provided. If the study items are partially exempted, sufficient reasons should be provided.

For those adopting traditional process and with application experience in humans, single-dose toxicity study and repeated-dose toxicity study data should be provided in general.

For those adopting non-traditional process but with clinical application data for reference, safety pharmacology, single-dose toxicity study and repeated-dose toxicity study data should be provided in general.

For those adopting non-traditional process and without application experience in humans, a comprehensive toxicology study should be carried out in general.

In case of identifying unexpected adverse reactions in the clinical trial or unexpected toxicity in the toxicology study, an additional study should be carried out.

For improved new TCMs, corresponding toxicology study data should be provided in accordance with the changes. If the purpose of modification lies in or includes improvement of safety, toxicological comparison study should be carried out, to make comparison with the original dosage form/administration route/process, so as to describe advantages of the modification.

When adding functions and indications of TCMs, for those requiring prolonging of administration period or increasing dose, it should be described whether the original toxicology study data can support such prolonged period or increased dose, and otherwise toxicology study data supporting such prolonged administration period or increased dose should be provided.

Generally speaking, safety pharmacology, single-dose toxicity, repeated-dose toxicity and genotoxicity study data supporting corresponding clinical trial period, allergy, irritation and hemolysis study data or literature data should be provided when applying for clinical trials. In the follow-up period, repeated-dose toxicity studies supporting different administration periods of clinical trial or supporting marketing should be provided in accordance with the progress of the clinical trial. The reproductive toxicity study should be provided in different development stages of clinical trials in accordance with the risk degree. Generally, carcinogenic study data can be provided when applying for marketing authorization.

During the drug R&D process, in case of changes in manufacturing process of the test substance that may influence its safety, corresponding toxicology study should be carried out.

The design thought, implementation process, results and evaluation of the study should be listed in the toxicology study data.

Toxicology study reports should be submitted in the following sequence:

4.3.1 Single-dose toxicity study

4.3.2 Repeated-dose toxicity study

4.3.3 Genotoxicity study

4.3.4 Carcinogenicity study

4.3.5 Reproductive toxicity study

4.3.6 Preparation safety study (irritation, hemolysis, and allergy studies, etc.)

4.3.7 Other toxicity studies

(V) Clinical study data

5.1. Innovative TCMs

5.1.1 Innovative TCMs whose formula composition conforms to TCM theories and having application experience in humans

5.1.1.1 TCM theories

5.1.1.1.1 Formula composition, functions and indications

5.1.1.1.2 Basic understanding of indications in TCM theories

5.1.1.1.3 TCM theories of the proposed formula

5.1.1.1.4 Rationality evaluation of formula

5.1.1.1.5 Safety analysis of formula

5.1.1.1.6 Comparison with same variety of TCMs having existing national drug standards or national drug registration standards

5.1.1.2 Application experience in humans

5.1.1.2.1 Certificates

5.1.1.2.2 Outline of previous clinical applications

5.1.1.2.3 Literature review

5.1.1.2.4 Summary report of previous clinical applications

5.1.1.2.5 Outline of proposed indications, available treatments, and unmet clinical needs

5.1.1.2.6 Evaluation of support of application experience in humans for proposed functions and indications

Specific drafting requirements for TCM theories and application experience in humans may refer to relevant technical requirements and guidelines.

5.1.1.3 Clinical trials

If clinical trials are necessary, the following data should be submitted:

5.1.1.3.1 Clinical trial plan and protocol as well as the appendixes

5.1.1.3.1.1 Clinical trial plan and protocol

5.1.1.3.1.2 Sample of informed consent form

5.1.1.3.1.3 Investigator's Brochure

5.1.1.3.1.4 Statistical analysis plan

5.1.1.3.2 Clinical trial report and the appendixes (submitted after completion of clinical trials)

5.1.1.3.2.1 Clinical trial report

5.1.1.3.2.2 Sample of case report form and patient log, etc.

5.1.1.3.2.3 Key standard operating procedures for primary efficacy and safety data of clinical trials

5.1.1.3.2.4 Description of changes in the clinical trial protocol

5.1.1.3.2.5 Approval documents from Ethics Committee

5.1.1.3.2.6 Statistical analysis plan

5.1.1.3.2.7 Electronic documents of clinical trial database

When applying for drug marketing authorization after completing clinical trials, the applicant should submit the clinical trial database in the form of CD. Specific requirements for database format and relevant documents, etc. may refer to relevant guidelines for submitting clinical trial data.

5.1.1.3.3 References

Provide full texts of related references, and for foreign literatures, Chinese translation of the abstract and citations should also be provided.

5.1.1.4 Clinical value evaluation

Evaluate the clinical value of the product and support of the application dossiers for proposed functions and indications based on benefit-risk evaluation, TCM theories, application experience in humans and clinical trial results.

Note:

Based on TCM theories and application experience in humans, the applicant may have communications and exchanges with the Center for Drug Evaluation on requirements for clinical trials before submitting the application for clinical trials.

5.1.2 Innovative TCMs from other sources

5.1.2.1 Study background

5.1.2.1.1 Proposed functions and indications and clinical positioning

The applicant should, in accordance with the R&D conditions and the TCM theories on which the formula is based, describe the basis for determination of the proposed functions and indications and clinical positioning, including but not limited to literature analysis and pharmacology study, etc.

5.1.2.1.2 Outline of diseases, available treatments, and unmet clinical needs

Describe the basic information of the proposed indications, studies on available treatments both at home and abroad and relevant drug marketing conditions, main problems with existing treatments and unmet clinical needs, and also describe the expected safety and efficacy characteristics and the problems to be solved of this product.

5.1.2.2 Clinical trials

Data should be submitted in accordance with relevant requirements under "5.1.1.3 Clinical trials".

5.1.2.3 Clinical value evaluation

Based on benefit-risk evaluation and in connection with the study background and clinical trials, evaluate the clinical value of the product and support of the application dossiers for proposed functions and indications.

Note:

Based on the formula composition, administration route and non-clinical safety evaluation results, etc., the applicant may have communications and exchanges with the Center for Drug Evaluation on requirements for clinical trials before submitting the application for clinical trials.

5.2. Improved new TCMs

5.2.1 Study background

The purpose and basis for modification should be described. If application experience in humans is available, data should be submitted in accordance with relevant requirements under "5.1.1.2 Application experience in humans".

5.2.2 Clinical trials

Data should be submitted in accordance with relevant requirements under "5.1.1.3 Clinical trials".

5.2.3 Clinical value evaluation

In connection with the modification purpose and clinical trials, evaluate the clinical value of the product and support of the application dossiers for proposed changes.

Note:

In reference to relevant requirements for innovative TCMs, the applicant may have communications and exchanges with the Center for Drug Evaluation on requirements for clinical trials before submitting the application for clinical trials.

5.3 Compound preparations of TCMs originated from ancient classic formulas

5.3.1 Compound preparations of TCMs managed in accordance with the *Directory of Ancient Classic Formulas of Traditional Chinese Medicines*

Provide drafting instructions and basis of the drug package insert, and describe contents and basis of clinically relevant items in the drug package insert.

5.3.2 Other compound preparations of TCMs originated from ancient classic formulas

5.3.2.1 Discussion on the formula source and historical development, formula composition, functions and indications, usage and dosage and TCM theories of ancient classic formulas

5.3.2.2 For compound preparations of TCMs with addition or subtraction of ingredients based on ancient classic formulas, the cause and basis for such addition or subtraction, rationality evaluation of formula, and safety analysis of formula should also be provided.

5.3.2.3 Application experience in humans

5.3.2.3.1 Certificates

5.3.2.3.2 Outline of previous clinical applications

5.3.2.3.3 Literature review

5.3.2.3.4 Summary report of previous clinical applications

5.3.2.3.5 Evaluation of support of application experience in humans for proposed functions and indications

5.3.2.4 Clinical value evaluation

Based on benefit-risk evaluation and in connection with TCM theories, formula source and its addition or subtraction, and application experience in humans, evaluate the clinical value of the product and support of the application dossiers for proposed functions and indications.

5.3.2.5 Drafting instructions and basis of drug package insert

Describe contents and basis of clinically relevant items in the drug package insert.

Specific drafting requirements for TCM theories, application experience in humans and drug package insert may refer to relevant technical requirements and guidelines.

Note:

Implementation rules and technical requirements for registration application, review and approval and marketing regulation, etc. for such TCMs should be formulated separately.

5.4 TCMs with identical name and formula

5.4.1 Study background

Provide the basis for selecting references TCMs with identical name and formula.

5.4.2 Clinical trials

If clinical trials are necessary, data should be submitted in accordance with relevant requirements under "5.1.1.3 Clinical trials".

5.5 Changes during the clinical trial period (if applicable)

For drugs approved for carrying out clinical trials, if the scope of target population is to be enlarged (e.g., add the pediatric population), and the usage and dosage are to be changed (e.g., increase the dose or prolong the treatment course), etc., corresponding project purpose and basis, clinical trial plan and protocol and the appendixes should be provided in accordance with the changes; and if during clinical trials of drugs, there are changes in the clinical trial protocol of drugs, non-clinical or pharmaceutical changes or new findings, which need to be considered as supplementary application, then specific comparison and description of the changes in protocol as well as the cause and basis of the changes should be provided for clinical aspects.

In the meantime, it is also necessary to analyze and sort out the existing data on application experience in humans and clinical trials, so as to provide basis for changes, and attention should be paid to influences of the changes on efficacy and safety risks to the subjects.

中药注册分类及申报资料要求

—— 目　录 ——

一、中药注册分类

中药是指在我国中医药理论指导下使用的药用物质及其制剂。

1. **中药创新药**。指处方未在国家药品标准、药品注册标准及国家中医药主管部门发布的《古代经典名方目录》中收载，具有临床价值，且未在境外上市的中药新处方制剂。一般包含以下情形：

1.1 中药复方制剂，系指由多味饮片、提取物等在中医药理论指导下组方而成的制剂。

1.2 从单一植物、动物、矿物等物质中提取得到的提取物及其制剂。

1.3 新药材及其制剂，即未被国家药品标准、药品注册标准以及省、自治区、直辖市药材标准收载的药材及其制剂，以及具有上述标准药材的原动、植物新的药用部位及其制剂。

2. **中药改良型新药**。指改变已上市中药的给药途径、剂型，且具有临床应用优势和特点，或增加功能主治等的制剂。一般包含以下情形：

2.1 改变已上市中药给药途径的制剂，即不同给药途径或不同吸收部位之间相互改变的制剂。

2.2 改变已上市中药剂型的制剂，即在给药途径不变的情况下改变剂型的制剂。

2.3 中药增加功能主治。

2.4 已上市中药生产工艺或辅料等改变引起药用物质基础或药物吸收、利用明显改变的。

3. 古代经典名方中药复方制剂。古代经典名方是指符合《中华人民共和国中医药法》规定的，至今仍广泛应用、疗效确切、具有明显特色与优势的古代中医典籍所记载的方剂。古代经典名方中药复方制剂是指来源于古代经典名方的中药复方制剂。包含以下情形：

3.1 按古代经典名方目录管理的中药复方制剂。

3.2 其他来源于古代经典名方的中药复方制剂。包括未按古代经典名方目录管理的古代经典名方中药复方制剂和基于古代经典名方加减化裁的中药复方制剂。

4. 同名同方药。指通用名称、处方、剂型、功能主治、用法及日用饮片量与已上市中药相同，且在安全性、有效性、质量可控性方面不低于该已上市中药的制剂。

天然药物是指在现代医药理论指导下使用的天然药用物质及其制剂。天然药物参照中药注册分类。

其他情形，主要指境外已上市境内未上市的中药、天然药物制剂。

二、中药注册申报资料要求

本申报资料项目及要求适用于中药创新药、改良型新药、古代经典名方中药复方制剂以及同名同方药。申请人需要基于不同注册分类、不同申报阶段以及中药注册受理审查指南的要求提供相应资料。申报资料应按照项目编号提供，对应项目无相关信息或研究资料，项目编号和名称也应保留，可在项下注明"无相关研究内容"或"不适用"。如果申请人要求减免资料，应当充分说明理由。申报资料的撰写还应参考相关法规、技术要求及技术指导原则的相关规定。境外生产药品提供的境外药品管理机构证明文件及全部技术资料应当是中文翻译文本并附原文。

天然药物制剂申报资料项目按照本文件要求，技术要求按照天然药物研究技术要求。天然药物的用途以适应症表述。

境外已上市境内未上市的中药、天然药物制剂参照中药创新药提供相关研究资料。

（一）行政文件和药品信息

1.0 说明函（详见附：说明函）

主要对于本次申请关键信息的概括与说明。

1.1 目录

按照不同章节分别提交申报资料目录。

1.2 申请表

主要包括产品名称、剂型、规格、注册类别、申请事项等产品基本信息。

1.3 产品信息相关材料

1.3.1 说明书

1.3.1.1 研究药物说明书及修订说明（适用于临床试验申请）

1.3.1.2 上市药品说明书及修订说明（适用于上市许可申请）

应按照有关规定起草药品说明书样稿，撰写说明书各项内容的起草说明，并提供有关安全性和有效性等方面的最新文献。

境外已上市药品尚需提供境外上市国家或地区药品管理机构核准的原文说明书，并附中文译文。

1.3.2 包装标签

1.3.2.1 研究药物包装标签（适用于临床试验申请）

1.3.2.2 上市药品包装标签（适用于上市许可申请）

境外已上市药品尚需提供境外上市国家或地区使用的包装标签实样。

1.3.3 产品质量标准和生产工艺

产品质量标准参照《中国药典》格式和内容撰写。

生产工艺资料（适用于上市许可申请）参照相关格式和内容撰写要求撰写。

1.3.4 古代经典名方关键信息

古代经典名方中药复方制剂应提供古代经典名方的处方、药材基原、药用部位、炮制方法、剂量、用法用量、功能主治等关键信息。按古代经典名方目录管理的中药复方制剂应与国家发布的相关信息一致。

1.3.5 药品通用名称核准申请材料

未列入国家药品标准或者药品注册标准的，申请上市许可时应提交药品通用名称核准申请材料。

1.3.6 检查相关信息（适用于上市许可申请）

包括药品研制情况信息表、药品生产情况信息表、现场主文件清单、药品注册临床试验研究信息表、临床试验信息表以及检验报告。

1.3.7 产品相关证明性文件

1.3.7.1 药材／饮片、提取物等处方药味，药用辅料及药包材证明文件

药材／饮片、提取物等处方药味来源证明文件。

药用辅料及药包材合法来源证明文件，包括供货协议、发票等（适用于制剂未选用已登记原辅包情形）。

药用辅料及药包材的授权使用书（适用于制剂选用已登记原辅包情形）。

1.3.7.2 专利信息及证明文件

申请的药物或者使用的处方、工艺、用途等专利情况及其权属状态说明，以及对他人的专利不构成侵权的声明，并提供相关证明性资料和文件。

1.3.7.3 特殊药品研制立项批准文件

麻醉药品和精神药品需提供研制立项批复文件复印件。

1.3.7.4 对照药来源证明文件

1.3.7.5 药物临床试验相关证明文件（适用于上市许可申请）

《药物临床试验批件》/ 临床试验通知书、临床试验用药质量标准及临床试验登记号（内部核查）。

1.3.7.6 研究机构资质证明文件

非临床研究安全性评价机构应提供药品监督管理部门出具的符合《药物非临床研究质量管理规范》（简称 GLP）的批准证明或检查报告等证明性文件。临床研究机构应提供备案证明。

1.3.7.7 允许药品上市销售证明文件（适用于境外已上市的药品）

境外药品管理机构出具的允许药品上市销售证明文件、公证认证文书及中文译文。出口国或地区物种主管当局同意出口的证明。

1.3.8 其他产品信息相关材料

1.4 申请状态（如适用）

1.4.1 既往批准情况

提供该品种相关的历次申请情况说明及批准 / 未批准证明文件（内部核查）。

1.4.2 申请调整临床试验方案、暂停或者终止临床试验

1.4.3 暂停后申请恢复临床试验

1.4.4 终止后重新申请临床试验

1.4.5 申请撤回尚未批准的药物临床试验申请、上市注册许可申请

1.4.6 申请上市注册审评期间变更仅包括申请人更名、变更注册地址名称等不涉及技术审评内容的变更

1.4.7 申请注销药品注册证书

1.5 加快上市注册程序申请（如适用）

1.5.1 加快上市注册程序申请

包括突破性治疗药物程序、附条件批准程序、优先审评审批程序及特别审批程序

1.5.2 加快上市注册程序终止申请

1.5.3 其他加快注册程序申请

1.6 沟通交流会议（如适用）

1.6.1 会议申请

1.6.2 会议背景资料

1.6.3 会议相关信函、会议纪要以及答复

1.7 临床试验过程管理信息（如适用）

1.7.1 临床试验期间增加功能主治

1.7.2 临床试验方案变更、非临床或者药学的变化或者新发现等可能增加受试者安全性风险的

1.7.3 要求申办者调整临床试验方案、暂停或终止药物临床试验

1.8 药物警戒与风险管理（如适用）

1.8.1 研发期间安全性更新报告及附件

1.8.1.1 研发期间安全性更新报告

1.8.1.2 严重不良反应累计汇总表

1.8.1.3 报告周期内境内死亡受试者列表

1.8.1.4 报告周期内境内因任何不良事件而退出临床试验的受试者列表

1.8.1.5 报告周期内发生的药物临床试验方案变更或者临床方面的新发现、非临床或者药学的变化或者新发现总结表

1.8.1.6 下一报告周期内总体研究计划概要

1.8.2 其他潜在的严重安全性风险信息

1.8.3 风险管理计划

包括药物警戒活动计划和风险最小化措施等。

1.9 上市后研究（如适用）

包括Ⅳ期和有特定研究目的的研究等。

1.10 申请人 / 生产企业证明性文件

1.10.1 境内生产药品申请人 / 生产企业资质证明文件

申请人 / 生产企业机构合法登记证明文件（营业执照等）。申请上市许可时，申请人和生产企业应当已取得相应的《药品生产许可证》及变更记录页（内部核查）。

申请临床试验的，应提供临床试验用药物在符合药品生产质量管理规范的

条件下制备的情况说明。

1.10.2 境外生产药品申请人 / 生产企业资质证明文件

生产厂和包装厂符合药品生产质量管理规范的证明文件、公证认证文书及中文译文。

申请临床试验的，应提供临床试验用药物在符合药品生产质量管理规范的条件下制备的情况说明。

1.10.3 注册代理机构证明文件

境外申请人指定中国境内的企业法人办理相关药品注册事项的，应当提供委托文书、公证文书及其中文译文，以及注册代理机构的营业执照复印件。

1.11 小微企业证明文件（如适用）

说明：1. 标注"如适用"的文件是申请人按照所申报药品特点、所申报的申请事项并结合药品全生命周期管理要求选择适用的文件提交。2. 标注"内部核查"的文件是指监管部门需要审核的文件，不强制申请人提交。3. 境外生产的药品所提交的境外药品监督管理机构或地区出具的证明文件（包括允许药品上市销售证明文件、GMP 证明文件以及允许药品变更证明文件等）符合世界卫生组织推荐的统一格式原件的，可不经所在国公证机构公证及驻所在国中国使领馆认证。

附：说明函

关于 XX 公司申报的 XX 产品的 XX 申请

1. 简要说明

包括但不限于：产品名称（拟定）、功能主治、用法用量、剂型、规格。

2. 背景信息

简要说明该产品注册分类及依据、申请事项及相关支持性研究。

加快上市注册程序申请（包括突破性治疗药物程序、附条件批准程序、优先审评审批程序及特别审批程序等）及其依据（如适用）。

附加申请事项，如减免临床、非处方药或儿童用药等（如适用）。

3. 其他重要需特别说明的相关信息

（二）概要

2.1 品种概况

简述药品名称和注册分类，申请阶段。

简述处方、辅料、制成总量、规格、申请的功能主治、拟定用法用量（包括剂量和持续用药时间信息），人日用量（需明确制剂量、饮片量）。

简述立题依据、处方来源、人用经验等。改良型新药应提供原制剂的相关信息（如上市许可持有人、药品批准文号、执行标准等），简述与原制剂在处方、工艺以及质量标准等方面的异同。同名同方药应提供同名同方的已上市中药的相关信息（如上市许可持有人、药品批准文号、执行标准等）以及选择依据，简述与同名同方的已上市中药在处方、工艺以及质量控制等方面的对比情况，并说明是否一致。

申请临床试验时，应简要介绍申请临床试验前沟通交流情况。

申请上市许可时，应简要介绍与国家药品监督管理局药品审评中心的沟通交流情况；说明临床试验批件／临床试验通知书情况，并简述临床试验批件／临床试验通知书中要求完成的研究内容及相关工作完成情况；临床试验期间发生改变的，应说明改变的情况，是否按照有关法规要求进行了申报及批准情况。

申请古代经典名方中药复方制剂，应简述古代经典名方的处方、药材基原、药用部位、炮制方法、剂量、用法用量、功能主治等关键信息。按古代经典名方目录管理的中药复方制剂，应说明与国家发布信息的一致性。

2.2 药学研究资料总结报告

药学研究资料总结报告是申请人对所进行的药学研究结果的总结、分析与评价，各项内容和数据应与相应的药学研究资料保持一致，并基于不同申报阶段撰写相应的药学研究资料总结报告。

2.2.1 药学主要研究结果总结

（1）临床试验期间补充完善的药学研究（适用于上市许可申请）

简述临床试验期间补充完善的药学研究情况及结果。

（2）处方药味及药材资源评估

说明处方药味质量标准出处。简述处方药味新建立的质量控制方法及限度。未被国家药品标准、药品注册标准以及省、自治区、直辖市药材标准收载的处方药味，应说明是否按照相关技术要求进行了研究或申报，简述结果。

简述药材资源评估情况。

（3）饮片炮制

简述饮片炮制方法。申请上市许可时，应明确药物研发各阶段饮片炮制方法的一致性。若有改变，应说明相关情况。

（4）生产工艺

简述处方和制法。若为改良型新药或同名同方药，还需简述工艺的变化情况。

简述剂型选择及规格确定的依据。

简述制备工艺路线、工艺参数及确定依据。说明是否建立了中间体的相关质量控制方法，简述检测结果。

申请临床试验时，应简述中试研究结果和质量检测结果，评价工艺的合理性，分析工艺的可行性。申请上市许可时，应简述放大生产样品及商业化生产的批次、规模、质量检测结果等，说明工艺是否稳定、可行。

说明辅料执行标准情况。申请上市许可时，还应说明辅料与药品关联审评审批情况。

（5）质量标准

简述质量标准的主要内容及其制定依据、对照品来源、样品的自检结果。

申请上市许可时，简述质量标准变化情况。

（6）稳定性研究

简述稳定性考察条件及结果，评价样品的稳定性，拟定有效期及贮藏条件。

明确直接接触药品的包装材料和容器及其执行标准情况。申请上市许可时，还应说明包材与药品关联审评审批情况。

2.2.2 药学研究结果分析与评价

对处方药味研究、药材资源评估、剂型选择、工艺研究、质量控制研究、稳定性考察的结果进行总结，综合分析、评价产品质量控制情况。申请临床试验时，应结合临床应用背景、药理毒理研究结果及相关文献等，分析药学研究结果与药品的安全性、有效性之间的相关性，评价工艺合理性、质量可控性，初步判断稳定性。申请上市许可时，应结合临床试验结果等，分析药学研究结果与药品的安全性、有效性之间的相关性，评价工艺可行性、质量可控性和药品稳定性。

按古代经典名方目录管理的中药复方制剂应说明药材、饮片、按照国家发布的古代经典名方关键信息及古籍记载制备的样品、中间体、制剂之间质量的相关性。

2.2.3 参考文献

提供有关的参考文献，必要时应提供全文。

2.3 药理毒理研究资料总结报告

药理毒理研究资料总结报告应是对药理学、药代动力学、毒理学研究的综合性和关键性评价。应对药理毒理试验策略进行讨论并说明理由。应说明所提交试验的 GLP 依从性。

对于申请临床试验的药物，需综合现有药理毒理研究资料，分析说明是否支持所申请进行的临床试验。在临床试验过程中，若为支持相应临床试验阶段或开发进程进行了药理毒理研究，需及时更新药理毒理研究资料，提供相关研究试验报告。临床试验期间若进行了变更（如工艺变更），需根据变更情况确定所需要进行的药理毒理研究，并提供相关试验报告。对于申请上市许可的药物，需说明临床试验期间进行的药理毒理研究，并综合分析现有药理毒理研究资料是否支持本品上市申请。

撰写按照以下顺序：药理毒理试验策略概述、药理学研究总结、药代动力学研究总结、毒理学研究总结、综合评估和结论、参考文献。

对于申请上市许可的药物，说明书样稿中【药理毒理】项应根据所进行的药理毒理研究资料进行撰写，并提供撰写说明及支持依据。

2.3.1 药理毒理试验策略概述

结合申请类别、处方来源或人用经验资料、所申请的功能主治等，介绍药理毒理试验的研究思路及策略。

2.3.2 药理学研究总结

简要概括药理学研究内容。按以下顺序进行撰写：概要、主要药效学、次要药效学、安全药理学、药效学药物相互作用、讨论和结论，并附列表总结。

应对主要药效学试验进行总结和评价。如果进行了次要药效学研究，应按照器官系统/试验类型进行总结并评价。应对安全药理学试验进行总结和评价。如果进行了药效学药物相互作用研究，则在此部分进行简要总结。

2.3.3 药代动力学研究总结

简要概括药代动力学研究内容，按以下顺序进行撰写：概要、分析方法、吸收、分布、代谢、排泄、药代动力学药物相互作用、其他药代动力学试验、讨论和结论，并附列表总结。

2.3.4 毒理学研究总结

简要概括毒理学试验结果，并说明试验的 GLP 依从性，说明毒理学试验受试物情况。

按以下顺序进行撰写：概要、单次给药毒性试验、重复给药毒性试验、遗传毒性试验、致癌性试验、生殖毒性试验、制剂安全性试验（刺激性、溶血性、过敏性试验等）、其他毒性试验、讨论和结论，并附列表总结。

2.3.5 综合分析与评价

对药理学、药代动力学、毒理学研究进行综合分析与评价。

分析主要药效学试验的量效关系（如起效剂量、有效剂量范围等）及时效关系（如起效时间、药效持续时间或最佳作用时间等），并对药理作用特点及其与拟定功能主治的相关性和支持程度进行综合评价。

安全药理学试验属于非临床安全性评价的一部分，可结合毒理学部分的毒理学试验结果进行综合评价。

综合各项药代动力学试验，分析其吸收、分布、代谢、排泄、药物相互作用特征。包括受试物和 / 或其活性代谢物的药代动力学特征，如吸收程度和速率、动力学参数、分布的主要组织、与血浆蛋白的结合程度、代谢产物和可能的代谢途径、排泄途径和程度等。需关注药代研究结果是否支持毒理学试验动物种属的选择。分析各项毒理学试验结果，综合分析及评价各项试验结果之间的相关性，种属和性别之间的差异性等。

分析药理学、药代动力学与毒理学结果之间的相关性。

结合药学、临床资料进行综合分析与评价。

2.3.6 参考文献

提供有关的参考文献，必要时应提供全文。

2.4 临床研究资料总结报告

2.4.1 中医药理论或研究背景

根据注册分类提供相应的简要中医药理论或研究背景。如为古代经典名方中药复方制剂的，还应简要说明处方来源、功能主治、用法用量等关键信息及其依据等。

2.4.2 人用经验

如有人用经验的，需提供简要人用经验概述，并分析说明人用经验对于拟定功能主治或后续所需开展临床试验的支持情况。

2.4.3 临床试验资料综述

可参照《中药、天然药物综述资料撰写的格式和内容的技术指导原则——临床试验资料综述》的相关要求撰写。

2.4.4 临床价值评估

基于风险获益评估，结合注册分类，对临床价值进行简要评估。

2.4.5 参考文献

提供有关的参考文献，必要时应提供全文。

2.5 综合分析与评价

根据研究结果，结合立题依据，对安全性、有效性、质量可控性及研究工作的科学性、规范性和完整性进行综合分析与评价。

申请临床试验时，应根据研究结果评估申报品种对拟选适应病症的有效性和临床应用的安全性，综合分析研究结果之间的相互关联，权衡临床试验的风险 / 获益情况，为是否或如何进行临床试验提供支持和依据。

申请上市许可时，应在完整地了解药品研究结果的基础上，对所选适用人群的获益情况及临床应用后可能存在的问题或风险作出综合评估。

（三）药学研究资料

申请人应基于不同申报阶段的要求提供相应药学研究资料。相应技术要求见相关中药药学研究技术指导原则。

3.1 处方药味及药材资源评估

3.1.1 处方药味

中药处方药味包括饮片、提取物等。

3.1.1.1 处方药味的相关信息

提供处方中各药味的来源（包括生产商/供货商等）、执行标准以及相关证明性信息。

饮片：应提供药材的基原（包括科名、中文名、拉丁学名）、药用部位（矿物药注明类、族、矿石名或岩石名、主要成份）、药材产地、采收期、饮片炮制方法、药材是否种植养殖（人工生产）或来源于野生资源等信息。对于药材基原易混淆品种，需提供药材基原鉴定报告。多基原的药材除必须符合质量标准的要求外，必须固定基原，并提供基原选用的依据。药材应固定产地。涉及濒危物种的药材应符合国家的有关规定，应保证可持续利用，并特别注意来源的合法性。

按古代经典名方目录管理的中药复方制剂所用饮片的药材基原、药用部位、炮制方法等应与国家发布的古代经典名方关键信息一致。应提供产地选择的依据，尽可能选择道地药材和/或主产区的药材。

提取物：外购提取物应提供其相关批准（备案）情况、制备方法及生产商/供应商等信息。自制提取物应提供所用饮片的相关信息，提供详细制备工艺及其工艺研究资料（具体要求同"3.3 制备工艺"部分）。

3.1.1.2 处方药味的质量研究

提供处方药味的检验报告。

自拟质量标准或在原质量标准基础上进行完善的，应提供相关研究资料（相关要求参照"3.4 制剂质量与质量标准研究"），提供质量标准草案及起草说明、药品标准物质及有关资料等。

按古代经典名方目录管理的中药复方制剂还应提供多批药材/饮片的质量研究资料。

3.1.1.3 药材生态环境、形态描述、生长特征、种植养殖（人工生产）技术等申报新药材的需提供。

3.1.1.4 植物、动物、矿物标本，植物标本应当包括全部器官，如花、果

实、种子等

申报新药材的需提供。

3.1.2 药材资源评估

药材资源评估内容及其评估结论的有关要求见相关技术指导原则。

3.1.3 参考文献

提供有关的参考文献，必要时应提供全文。

3.2 饮片炮制

3.2.1 饮片炮制方法

明确饮片炮制方法，提供饮片炮制加工依据及详细工艺参数。按古代经典名方目录管理的中药复方制剂所用饮片的炮制方法应与国家发布的古代经典名方关键信息一致。

申请上市许可时，应说明药物研发各阶段饮片炮制方法的一致性，必要时提供相关研究资料。

3.2.2 参考文献

提供有关的参考文献，必要时应提供全文。

3.3 制备工艺

3.3.1 处方

提供 1000 个制剂单位的处方组成。

3.3.2 制法

3.3.2.1 制备工艺流程图

按照制备工艺步骤提供完整、直观、简洁的工艺流程图，应涵盖所有的工艺步骤，标明主要工艺参数和所用提取溶剂等。

3.3.2.2 详细描述制备方法

对工艺过程进行规范描述（包括包装步骤），明确操作流程、工艺参数和范围。

3.3.3 剂型及原辅料情况

药味及辅料	用量	作用	执行标准
制剂工艺中使用到并最终去除的溶剂			

（1）说明具体的剂型和规格。以表格的方式列出单位剂量产品的处方组成，列明各药味（如饮片、提取物）及辅料在处方中的作用，执行的标准。对于制剂工艺中使用到但最终去除的溶剂也应列出。

（2）说明产品所使用的包装材料及容器。

3.3.4 制备工艺研究资料

3.3.4.1 制备工艺路线筛选

提供制备工艺路线筛选研究资料，说明制备工艺路线选择的合理性。处方来源于医院制剂、临床验方或具有人用经验的，应详细说明在临床应用时的具体使用情况（如工艺、剂型、用量、规格等）。

改良型新药还应说明与原制剂生产工艺的异同及参数的变化情况。

按古代经典名方目录管理的中药复方制剂应提供按照国家发布的古代经典名方关键信息及古籍记载进行研究的工艺资料。

同名同方药还应说明与同名同方的已上市中药生产工艺的对比情况，并说明是否一致。

3.3.4.2 剂型选择

提供剂型选择依据。

按古代经典名方目录管理的中药复方制剂应提供剂型（汤剂可制成颗粒剂）与古籍记载一致性的说明资料。

3.3.4.3 处方药味前处理工艺

提供处方药味的前处理工艺及具体工艺参数。申请上市许可时，还应明确关键工艺参数控制点。

3.3.4.4 提取、纯化工艺研究

描述提取纯化工艺流程、主要工艺参数及范围等。

提供提取纯化工艺方法、主要工艺参数的确定依据。生产工艺参数范围的确定应有相关研究数据支持。申请上市许可时，还应明确关键工艺参数控制点。

3.3.4.5 浓缩工艺

描述浓缩工艺方法、主要工艺参数及范围、生产设备等。

提供浓缩工艺方法、主要工艺参数的确定依据。生产工艺参数范围的确定应有相关研究数据支持。申请上市许可时，还应明确关键工艺参数控制点。

3.3.4.6 干燥工艺

描述干燥工艺方法、主要工艺参数及范围、生产设备等。

提供干燥工艺方法以及主要工艺参数的确定依据。生产工艺参数范围的确

定应有相关研究数据支持。申请上市许可时，还应明确关键工艺参数控制点。

3.3.4.7 制剂成型工艺

描述制剂成型工艺流程、主要工艺参数及范围等。

提供中间体、辅料研究以及制剂处方筛选研究资料，明确所用辅料的种类、级别、用量等。

提供成型工艺方法、主要工艺参数的确定依据。生产工艺参数范围的确定应有相关研究数据支持。对与制剂性能相关的理化性质进行分析。申请上市许可时，还应明确关键工艺参数控制点。

3.3.5 中试和生产工艺验证

3.3.5.1 样品生产企业信息

申请临床试验时，根据实际情况填写。如不适用，可不填。

申请上市许可时，需提供样品生产企业的名称、生产场所的地址等。提供样品生产企业合法登记证明文件、《药品生产许可证》复印件。

3.3.5.2 批处方

以表格的方式列出（申请临床试验时，以中试放大规模；申请上市许可时，以商业规模）产品的批处方组成，列明各药味（如饮片、提取物）及辅料执行的标准，对于制剂工艺中使用到但最终去除的溶剂也应列出。

药味及辅料	用量	执行标准
制剂工艺中使用到并最终去除的溶剂		

3.3.5.3 工艺描述

按单元操作过程描述（申请临床试验时，以中试批次；申请上市许可时，以商业规模生产工艺验证批次）样品的工艺（包括包装步骤），明确操作流程、工艺参数和范围。

3.3.5.4 辅料、生产过程中所用材料

提供所用辅料、生产过程中所用材料的级别、生产商/供应商、执行的标准以及相关证明文件等。如对辅料建立了内控标准，应提供。提供辅料、生产过程中所用材料的检验报告。

如所用辅料需要精制的，提供精制工艺研究资料、内控标准及其起草说明。

申请上市许可时，应说明辅料与药品关联审评审批情况。

3.3.5.5 主要生产设备

提供中试（适用临床试验申请）或工艺验证（适用上市许可申请）过程中所用主要生产设备的信息。申请上市许可时，需关注生产设备的选择应符合生产工艺的要求。

3.3.5.6 关键步骤和中间体的控制

列出所有关键步骤及其工艺参数控制范围。提供研究结果支持关键步骤确定的合理性以及工艺参数控制范围的合理性。申请上市许可时，还应明确关键工艺参数控制点。

列出中间体的质量控制标准，包括项目、方法和限度，必要时提供方法学验证资料。明确中间体（如浸膏等）的得率范围。

3.3.5.7 生产数据和工艺验证资料

提供研发过程中代表性批次（申请临床试验时，包括但不限于中试放大批等；申请上市许可时，应包括但不限于中试放大批、临床试验批、商业规模生产工艺验证批等）的样品情况汇总资料，包括：批号、生产时间及地点、生产数据、批规模、用途（如用于稳定性试验等）、质量检测结果（例如含量及其他主要质量指标）。申请上市许可时，提供商业规模生产工艺验证资料，包括工艺验证方案和验证报告，工艺必须在预定的参数范围内进行。

生产工艺研究应注意实验室条件与中试和生产的衔接，考虑大生产设备的可行性、适应性。生产工艺进行优化的，应重点描述工艺研究的主要变更（包括批量、设备、工艺参数等的变化）及相关的支持性验证研究。

按古代经典名方目录管理的中药复方制剂应提供按照国家发布的古代经典名方关键信息及古籍记载制备的样品、中试样品和商业规模样品的相关性研究资料。

临床试验期间，如药品规格、制备工艺等发生改变的，应根据实际变化情况，参照相关技术指导原则开展研究工作，属重大变更以及引起药用物质或制剂吸收、利用明显改变的，应提出补充申请。申请上市许可时，应详细描述改变情况（包括设备、工艺参数等的变化）、改变原因、改变时间以及相关改变是否获得国家药品监督管理部门的批准等内容，并提供相关研究资料。

3.3.6 试验用样品制备情况

3.3.6.1 毒理试验用样品

应提供毒理试验用样品制备信息。一般应包括：

（1）毒理试验用样品的生产数据汇总，包括批号、投料量、样品得量、用途等。毒理学试验样品应采用中试及中试以上规模的样品。

（2）制备毒理试验用样品所用处方药味的来源、批号以及自检报告等。

（3）制备毒理试验用样品用主要生产设备的信息。

（4）毒理试验用样品的质量标准、自检报告及相关图谱等。

3.3.6.2 临床试验用药品（适用于上市许可申请）

申请上市许可时，应提供用于临床试验的试验药物和安慰剂（如适用）的制备信息。

（1）用于临床试验的试验药物

提供用于临床试验的试验药物的批生产记录复印件。批生产记录中需明确生产厂房/车间和生产线。

提供用于临床试验的试验药物所用处方药味的基原、产地信息及自检报告。

提供生产过程中使用的主要设备等情况。

提供用于临床试验的试验药物的自检报告及相关图谱。

（2）安慰剂

提供临床试验用安慰剂的批生产记录复印件。

提供临床试验用安慰剂的配方，以及配方组成成份的来源、执行标准等信息。

提供安慰剂与试验样品的性味对比研究资料，说明安慰剂与试验样品在外观、大小、色泽、重量、味道和气味等方面的一致性情况。

3.3.7 "生产工艺"资料（适用于上市许可申请）

申请上市许可的药物，应参照中药相关生产工艺格式和内容撰写要求提供"生产工艺"资料。

3.3.8 参考文献

提供有关的参考文献，必要时应提供全文。

3.4 制剂质量与质量标准研究

3.4.1 化学成份研究

提供化学成份研究的文献资料或试验资料。

3.4.2 质量研究

提供质量研究工作的试验资料及文献资料。

按古代经典名方目录管理的中药复方制剂应提供药材、饮片按照国家发布的古代经典名方关键信息及古籍记载制备的样品、中间体、制剂的质量相关性研究资料。

同名同方药应提供与同名同方的已上市中药的质量对比研究结果。

3.4.3 质量标准

提供药品质量标准草案及起草说明，并提供药品标准物质及有关资料。对于药品研制过程中使用的对照品，应说明其来源并提供说明书和批号。对于非法定来源的对照品，申请临床试验时，应说明是否按照相关技术要求进行研究，提供相关研究资料；申请上市许可时，应说明非法定来源的对照品是否经法定部门进行标定，提供相关证明性文件。

境外生产药品提供的质量标准的中文本须按照中国国家药品标准或药品注册标准的格式整理报送。

3.4.4 样品检验报告

申请临床试验时，提供至少 1 批样品的自检报告。

申请上市许可时，提供连续 3 批样品的自检及复核检验报告。

3.4.5 参考文献

提供有关的参考文献，必要时应提供全文。

3.5 稳定性

3.5.1 稳定性总结

总结稳定性研究的样品情况、考察条件、考察指标和考察结果，并拟定贮存条件和有效期。

3.5.2 稳定性研究数据

提供稳定性研究数据及图谱。

3.5.3 直接接触药品的包装材料和容器的选择

阐述选择依据。提供包装材料和容器执行标准、检验报告、生产商 / 供货商及相关证明文件等。提供针对所选用包装材料和容器进行的相容性等研究资料（如适用）。

申请上市许可时，应说明包装材料和容器与药品关联审评审批情况。

3.5.4 上市后的稳定性研究方案及承诺（适用于上市许可申请）

申请药品上市许可时，应承诺对上市后生产的前三批产品进行长期稳定性考察，并对每年生产的至少一批产品进行长期稳定性考察，如有异常情况应及时通知药品监督管理部门。

提供后续稳定性研究方案。

3.5.5 参考文献

提供有关的参考文献，必要时应提供全文。

（四）药理毒理研究资料

申请人应基于不同申报阶段的要求提供相应药理毒理研究资料。相应要求详见相关技术指导原则。

非临床安全性评价研究应当在经过 GLP 认证的机构开展。

天然药物的药理毒理研究参考相应研究技术要求进行。

4.1 药理学研究资料

药理学研究是通过动物或体外、离体试验来获得非临床有效性信息，包括药效学作用及其特点、药物作用机制等。药理学申报资料应列出试验设计思路、试验实施过程、试验结果及评价。

中药创新药，应提供主要药效学试验资料，为进入临床试验提供试验证据。药物进入临床试验的有效性证据包括中医药理论、临床人用经验和药效学研究。根据处方来源及制备工艺等不同，以上证据所占有权重不同，进行试验时应予综合考虑。

药效学试验设计时应考虑中医药特点，根据受试物拟定的功能主治，选择合适的试验项目。

提取物及其制剂，提取物纯化的程度应经筛选研究确定，筛选试验应与拟定的功能主治具有相关性，筛选过程中所进行的药理毒理研究应体现在药理毒理申报资料中。如有同类成份的提取物及其制剂上市，则应当与其进行药效学及其他方面的比较，以证明其优势和特点。

中药复方制剂，根据处方来源和组成、临床人用经验及制备工艺情况等可适当减免药效学试验。

具有人用经验的中药复方制剂，可根据人用经验对药物有效性的支持程度，适当减免药效学试验；若人用经验对有效性具有一定支撑作用，处方组成、工艺路线、临床定位、用法用量等与既往临床应用基本一致的，则可不提供药效学试验资料。

依据现代药理研究组方的中药复方制剂，需采用试验研究的方式来说明组方的合理性，并通过药效学试验来提供非临床有效性信息。

中药改良型新药，应根据其改良目的、变更的具体内容来确定药效学资料的要求。若改良目的在于或包含提高有效性，应提供相应的对比性药效学研究资料，以说明改良的优势。中药增加功能主治，应提供支持新功能主治的药效学试验资料，可根据人用经验对药物有效性的支持程度，适当减免药效学试验。

安全药理学试验属于非临床安全性评价的一部分，其要求见"4.3 毒理学研究资料"。

药理学研究报告应按照以下顺序提交：

4.1.1 主要药效学

4.1.2 次要药效学

4.1.3 安全药理学

4.1.4 药效学药物相互作用

4.2 药代动力学研究资料

非临床药代动力学研究是通过体外和动物体内的研究方法，揭示药物在体内的动态变化规律，获得药物的基本药代动力学参数，阐明药物的吸收、分布、代谢和排泄的过程和特征。

对于提取的单一成份制剂，参考化学药物非临床药代动力学研究要求。

其他制剂，视情况（如安全性风险程度）进行药代动力学研究或药代动力学探索性研究。

缓、控释制剂，临床前应进行非临床药代动力学研究，以说明其缓、控释特征；若为改剂型品种，还应与原剂型进行药代动力学比较研究；若为同名同方药的缓、控释制剂，应进行非临床药代动力学比较研究。

在进行中药非临床药代动力学研究时，应充分考虑其成份的复杂性，结合其特点选择适宜的方法开展体内过程或活性代谢产物的研究，为后续研发提供参考。

若拟进行的临床试验中涉及到与其他药物（特别是化学药）联合应用，应考虑通过体外、体内试验来考察可能的药物相互作用。

药代动力学研究报告应按照以下顺序提交：

4.2.1 分析方法及验证报告

4.2.2 吸收

4.2.3 分布（血浆蛋白结合率、组织分布等）

4.2.4 代谢（体外代谢、体内代谢、可能的代谢途径、药物代谢酶的诱导或抑制等）

4.2.5 排泄

4.2.6 药代动力学药物相互作用（非临床）

4.2.7 其他药代试验

4.3 毒理学研究资料

毒理学研究包括：单次给药毒性试验，重复给药毒性试验，遗传毒性试验，生殖毒性试验，致癌性试验，依赖性试验，刺激性、过敏性、溶血性等与局部、全身给药相关的制剂安全性试验，其他毒性试验等。

中药创新药，应尽可能获取更多的安全性信息，以便于对其安全性风险进行评价。根据其品种特点，对其安全性的认知不同，毒理学试验要求会有所差异。

新药材及其制剂，应进行全面的毒理学研究，包括安全药理学试验、单次给药毒性试验、重复给药毒性试验、遗传毒性试验、生殖毒性试验等，根据给药途径、制剂情况可能需要进行相应的制剂安全性试验，其余试验根据品种具体情况确定。

提取物及其制剂，根据其临床应用情况，以及可获取的安全性信息情况，确定其毒理学试验要求。如提取物立题来自于试验研究，缺乏对其安全性的认知，应进行全面的毒理学试验。如提取物立题来自于传统应用，生产工艺与传统应用基本一致，一般应进行安全药理学试验、单次给药毒性试验、重复给药毒性试验，以及必要时其他可能需要进行的试验。

中药复方制剂，根据其处方来源及组成、人用安全性经验、安全性风险程度的不同，提供相应的毒理学试验资料，若减免部分试验项目，应提供充分的理由。

对于采用传统工艺，具有人用经验的，一般应提供单次给药毒性试验、重复给药毒性试验资料。

对于采用非传统工艺，但具有可参考的临床应用资料的，一般应提供安全药理学、单次给药毒性试验、重复给药毒性试验资料。

对于采用非传统工艺，且无人用经验的，一般应进行全面的毒理学试验。

临床试验中发现非预期不良反应时，或毒理学试验中发现非预期毒性时，应考虑进行追加试验。

中药改良型新药，根据变更情况提供相应的毒理学试验资料。若改良目的在于或包含提高安全性的，应进行毒理学对比研究，设置原剂型/原给药途径/原工艺进行对比，以说明改良的优势。

中药增加功能主治，需延长用药周期或者增加剂量者，应说明原毒理学试验资料是否可以支持延长周期或增加剂量，否则应提供支持用药周期延长或剂量增加的毒理学研究资料。

一般情况下，安全药理学、单次给药毒性、支持相应临床试验周期的重复给药毒性、遗传毒性试验资料、过敏性、刺激性、溶血性试验资料或文献资料应在申请临床试验时提供。后续需根据临床试验进程提供支持不同临床试验给药期限或支持上市的重复给药毒性试验。生殖毒性试验根据风险程度在不同的临床试验开发阶段提供。致癌性试验资料一般可在申请上市时提供。

药物研发的过程中，若受试物的工艺发生可能影响其安全性的变化，应进行相应的毒理学研究。

毒理学研究资料应列出试验设计思路、试验实施过程、试验结果及评价。毒理学研究报告应按照以下顺序提交：

4.3.1 单次给药毒性试验

4.3.2 重复给药毒性试验

4.3.3 遗传毒性试验

4.3.4 致癌性试验

4.3.5 生殖毒性试验

4.3.6 制剂安全性试验（刺激性、溶血性、过敏性试验等）

4.3.7 其他毒性试验

（五）临床研究资料

5.1 中药创新药

5.1.1 处方组成符合中医药理论、具有人用经验的创新药

5.1.1.1 中医药理论

5.1.1.1.1 处方组成，功能、主治病证

5.1.1.1.2 中医药理论对主治病证的基本认识

5.1.1.1.3 拟定处方的中医药理论

5.1.1.1.4 处方合理性评价

5.1.1.1.5 处方安全性分析

5.1.1.1.6 和已有国家标准或药品注册标准的同类品种的比较

5.1.1.2 人用经验

5.1.1.2.1 证明性文件

5.1.1.2.2 既往临床应用情况概述

5.1.1.2.3 文献综述

5.1.1.2.4 既往临床应用总结报告

5.1.1.2.5 拟定主治概要、现有治疗手段、未解决的临床需求

5.1.1.2.6 人用经验对拟定功能主治的支持情况评价

中医药理论和人用经验部分的具体撰写要求，可参考相关技术要求、技术指导原则。

5.1.1.3 临床试验

需开展临床试验的，应提交以下资料：

5.1.1.3.1 临床试验计划与方案及其附件

5.1.1.3.1.1 临床试验计划和方案

5.1.1.3.1.2 知情同意书样稿

5.1.1.3.1.3 研究者手册

5.1.1.3.1.4 统计分析计划

5.1.1.3.2 临床试验报告及其附件（完成临床试验后提交）

5.1.1.3.2.1 临床试验报告

5.1.1.3.2.2 病例报告表样稿、患者日志等

5.1.1.3.2.3 与临床试验主要有效性、安全性数据相关的关键标准操作规程

5.1.1.3.2.4 临床试验方案变更情况说明

5.1.1.3.2.5 伦理委员会批准件

5.1.1.3.2.6 统计分析计划

5.1.1.3.2.7 临床试验数据库电子文件

申请人在完成临床试验提出药品上市许可申请时，应以光盘形式提交临床试验数据库。数据库格式以及相关文件等具体要求见临床试验数据递交相关技术指导原则。

5.1.1.3.3 参考文献

提供有关的参考文献全文，外文文献还应同时提供摘要和引用部分的中文译文。

5.1.1.4 临床价值评估

基于风险获益评估，结合中医药理论、人用经验和临床试验，评估本品的临床价值及申报资料对于拟定功能主治的支持情况。

说明：

申请人可基于中医药理论和人用经验，在提交临床试验申请前，就临床试验要求与药审中心进行沟通交流。

5.1.2 其他来源的创新药

5.1.2.1 研究背景

5.1.2.1.1 拟定功能主治及临床定位

应根据研发情况和处方所依据的理论，说明拟定功能主治及临床定位的确定依据，包括但不限于文献分析、药理研究等。

5.1.2.1.2 疾病概要、现有治疗手段、未解决的临床需求

说明拟定适应病证的基本情况、国内外现有治疗手段研究和相关药物上市情况，现有治疗存在的主要问题和未被满足的临床需求，以及说明本品预期的

安全性、有效性特点和拟解决的问题。

5.1.2.2 临床试验

应按照"5.1.1.3 临床试验"项下的相关要求提交资料。

5.1.2.3 临床价值评估

基于风险获益评估，结合研究背景和临床试验，评估本品的临床价值及申报资料对于拟定功能主治的支持情况。

说明：

申请人可基于处方组成、给药途径和非临床安全性评价结果等，在提交临床试验申请前，就临床试验要求与药审中心进行沟通交流。

5.2 中药改良型新药

5.2.1 研究背景

应说明改变的目的和依据。如有人用经验，可参照"5.1.1.2 人用经验"项下的相关要求提交资料。

5.2.2 临床试验

应按照"5.1.1.3 临床试验"项下的相关要求提交资料。

5.2.3 临床价值评估

结合改变的目的和临床试验，评估本品的临床价值及申报资料对于拟定改变的支持情况。

说明：

申请人可参照中药创新药的相关要求，在提交临床试验申请前，就临床试验要求与药审中心进行沟通交流。

5.3 古代经典名方中药复方制剂

5.3.1 按古代经典名方目录管理的中药复方制剂

提供药品说明书起草说明及依据，说明药品说明书中临床相关项草拟的内容及其依据。

5.3.2 其他来源于古代经典名方的中药复方制剂

5.3.2.1 古代经典名方的处方来源及历史沿革、处方组成、功能主治、用法用量、中医药理论论述

5.3.2.2 基于古代经典名方加减化裁的中药复方制剂，还应提供加减化裁的理由及依据、处方合理性评价、处方安全性分析。

5.3.2.3 人用经验

5.3.2.3.1 证明性文件

5.3.2.3.2 既往临床实践情况概述

5.3.2.3.3 文献综述

5.3.2.3.4 既往临床实践总结报告

5.3.2.3.5 人用经验对拟定功能主治的支持情况评价

5.3.2.4 临床价值评估

基于风险获益评估，结合中医药理论、处方来源及其加减化裁、人用经验，评估本品的临床价值及申报资料对于拟定功能主治的支持情况。

5.3.2.5 药品说明书起草说明及依据

说明药品说明书中临床相关项草拟的内容及其依据。

中医药理论、人用经验部分以及药品说明书的具体撰写要求，可参考相关技术要求、技术指导原则。

说明：

此类中药的注册申请、审评审批、上市监管等实施细则和技术要求另行制定。

5.4 同名同方药

5.4.1 研究背景

提供对照同名同方药选择的合理性依据。

5.4.2 临床试验

需开展临床试验的，应按照"5.1.1.3 临床试验"项下的相关要求提交资料。

5.5 临床试验期间的变更（如适用）

获准开展临床试验的药物拟增加适用人群范围（如增加儿童人群）、变更用法用量（如增加剂量或延长疗程）等，应根据变更事项提供相应的立题目的和依据、临床试验计划与方案及其附件；药物临床试验期间，发生药物临床试验方案变更、非临床或者药学的变化或者有新发现，需按照补充申请申报的，临床方面应提供方案变更的详细对比与说明，以及变更的理由和依据。

同时，还需要对已有人用经验和临床试验数据进行分析整理，为变更提供依据，重点关注变更对受试者有效性及安全性风险的影响。

Guideline for Quality Control Study of TCM Crude Drugs of New Traditional Chinese Medicines (TCMs) (Trial)

I. Overview

TCM crude drugs serve as the foundation for research and development (R&D) as well as the production of new TCMs. The quality of these materials plays a crucial role in ensuring the safety, efficacy, and quality control of new TCMs. In order to improve the quality control system of TCM preparations, strengthen the traceability of drug quality, and provide safe and effective TCM crude drugs with stable quality for TCM preparations, based on the concept of whole-process quality control and risk control, this guideline are developed for the key links and key quality control points in the production of TCM crude drugs.

The guideline primarily focus on the origins and medicinal parts of TCM crude drugs, their places of origin, cultivation and breeding, harvesting and on-site processing, packaging and storage, and quality standards, so as to provide a reference for the studies on quality control of TCM crude drugs for new TCMs.

II. Basic Principles

(I) Respect the TCM traditions and characteristics

The studies on quality control of TCM crude drugs should adhere to the principles of TCM theories and respect the TCM traditional experience and characteristics. The traditional experience should be respected in aspects such as suitable places of origin, production methods, growth years, harvesting time, on-site processing methods, and quality evaluation of TCM crude drugs. The preservation of traditional experience and techniques, as well as the integration of modern science and technology are encouraged to enhance traditional quality evaluation practices and indicators.

(II) Meet the design requirements for study on new TCMs

Based on the design requirements for study on new TCMs and the characteristics of different TCM crude drugs, the key factors and risk control points affecting the quality stability of TCM crude drugs and TCM preparations should be studied to meet the requirements for quality control of these preparations. Take necessary measures, such as fixing the origins, the medicinal parts and places of origins, etc. to ensure that the quality of TCM crude drugs of new TCMs is basically stable.

(III) Strengthen the quality control throughout the entire production process

Studies on quality control of the entire production process of TCM crude drugs, including their origins, places of origin, cultivation and breeding, harvesting and processing, packaging, and storage, should be strengthened. Encourage the cultivation and breeding of TCM crude drugs in accordance with the requirements of Good Agricultural Practices (GAP) for TCM crude drugs, and establish corresponding quality control and management measures for the harvesting, on-site processing, packaging, and storage of wild TCM crude drugs. The traceability of the source of TCM crude drugs should be guaranteed, and the use of modern information technology to establish a traceability system should be encouraged.

(IV) Pay attention to the sustainable utilization of TCM crude drugs resources

The relationship between the rational utilization of TCM crude drugs and resource protection should be properly managed. Resource assessment should be conducted to ensure the sustainable utilization of TCM crude drugs resources. The use of TCM crude drugs derived from wild animals and plants should comply with the relevant national regulations and requirements for the management of wild animals and plants. For new TCMs, the use of TCM crude drugs derived from wild animals should be strictly restricted. In principle, TCM crude drugs derived from valuable, rare and endangered wild animals and plants should not be used. If such use is indeed necessary, strict requirements should be implemented, and studies on cultivation, breeding, or wild tending should be conducted as soon as possible to ensure the sustainable utilization of such resources. In addition, the use of paleontological fossil TCM crude drugs should comply with the relevant national regulations and requirements on the protection and management of paleontological fossils.

III. Main Contents

(I) Origins and medicinal parts

Accurate origins are the basis for ensuring the quality of TCM crude drugs. The Chinese names and Latin names of the original plants or animals and the medicinal parts of TCM crude drugs should be clearly defined. For TCM crude drugs with multiple origins, one of the origins should be fixed. If multiple origins of TCM crude drugs need to be used, sufficient basis should be provided, and the use ratio should be fixed to guarantee the stable quality of relevant preparations. Where there are clearly selected varieties for cultivation and breeding of TCM crude drugs, the variety information should be described in a general manner. For mineral TCM crude drugs, the classes, families, ore names, rock names, and main components of the minerals should be specified.

Measures should be taken to guarantee the accuracy of the origins and medicinal parts when using TCM crude drugs. In principle, it should be mandatory to collect voucher specimens of the original plants, animals, or minerals for new TCM crude drugs, easily confused TCM crude drugs, and TCM crude drugs with difficult-to-determine origins. These specimens should be identified by experts or qualified institutions, and both the specimens and related materials, including photos, should be preserved. If necessary, it is also required to conduct comparative study with counterfeit products to confirm the origins of TCM crude drugs, in combination with the survey at the places of origin. For new TCM crude drugs, it is important to provide detailed descriptions of relevant information, including the morphological characteristics and medicinal parts of the original plants/animals. Additionally, information about the growing environment, habits, places of origin, distribution, and available resources should also be included. If wild TCM crude drugs have species that are easy to be confused in the same growing areas and the same harvesting periods, the identification of origins and the difference from confusing substances should be studied.

(II) Place of origin

The place of origin is one of the important factors affecting the quality of TCM crude drugs, and fixed place of origin is an important measure to guarantee the relative stable quality of TCM crude drugs. Through literature studies, surveys of place of origin, and other methods, we can gain an understanding of the Daodi (geo-authentic) areas, main production areas, core distribution areas, and suitable growth areas of TCM crude drugs. This allows us to comprehend the variations in quality of TCM crude drugs in different regions and consequently enhance our studies on the quality patterns of TCM crude drugs in various places of origin. The geological environment and associated minerals in the place of origin of the mineral TCM crude drugs are closely related to heavy metals and other impurities in the TCM crude drugs. Therefore, targeted studies should be conducted.

The places of origin of TCM crude drugs should be carefully selected by taking into account factors such as growth habits, clinical medication experience, traditional practices, quality of TCM crude drugs, resource availability, and cultivation and breeding conditions. It is encouraged to use the Daodi areas as the places of origins of the TCM crude drugs, as the planting areas, and the places with similar ecological environment can also be chosen for the same purposes.

The places of origins are generally the specific growth areas of TCM crude drugs with similar ecological environment, and the ranges should be determined according to changes in the quality of the TCM crude drugs. The quality of TCM crude drugs growing in the same places of origins should generally be relatively stable. Under the premise of ensuring the stable quality of TCM crude drugs, multiple places of origins can be selected.

(III) Cultivation and breeding

For the cultivation and breeding of TCM crude drugs, it is required to understand the growth and development patterns or living habits of medicinal plants or animals. Considering the characteristics of TCMs and the R&D regularities of new TCMs, it is crucial to emphasize the management of all aspects of the cultivation and breeding of TCM crude drugs after marketing of new TCMs. Attention should be paid to the following aspects:

1. Seeds and seedlings

The sources of seeds and seedlings should be clarified to ensure that their quality remains stable. Encourage the selection of seeds and seedlings from germplasm or excellent varieties propagated in Daodi areas. If the varieties are changed, sufficient risk assessment and study should be carried out to prove their safety, efficacy and quality control, and to ensure that the quality of TCM crude drugs before and after the change is consistent.

2. Agricultural inputs

During the process of cultivation of medicinal plants, the management of inputs such as pesticides and fertilizers should be strengthened. The selection of pesticide types, dosages, and application methods should be based on the growth characteristics of TCM crude drugs, the effectiveness in controlling pests and diseases, the potential for residues, and the risk of pollution. Whenever possible, it is advisable to use the lowest dose and minimize the number of applications. The use of pesticides should comply with relevant national regulations, and it is necessary to timely pay attention to the list of prohibited and restricted pesticides issued by relevant national departments. During the process of breeding medicinal animals, the regulations of relevant national departments on animal breeding and the safe use of veterinary drugs should be strictly followed.

The management of documents on the cultivation and breeding of TCM crude drugs should be strengthened. Detailed records of agricultural inputs such as pesticides, fertilizers or veterinary drugs used should be kept, including names, dosages, frequency, time, and safe interval of use, etc.

3. Studies on cultivation and breeding

Encourage studies on cultivation and breeding of TCM crude drugs such as ecological cultivation, wild tending, and biomimetic cultivation techniques, explore the law of quality and yield formation of TCM crude drugs, study the key technologies affecting the quality of TCM crude drugs, and study and establish quality control methods. According to the needs of quality control and risk management during the cultivation and breeding process, the quality of TCM crude drugs and harmful pollutants such as pesticides should be tracked and monitored. The causes of problems, if identified, should be found in time and effective measures should be taken to rectify such problems. During the long-term cultivation and breeding of medicinal plants or animals, there should be measures to ensure the stability of germplasm and prevent the variation and degradation of the germplasm of TCM crude drugs.

(IV) Harvesting and on-site processing

Harvesting and on-site processing are important factors that impact the quality of TCM crude drugs. Generally, the traditional experience should be respected, and the principle of "Quality first with output considered" should be adhered to. Attention should be paid to the following contents:

1. Harvesting

In the process of harvesting of TCM crude drugs, the growth years, harvesting periods and harvesting methods should be determined according to the characteristics and growth phenological period of the TCM crude drugs. When the growth years and harvesting periods are inconsistent with traditional experience, it should be necessary to provide sufficient reasons.

For the harvesting of wild TCM crude drugs, it is important to develop scientific and well-planned harvesting strategies to ensure the sustainable utilization of TCM resources. During the harvesting process, mixed harvesting and mixing with non-medicinal parts or impurities should be avoided. The training of harvesting personnel and the management of information, such as harvesting locations, time, and quantity, etc., should be strengthened.

The mining of mineral TCM crude drugs should comply with the relevant national regulations, pay attention to the studies on the places of origins, and also pay special attention to the geological environment and associated minerals in order to avoid the mixing of impurities.

2. On-site processing

For the on-site processing of TCM crude drugs, it is generally recommended to follow traditional experience, conduct studies and determine appropriate on-site processing methods based on the characteristics of TCM crude drugs and the requirements of preparations. Additionally, it is important to specify the key process parameters. Encourage the adoption of high-efficiency and intensive on-site processing techniques that have a scientific basis and have been proven by production practice. The secondary pollution or degradation of the quality of TCM crude drugs should be avoided during on-site processing.

(V) Packaging and storage

The packaging and storage of TCM crude drugs have a significant impact on their quality. The packaging of TCM crude drugs should be able to protect their quality and facilitate their distribution.

1. Packaging and labels

The packaging materials should comply with relevant national regulations and maintain the stable quality of TCM crude drugs and prevent pollution. Appropriate packaging materials should be selected based on the characteristics of TCM crude drugs. Special attention should be given to the packaging of TCM crude drugs that are easily volatile, and prone to contamination, damp, or deterioration. The origins, places of origin, and harvesting periods of the TCM crude drugs in the same package should be consistent. Labels should be printed or affixed to the package in accordance with the provisions, and the label contents should comply with the requirements of laws and regulations.

2. Storage conditions

The storage of TCM crude drugs should meet the maintenance requirements of TCMs. Studies should be conducted on the impact of storage conditions (such as temperature, humidity, and illumination, etc.) and storage time on the quality of TCM crude drugs, taking into consideration their characteristics and traditional experience. In particular, for TCM crude drugs that are prone to moth infestation, mold growth, spoilage, and oil leakage, it is important to establish appropriate quality control indicators based on study findings, determine suitable storage conditions, and enhance quality control measures. The study and application of new storage techniques that contribute to advancing the quality of TCM crude drugs are encouraged.

(VI) Quality studies and quality standards

The quality standards of the TCM crude drugs for new TCMs should be studied and improved according to the needs of quality control for preparations. The quality standards for TCM crude drugs should conform to the characteristics of TCMs, reflect their quality status, embody the overall quality control concept, and help ensure the stable quality of TCM crude drugs. It is important to focus on the integration of science and practicality, the combination of traditional methods and new techniques/methods, and the exploration of the relationship between traditional quality evaluation experience and modern test indicators. Attention should be paid to the following contents:

1. Guarantee accurate origins

The specific identification methods for TCM crude drugs should be established to ensure their accurate origins and avoid easily confusing products, adulteration and fake. Appropriate reference TCM crude drugs, reference extracts and standard spectra, etc can be selected as controls. When necessary, comparative studies with counterfeit products are required to demonstrate the specificity of the method. The use of effective traditional identification methods should be encouraged. The study and establishment of effective origin identification methods should be based on the achievements of scientific research and investigating research results in the works of National Post-market Drug Surveillance.

2. Control safety risks

For TCM crude drugs traditionally known as highly toxic and toxic, as well as toxic TCM crude drugs found by modern studies (e.g., TCM crude drugs of Aristolochiaceae family), the basic studies on toxic components should be strengthened, and reasonable quality control indicators and limit requirements should be determined based on the safety and risk assessment results of preparations. Attention should be paid to conducting relevant studies on TCM crude drugs that contain components belonging to the same family and genus as known toxic components.

Where purchased TCM crude drugs have problems such as weight gain , dyeing, adulteration and fake, studies should be strengthened, and according to the needs of risk management, add targeted test items in reference to the national supplementary test methods or relevant studies, the test items can be added in internal control standards when necessary.

The studies on exogenous pollutants in TCM crude drugs should be strengthened. According to the use of pesticides, veterinary drugs and fumigants, etc. in the production process of TCM crude drugs, as well as the risk of possible contamination by heavy metals, harmful elements and mycotoxins, etc., comprehensive assessment should be performed in combination with the processing method and manufacturing process of corresponding preparations, and the test items for related exogenous pollutants should be established in quality standards when necessary. The relevant specifications for exogenous pollutants should be set up based on regions and TCM crude drugs varieties according to the study results. For mineral TCM crude drugs, attention should be paid to the geological environment of mineral deposits, the standardization of harvesting and processing methods, and it is also required to strengthen the control of associated heavy metals and harmful elements. In addition, for animal TCM crude drugs, attention should be paid to problems such as carrying pathogenic microorganisms to prevent biosafety risks, especially for those derived from wild animals.

3. Stable and controllable quality

Quality standards should reflect the overall quality attributes of TCM crude drugs, and attention should be paid to the correlation between the test items and indicators, and the key quality attributes of preparations. Reasonable quality requirements should be studied and established based on the quality status of TCM crude drugs and the design requirements for studies on new TCMs. Moreover, it is encouraged to study and develop test methods of multiple markers, such as extractive determination methods, fingerprint/characteristic chromatogram methods, assays for major chemical classes, and assays for multiple components, which will help control the overall quality of TCM crude drugs and ensure quality stability of relevant preparations.

Ⅳ. References

1. State Food and Drug Administration. *Technical Guidelines for Pre-treatment of Raw TCM Materials and Natural Medicines*, 2005.

2. State Food and Drug Administration. *Technical Requirements for Study on New Natural Medicines*, 2013.

中药新药用药材质量控制研究
技术指导原则（试行）

一、概述

药材是中药新药研发和生产的源头，其质量是影响中药新药安全、有效和质量可控的关键因素。为完善中药制剂质量控制体系，加强药品质量的可追溯性，为中药制剂提供安全有效、质量稳定的药材，基于全过程质量控制和风险管控的理念，针对药材生产的关键环节和关键质控点，制定本技术指导原则。

本指导原则主要包括药材基原与药用部位、产地、种植养殖、采收与产地加工、包装与贮藏及质量标准等内容，旨在为中药新药用药材的质量控制研究提供参考。

二、基本原则

（一）尊重中医药传统和特色

药材质量控制研究应遵循中医药理论，尊重中医药传统经验和特色。药材的适宜产地、生产方式、生长年限、采收时间、产地加工方法及药材的质量评价等应尊重传统经验。鼓励传承传统经验和技术，鼓励应用现代科学技术表征传统质量评价经验和指标。

（二）满足中药新药研究设计需要

应基于中药新药研究设计的需要，根据不同药材的特点，研究影响药材及制剂质量稳定的关键因素和风险控制点，满足制剂质量控制的需要。采取必要的措施如固定基原、药用部位、产地等以保证中药新药用药材质量基本稳定。

（三）加强生产全过程质量控制

应加强药材的基原、产地、种植养殖、采收加工、包装贮藏等生产全过程的质量控制研究。鼓励参照中药材生产质量管理规范（GAP）的要求进行药材种植养殖，建立野生药材的采收、产地加工、包装贮藏等相应的质量控制和管理措施。应保证药材来源可追溯，鼓励运用现代信息技术建立药材追溯体系。

（四）关注药材资源可持续利用

应处理好药材合理利用与资源保护的关系，开展资源评估，保证药材资源的可持续利用。使用源自野生动植物的药材，应符合国家关于野生动植物管理的相关法规及要求。中药新药应严格限定使用源自野生动物的药材，原则上不使用源自珍稀濒危野生动植物的药材，如确需使用，应严格要求，尽早开展种植养殖或野生抚育研究，保证资源可持续利用。使用古生物化石类药材的，应符合国家关于古生物化石保护管理的相关法规及要求。

三、主要内容

（一）基原与药用部位

基原准确是保证药材质量的基础。应明确药材的原植/动物中文名、拉丁学名及药用部位。对于多基原药材，一般应固定使用其中一个基原，若需使用多个基原的，应提供充分的依据，并固定使用比例，保证制剂质量的稳定。种植养殖药材有明确选育品种的，一般应说明品种信息。矿物药应明确该矿物的类、族、矿石名或岩石名以及主要成份。

应采取措施保证所用药材基原和药用部位准确。新药材、易混淆药材、难以确定基原的药材，原则上应采集原植/动/矿物的凭证标本，由专家或有资质的机构进行物种鉴定，并保留标本、照片及相关资料。必要时还需与伪品进行对比研究，并结合产地调研等，确认药材基原。新药材应详细描述药材的相关信息，如原植/动物形态特征和药用部位，说明原植/动物的生长环境、习性、产地、分布及资源等。野生药材在相同生长区域、相同采收期有易混淆物种的，应进行基原鉴别及与易混淆品区别的研究。

（二）产地

产地是影响药材质量的重要因素之一，固定产地是保证药材质量相对稳定的重要措施。通过文献研究、产地考察等方法，了解药材的道地产区、主产区、核心分布区及适生区等情况，了解不同产地药材的质量差异，加强不同产地药材质量规律的研究。矿物药产地的地质环境及伴生矿等情况与药材中重金属及其他杂质密切相关，应加强针对性的研究。

应综合考虑药材的生长习性、临床用药经验和传统习惯、药材质量、资源状况及种植养殖条件等合理选择药材产地。鼓励以道地产区作为药材产地，药材种植也可选择适宜生长区内生态环境与道地产区相似的地区。

产地一般为生态环境相似的特定药材生长区域，产地范围应根据所产药材质量变化情况而定，同一产地内所产药材的质量一般应相对稳定。在保证药材质量稳定的前提下，可以选择多个产地。

（三）种植养殖

药材的种植养殖应了解药用植/动物的生长发育规律或生活习性。考虑中药特点和中药新药研发规律，尤其在中药新药上市后应关注药材种植养殖各环节的管理，重点关注以下内容：

1. 种子种苗

应明确种子种苗的来源，保证其质量稳定。鼓励选用来源于道地产区种质或优良品种繁育的种子种苗。如变更品种，应进行充分的风险评估和研究，证明其安全、有效和质量可控，保证变更前后药材质量一致。

2. 农业投入品

药用植物种植过程中应加强农药化肥等投入品的管理。应结合药材生长特点、对病虫害的防治效果、残留情况及污染风险等合理确定农药种类、用量和使用方法，尽可能按最低剂量及最少次数使用。农药使用应符合国家有关规定，及时关注国家相关部门发布的农药禁限用名单。药用动物养殖过程中应严格遵守国家相关部门关于动物养殖、兽药安全使用等规定。

应加强种植养殖药材的文件管理。详细记录所用农药、化肥或兽药等农业投入品，内容包括名称、用量、次数、时间、使用安全间隔期等。

3. 种植养殖研究

鼓励开展药材生态种植、野生抚育和仿生栽培技术等种植养殖研究，探索药材质量和产量形成的规律，研究影响药材质量的关键技术，研究建立质量控制方法。应根据种植养殖过程中质量控制及风险管理的需要，对药材质量及农药等有害污染物进行跟踪监测，发现问题应及时查找原因，并采取有效措施整改。药用植/动物的长期种植养殖过程中，应有保证种质稳定的措施，防范药材种质变异和退化。

（四）采收与产地加工

采收和产地加工是影响药材质量的重要环节。一般应尊重传统经验，坚持质量优先、兼顾产量的原则。重点关注以下内容：

1. 采收

药材的采收应根据药材的特点和生长物候期，确定生长年限、采收期及采收方法。生长年限和采收期等与传统经验不一致时，应有充分的依据。

野生药材的采收应制定科学合理的采收方案，保证资源可持续利用。采收过程中应避免混采混收、非药用部位或杂质的混入。应加强对采收人员的培训及采收地点、时间、数量等信息的管理。

矿物药的采挖应符合国家相关规定，注意对产地的研究，特别关注地质环境及伴生矿等情况，避免杂质混入。

2. 产地加工

药材的产地加工一般应遵循传统经验，根据药材的特点和制剂需要，研究确定适宜的产地加工方法，明确关键工艺参数。鼓励采用有科学依据并经生产实践证明高效、集约化的产地加工技术。产地加工过程中应避免造成药材的二次污染或质量下降。

（五）包装与贮藏

药材的包装与贮藏对其质量有着重要的影响。药材的包装应能够保护药材的质量并便于流通。

1. 包装及标签

包装材料应符合国家相关规定，有利于保持药材质量稳定、不污染药材。应根据药材特点选择合适的包装材料，关注易挥发、污染、受潮、变质等特殊药材的包装。同一包装内药材的基原、产地、采收期等应一致。包装上应按照规定印有或者贴有标签，标签内容应符合法律、法规的要求。

2. 贮藏条件

药材的贮藏应符合中药养护要求，应结合药材的特点及传统经验，开展贮藏条件（如温度、湿度、光照等）和贮藏时间对药材质量影响的研究，特别是对易虫蛀、霉变、腐烂、走油等药材，应根据研究结果建立合理的质量控制指标，确定合理的贮藏条件，加强质量控制。鼓励有利于保证药材质量的贮藏新技术的研究和应用。

（六）质量研究与质量标准

中药新药用药材的质量标准应根据制剂质量控制需要进行研究完善。药材质量标准应符合中药特点，反映药材的质量状况，体现整体质量控制理念，有利于保证药材质量稳定。应注重科学性和实用性相结合，传统方法和新技术、新方法相结合，并探索传统质量评价经验与现代检测指标之间的相关性。重点关注以下内容：

1. 保证基原准确

应建立药材的专属性鉴别方法，保证药材来源准确，避免出现易混淆品、掺杂使假等问题。可选择适宜的对照药材、对照提取物、标准图谱等作为对照，必要时还需与伪品进行对比研究，说明方法的专属性。注意加强传统鉴别中有效方法的使用。鼓励根据基础科学研究进展和国家药品抽检探索性研究结果研究建立有效的基原鉴别方法。

2. 控制安全风险

对于传统认识为大毒（剧毒）、有毒的药材，以及现代研究发现的毒性药材（如马兜铃科药材等），应加强毒性成份的基础研究，结合制剂安全性及风险评估结果确定合理的质控指标及限度要求。对含有与已发现有毒成份同科属的药材应注意进行相关研究。

外购药材存在染色增重、掺杂使假等常见问题的，应加强研究，根据风险管理的需要，参照国家相关补充检验方法或研究增加针对性的检测项目，必要时列入内控标准。

应加强药材外源性污染物的研究。根据药材生产过程中农药、兽药、熏蒸剂等的使用情况，以及可能被重金属及有害元素、真菌毒素等污染的风险，结合炮制及相应制剂的生产工艺进行综合评估，必要时在质量标准中建立相关外源性污染物的检测项目，并根据研究结果，分区域、分品种制定外源性污染物控制标准。矿物药应关注矿床地质环境、采收和加工方法的规范性，加强伴生重金属及有害元素的控制。动物类药材应关注携带病原微生物等问题，防范生物安全风险，尤其是源自野生动物的药材。

3. 质量稳定可控

质量标准应能反映药材的整体质量属性，应关注检测项目和指标与制剂关键质量属性的相关性。应根据药材质量状况和中药新药研究设计要求，研究确定合理的质量要求。鼓励研究建立多指标检验检测方法，如浸出物测定、指纹/特征图谱、大类成份含量测定、多指标成份含量测定，以整体控制药材质量，保证制剂质量稳定。

四、参考文献

1. 国家食品药品监督管理局.《中药、天然药物原料的前处理技术指导原则》，2005 年.

2. 国家食品药品监督管理局.《天然药物新药研究技术要求》，2013 年.

Guideline for the Evaluation of Traditional Chinese Medicine (TCM) Resources

I. Overview

The Guideline is formulated in accordance with the *Drug Administration Law of the People's Republic of China* and the *Provisions for Drug Registration* to protect TCM resources, achieve their sustainable utilization, and guarantee their stable supply and quality control of TCM products.

The TCM resources mentioned in the Guideline refer to plants, animals, and mineral resources used exclusively for producing Chinese proprietary medicines (CPMs) and prepared slices/decoction pieces. The evaluation of TCM resources mentioned in the Guideline refers to the process in which marketing authorization holders of medicines (hereinafter referred to as the "MAHs") or TCM manufacturers compare the estimated consumption and estimated available amount of TCM resources in the next five years, and scientifically evaluate the possible impact of the manufacturing of TCM products on the sustainable utilization of TCM resources.

II. Basic Principles

(I) Principle of the combination of resource protection and industrial development

The evaluation of TCM resources should be in line with the "basic state policy of resource conservation and environmental protection", and the sustainable utilization of TCM resources should be actively promoted while strengthening TCM resource protection.

(II) Principle of the balance between the supply and consumption of TCM crude drug resources

The MAHs or manufacturers using TCM crude drug resources should provide evaluation data that demonstrate a balance between the estimated annual consumption and the available amount of TCM crude drug resources. If wild TCM crude drugs are used, the annual consumption of TCM crude drugs should be ensured below the annual growth volume of TCM crude drugs from the specified production areas available to the MAHs or manufacturers. The awareness of quality first should be strengthened, and sustainable yield should be comprehensively evaluated from both the quality and supply while ensuring that the quality meets the requirements of the product.

(III) Principle of dynamic evaluation

TCM crude drug resources should be evaluated at all the stages: project approval, R&D, and post-marketing of TCM products. The evaluation report should be updated timely if there are changes in the estimated consumption and estimated available amount of TCM resources.

In principle, for the marketed TCM products, TCM resources should be re-evaluated every five years. At the time of re-registration of CPMs, if the formula contains endangered wild TCM crude drugs and their production may lead to the depletion of corresponding TCM crude drug resources, the MAHs or manufacturers should conduct a TCM resource evaluation before such re-registration.

III. Evaluation Contents of TCM Resources

TCM resource evaluation mainly includes three aspects: estimated consumption, potential risks, and sustainable utilization measures. For compound CPMs, resource evaluation should be performed separately for each ingredient contained in the formula.

(I) Background information

Background information for TCM resource evaluation includes :

1. Market size analysis: CPMs should be discussed from the following aspects: product indications, target population, incidence rate of the treated disease, average dosage and biomass of the medicine necessary for each patient to achieve the therapeutic effect, and the potential market size of the product.

Decoction pieces should be discussed from the coverage of target market of sales.

2. Formula and actual feeding amount: List the name and prescribed amount of each ingredient, and specify the actual feeding amount of each ingredient.

3. Basic information on TCM resources: Clarify the origin species and their biological characteristics of TCM resources used by the MAHs or manufacturers, the medicinal parts and initial processing information at the places of origins of the used TCM resources, and the sources of wild or cultivated and bred resources.

4. Basic information on the places of origins: Geographic location of the places of origins of TCM crude drugs (providing the source regions of wild TCM crude drugs), area of cultivation and breeding bases, and methods of production and organization. Certificate of origin and relevant information on the importer should be provided for imported TCM crude drugs.

5. Quality information on TCM crude drugs: The primary basis for selecting the species of TCM resources, the location of the base, or the source region; and also relevant studies on the quality of TCM crude drugs.

(II) Estimated consumption

The estimated consumption of TCM resources refers to the total amount of TCM crude drugs that are estimated to be consumed during the evaluation period.

1. CPMs

For CPMs, the estimated consumption of the evaluated product is calculated based on the formula and the estimated annual sales. The calculation equation is as follows:

Estimated consumption (tons) = Amount of TCM crude drugs consumed per minimum packaging unit (g) × Estimated total number of minimum packaging units sold annually × 1/1000000.

Where: ① The amount of TCM crude drugs consumed per minimum packaging unit in grams is calculated based on Paragraph 2 under "Background information". ② The estimated total number of minimum packaging units sold annually can refer to the annual sales volume of similar marketed products in the past five years, or calculated based on the previous sales volume of the product. This information is mainly obtained from Paragraph 1 under "Background information".

2. Decoction pieces

Each product can be estimated based on the cumulative sales volume of all sales terminals (hospitals and pharmacies, etc.) or by referring to the sales volume of similar products each year. The information is primarily obtained from Paragraphs 1 & 2 under "Background information".

(III) Estimated available amount

This section is mainly intended to describe the way to obtain specific TCM crude drug resources by TCM manufacturers and the relevant available amount.

For TCM crude drug varieties that come from artificial cultivation and breeding, the scope of the base and annual yield of the base should be described; for wild TCM crude drug varieties, the scope of their source regions and available amounts should be stated.

(IV) Potential risks

Potential risks of TCM resources can be analyzed based on regeneration ability, medicine formation period, distribution regions, endangered category, and special values of TCM crude drugs. Relevant contents are available in Paragraphs 3 & 4 under "Background information".

1. Regeneration ability

It is required to describe whether the TCM crude drugs used are regenerative resources and the restrictions on regeneration, including whether there are barriers to breeding and special habitat requirements.

2. Medicine formation period of TCM crude drugs

The time required for TCM resources to grow from seedlings to maturity of reproductive organs and the time needed for producing TCM crude drugs that meet drug standards should be described. Literature data or actual measurement data can be cited.

3. Distribution regions

The distribution range of the used TCM resources should be described, especially from the perspective of Daodi (geo-authenticity) and quality variation. Literature data or actual measurement data can be cited.

4. Endangered category

Attention should be paid to updates on national, local, or international lists of valuable, rare, and endangered species under protection, and it should be indicated whether the TCM resource used is listed as a protected object or included in relevant protection lists.

5. Special values

It is required to describe the unique roles and values of the used TCM resources in the ecosystem and biodiversity. For example, glycyrrhiza and ephedra have crucial ecological value in wind prevention and sand fixation, and excessive harvesting may lead to soil desertification.

6. Special risk warning

In any of the following situations, a special warning about the risks associated with the TCM resources used must be included in the conclusion part of the evaluation report:

① Artificial cultivation and breeding are not feasible: The growth conditions or cultivation and breeding mechanisms of this type of TCM crude drugs are not yet clear, so artificial cultivation and breeding cannot be carried out, which poses obstacles to the sustainable supply of TCM crude drugs.

② The medicine formation period of TCM crude drugs is over five years (including five years): The time from seedling cultivation and breeding to TCM crude drugs meeting drug standards is over five years. A long production period results in large fluctuations in yield, making a dynamic match of supply and demand difficult.

③ Habitat requirements are special, and the distribution is narrow: TCM crude drugs of this type are only distributed in specific regions, and their production is difficult to expand. Excessive harvesting is likely to cause the species to be endangered.

④ Valuable, rare, and endangered wild resources: This type of TCM crude drugs has already encountered resource issues and has already been listed as valuable, rare, and endangered wild resources. Both domestic and international laws and regulations have restrictions on the use of such resources.

⑤ Unstable quality: TCM crude drugs of this type vary in quality across regions, or the varieties are likely to be mixed, leading to quality problems.

⑥ Existence of serious successive cropping obstacles: Due to factors such as plant diseases, insect pests, and nutrition, TCM crude drugs of this type cannot be repeatedly planted in the same plot of land and require constant change of the cultivated land, making quality management difficult.

⑦ Other risks that may cause problems with the amount or quality of resources: e.g. imported TCM crude drugs, changes in the place of origin, climate changes, environmental pollution, etc.

(V) Sustainable utilization and quality stabilization measures

The evaluation of sustainable utilization measures for TCM resources should focus on the following areas:

1. Sustainable availability

For the TCM crude drug varieties that come from artificial cultivation and breeding, a 5-year development plan for the base should be provided; for wild TCM crude drug varieties, the annual yield should be specified, and 5-year natural renewal, wild tending, and transformation of wild tending into artificial cultivation and breeding should be described.

2. Quality stabilization measures

The origin, places of origins, harvesting time, and initial processing method at the places of origins of TCM crude drugs should be clearly defined and fixed. If the TCM crude drugs come from artificial cultivation and breeding, the measures taken for ensuring compliance of cultivation and breeding with the requirements of the *Good Agricultural Practice* (GAP) should be described.

IV. Decision–making and Dynamic Adjustment of TCM Resource Evaluation

Whether sustainable utilization measures can effectively prevent potential risks should be analyzed. A decision of TCM resource evaluation can be made based on the match between the estimated consumption and estimated available amount.

If sustainable utilization measures can effectively prevent potential risks, and the estimated consumption matches the estimated available amount, it indicates that TCM products have a relatively lower risk in terms of the sustainable utilization of TCM resources.

If sustainable utilization measures are ineffective in preventing potential risks and the estimated consumption does not match the estimated available amount, the TCM products have a relatively higher risk in terms of the sustainable utilization of TCM resources. Therefore, the R&D or marketing of the products should be carefully considered, and adjustments to the estimated consumption or sustainable utilization measures may be necessary.

If, after adjustment, it is still unable to prevent potential risks effectively and the estimated consumption does not match the estimated available amount, the production of TCM products may result in the depletion of related TCM resources.

Annexes: 1. Format Requirements for TCM Resource Evaluation Report

2. Reference List of TCM crude drugs for Cultivation (Plants)

Annex 1

Format Requirements for TCM Resource Evaluation Report

A complete evaluation report of TCM resources is composed of an overview and a resource evaluation sub-report of each TCM crude drug involved in the product.

1 Overview

The overview includes cover, statement, product description, evaluation process description, main evaluation conclusion, and instructions on trade secrets involved.

1.1 Cover

The cover should include: title (Product name + Name of the TCM crude drugs used + Resource Evaluation Report), name of the MAH or manufacturer, evaluation date, etc.

1.2 Statement

The evaluation report of TCM resources of this product should be true, complete, and legally sourced, and should not infringe on any rights and interests of others. In case of any inaccuracies, we will assume all the resulting legal consequences.

1.3 Product description

Describe TCM crude drug varieties involved in the product, the registration application stage of the product, or the production and sales after marketing.

(1) Summary of the R&D process: Briefly describe the R&D background and purpose of the product and provide an overview of the product R&D process.

(2) Market size analysis: Analyze comprehensively the following aspects,

target population of the TCM products, the incidence of the treated diseases, the average dosage of the medicine necessary for each patient to achieve the therapeutic effect, and the market information of similar products, etc.

Manufacturers of decoction pieces should analyze the market size based on the coverage of target market of sales.

1.4 Overview of the evaluation process

Describe the organization and implementation processes for product resource evaluation.

1.5 Main evaluation conclusion

Summarize the evaluation conclusion for each of the TCM crude drug resources involved.

1.6 Instructions on trade secrets involved

Describe the content and scope of the trade secrets involved.

2 Sub-report of TCM resource evaluation

The sub-report of TCM resource evaluation consists of four main parts: cover, introduction, sub-report, and relevant annexes, and should be arranged in the order as follows.

2.1 Cover

The cover should include the following information: title of the report, the evaluation institution, the principal person in charge of the evaluation, and the evaluation time.

2.2 Introduction

2.2.1 Evaluate the source, reliability, completeness, and authenticity of the required data.

2.2.2 Evaluator information

Including the names, affiliations, professional titles, positions, and professional backgrounds of the principal personnel involved in the evaluation.

2.3 Sub-report

2.3.1 Title

Name of the TCM crude drugs (used in the TCM product) + Resource Evaluation Sub-report, e.g., Resource Evaluation Sub-report of Corni Fructus (for Use in Pills of Six Ingredients with Rehmannia).

2.3.2 Summary

Concisely summarize the sources of data used in the evaluation, evaluation methods, evaluation results, and evaluation conclusion, etc.

2.3.3 General background information

(1) Amount of TCM crude drugs necessary for the minimum packaging unit.

(2) Basic information on TCM resources: Including the information on the origin species of TCM resources used by the MAHs or manufacturers, the medicinal parts and initial processing information at the places of origins of the used TCM resources, and whether they are wild or from cultivation and breeding.

(3) Information on the place of origin: The place of origin, location (providing the source regions of wild TCM crude drugs), acreage, production and organization mode of the TCM resources used by the MAHs or manufacturers. For imported TCM crude drugs, it is necessary to provide relevant information on the country of origin and the importer.

(4) Quality information: Including the main basis for selecting TCM resource species, base location or source region, relevant studies on the quality of TCM crude drugs, quality standards adopted and the preparation basis for quality standards.

2.3.4 The evaluation of estimated consumption should include:

(1) Calculation process of the estimated consumption, and

(2) Description of various data sources.

2.3.5 Evaluation of the estimated available amount

Describe the calculation process and data sources of the estimated available amount.

2.3.6 The evaluation of potential risks should include:

(1) Regeneration ability,

(2) Medicine formation period of TCM crude drugs,

(3) Distribution region,

(4) Endangered category,

(5) Special value, and

(6) Special risk warning.

2.3.7 Sustainable utilization and quality stabilization measures of TCM resources should include:

(1) Sustainable availability measures,

(2) Quality stabilization measures, and

(3) Measure effectiveness evaluation.

2.3.8 Final conclusion

Describe the evaluation conclusion concisely and clearly based on the evaluation results.

2.3.9 Uncertainty analysis

Any uncertainties regarding materials and data (e.g., lack of knowledge, data limitations, and controversial issues) must be thoroughly discussed in this section, and the degree of influence of these uncertainties on the reliability of results should be detailed.

2.3.10 References

If literature and documents are cited in the evaluation report, sources of such cited literature and documents should be provided at the end of the report.

2.4 Relevant annexes

2.4.1 Certificates of bases related to cultivation and breeding of TCM crude drugs

For example: photocopies of the land certificate or land lease contract, the cooperation agreement, etc.

2.4.2 Technical procedures for standardized cultivation and breeding

2.4.3 Study/Research data on the quality of TCM crude drugs that meet the characteristics of TCM products

2.4.4 Other certificates related to this report

For example: Supply and marketing contracts and relevant test reports, etc.

2.4.5 Data summary table

Data Summary Table

Product name	(Name of CPM or decoction pieces)		
Name of TCM crude drugs	(Please refer to Note 1)		
Origin	(Please refer to Note 2)	Latin name	(Please refer to Note 2)
Medicinal part	☐ Plant (☐ Root ☐ Fruit and seed ☐ Whole plant ☐ Root and rhizome ☐ Flower ☐ Bark ☐ Leaf ☐ Woody stem ☐ Resins ☐ Physiological or pathological product) ☐ Animal (☐ Whole body ☐ Organs ☐ Physiological or pathological product ☐ Tissue ☐ Horn and bone ☐ Shell) ☐ Minerals ☐ Fungi ☐ Algae ☐ Lichens ☐ Others: _____		
Estimated amount of resources consumed	Year	Amount of TCM crude drugs consumed per minimum packaging unit * (g)	Estimated annual sales quantity of the minimum packaging unit *	Estimated annual consumption (tons)
	yyyy			
	yyyy			
	yyyy			
	yyyy			
	yyyy			
	Total			

continued

Risk profile evaluation	Artificial breeding		☐ N/A ☐ Immature ☐ Mature			
	Distribution region		☐ 1–2 provinces ☐ 3–6 provinces ☐ More than 6 provinces			
	Medicine formation period of TCM crude drugs (Please refer to Note 3)		Number of years of medicine formation period	☐ 1–2 years ☐ 3–5 years ☐ More than 5 years ☐ Others:_____		
			Harvesting period	☐ 1–2 years ☐ 3–5 years ☐ More than 5 years ☐ Others:_____		
	Endemic species in China		☐ Yes ☐ No			
	Valuable, rare and endangered wild species		☐ Yes ☐ No (Please refer to Note 4) Note:_____			
	Have special value		☐ Yes ☐ No (Please refer to Note 4) Note:_____			
	Risk warning required					
Sustainable utilization measures	**Cultivation of TCM crude drugs**	Location of the place of origin	Region (accurate to county level) Daodi places of origins (☐ Yes ☐ No ☐ Others:_____)			
		Area	$667m^2$ (a Chinese unit of land measurement)			
		Base location	Longitude:	Latitude:		Region:
		Production organization mode	☐ Self–built by company ☐ Cooperative base ☐ Others:_____			
		Standardized cultivation?	☐ Yes (GAP base: ☐ Yes ☐ No) ☐ No Others:_____			
		Initial processing mode at the place of origin				
		Estimated available amount	Year	Usable area ($667m^2$)	Yield per $667m^2$ ($Kg/667m^2$)	Estimated available amount (tons)
			yyyy			
			yyyy			
			yyyy			
			yyyy			
			yyyy			
			Total			

continued

Sustainable utilization measures	Estimated available amount	Base location	Longitud：		Latitude：	Region：
		Production organization mode	☐ Self–built by company ☐ Cooperative base ☐ Others： _____			
		Standardized breeding?	☐ Yes (GAP base: ☐ Yes ☐ No) ☐ No Others： _____			
		Initial processing mode at the place of origin				
		预计可获得量	Year	Breeding amount	Estimated available amount (tons)	
			yyyy			
			yyyy			
			yyyy			
			yyyy			
			yyyy			
			Total			
Sustainable utilization measure	Wild TCM crude drugs	Base location	Longitude:		Latitude:	Region:
		Area	667m^2			
		Acquisition route	☐ Self–harvested ☐ Purchased ☐ Others： _____			
		Restrictive measures	☐ Fenced ☐ Not fenced ☐ Others： _____			
		Harvesting time	XX 月—XX 月			
		Initial processing mode at the place of origin				
		Estimated available	Year	Usable region	Estimated available amount (tons)	
			yyyy			
			yyyy			
			yyyy			
			yyyy			
			yyyy			
			Total			
	Other measures					
Evaluation onclusion	Amount of resources		Estimated available amount ⩾ Estimated consumption ☐ Confirm			
	Quality of resources		Stable ☐ Confirm			

Note 1: In order to scientifically and completely obtain relevant data for TCM resource evaluation, the applicant should summarize the data according to the above table. A data summary table should be filled out for each TCM crude drug separately.

Note 2: The information on the origin species of TCM resources should mainly refer to the *Pharmacopoeia of the People's Republic of China*. For those not included in the *Pharmacopoeia of the People's Republic of China*, the names in the *Flora of China*, the *Fauna of China*, and other equivalent taxonomic monographs should prevail. If the names are updated, the latest ones should apply. The Latin name should follow the binomial nomenclature. Further details should be provided for infraspecific taxon or cultivars.

Note 3: The number of years of medicine formation period (taking the plant's TCM crude drugs as an example) refers to the time required from seedlings to the first harvest that meets medicinal requirements. The harvesting period (taking the plant's TCM crude drugs as an example) refers to the time between the last harvest and the next harvest for a TCM crude drug.

Note 4: List of protected wild TCM crude drugs: *Convention on International Trade in Endangered Species of Wild Fauna and Flora* (CITES) Annexes 1 and 2, *List of Important Wild Fauna Under State Protection*, *List of Important Wild Flora Under State Protection (First Batch)*, *List of Important Wild TCM crude drug Species Under State Protection*, and local protection lists.

Note 5: The part marked with an asterisk ("*") does not need to be filled out for decoction pieces.

Annex 2

Reference List of TCM crude drugs for Cultivation (Plants)

No.	Name of TCM crude drugs	Family	Category	Name of the origin plant	Latin name of the origin plant	Medicinal part	Remark
1	Anisi Stellati Fructus	Magnoliaceae	Plant	*Illicium verum* Hook. f.	*Illicium verum* Hook. f.	Dry mature fruit	
2	Ginseng Radix et Rhizoma	Araliaceae	Plant	*Panax ginseng* C. A. Mey.	*Panax ginseng* C. A. Mey.	Dry root and rhizome	
3	Ginseng Folium	Araliaceae	Plant	*Panax ginseng* C. A. Mey.	*Panax ginseng* C. A. Mey.	Dry leaf	
4	Canavaliae Semen	Leguminosae	Plant	*Canavalia gladiata* (Jacq.) DC.	*Canavalia gladiata* (Jacq.) DC.	Dry mature seed	
5	Notoginseng Radix et Rhizoma	Araliaceae	Plant	*Panax notoginseng* (Burk.) F. H. Chen	*Panax notoginseng* (Burk.) F. H. Chen	Dry root and rhizome	
6	Sparganii Rhizoma	Sparganiaceae	Plant	*Sparganium stoloniferum* Buch.–Ham.	*Sparganium stoloniferum* Buch.–Ham.	Dry tuber	
7	Zingiberis Rhizoma	Zingiberaceae	Plant	*Zingiber officinale* Rosc.	*Zingiber officinale* Rosc.	Dry rhizome	
8	Inulae Radix	Asteraceae	Plant	*Inula helenium* L.	*Inula helenium* L.	Dry root	

continued

No.	Name of TCM crude drugs	Family	Category	Name of the origin plant	Latin name of the origin plant	Medicinal part	Remark
9	Bolbostemmatis Rhizoma	Cucurbitaceae	Plant	*Bolbostemma paniculatum* (Maxim.) Franquet	*Bolbostemma paniculatum* (Maxim.) Franquet	Dry tuber	
10	Pseudolaricis Cortex	Pinaceae	Plant	*Pseudolarix amabilis* (Nelson) Rehd.	*Pseudolarix amabilis* (Nelson) Rehd.	Dry root or bark near the root	
11	Sojae Semen Germinatum	Leguminosae	Plant	*Glycine max* (L.) Merr.	*Glycine max* (L.) Merr.	Processed product of mature seeds that have sprouted and been dried	
12	Gleditsiae Sinensis Fructus	Leguminosae	Plant	*Gleditsia sinensis* Lam.	*Gleditsia sinensis* Lam.	Dry mature fruit	
13	Isatidis Folium	Cruciferae	Plant	*Isatis indigotica* Fort.	*Isatis indigotica* Fort.	Dry leaf	
14	Jujubae Fructus	Rhamnaceae	Plant	*Ziziphus jujuba* Mill.	*Ziziphus jujuba* Mill.	Dry mature fruit	
15	Rhei Radix et Rhizoma	Polygonaceae	Plant	*Rheum officinale* Baill. *Rheum palmatum* L.	*Rheum officinale* Baill. *Rheum palmatum* L.	Dry root and rhizome	Multiple origins
16	Allii Sativi Bulbus	Liliaceae	Plant	*Allium sativum* L.	*Allium sativum* L.	Bulb	
17	Arecae Pericarpium	Arecaceae	Plant	*Areca catechu* L.	*Areca catechu* L.	Dry pericarp	
18	Liriopes Radix	Liliaceae	Plant	*Liriope spicata* (Thunb.) Lour. var. *prolifera* Y. T. Ma	*Liriope spicata* (Thunb.) Lour. var. *prolifera* Y. T. Ma	Dry root tuber	Multiple origins
19	Corni Fructus	Cornaceae	Plant	*Cornus officinalis* Sieb. et Zucc.	*Cornus officinalis* Sieb. et Zucc.	Dry mature sarcocarp	
20	Dioscoreae Rhizoma	Dioscoreaceae	Plant	*Dioscorea opposita* Thunb.	*Dioscorea opposita* Thunb.	Dry rhizome	

continued

No.	Name of TCM crude drugs	Family	Category	Name of the origin plant	Latin name of the origin plant	Medicinal part	Remark
21	Kaempferiae Rhizoma	Zingiberaceae	Plant	Kaempferia galanga L.	Kaempferia galanga L.	Dry rhizome	
22	Lonicerae Flos	Caprifoliaceae	Plant	Lonicera fulvotomentosa Hsu et S. C. Cheng / Lonicera macranthoides Hand. –Mazz.	Lonicera fulvotomentosa Hsu et S. C. Cheng / Lonicera macranthoides Hand. –Mazz.	Dry flower bud or flower to blossom	Multiple origins
23	Crataegi Fructus	Rosaceae	Plant	Crataegus pinnatifida Bge. var. major N. E. Br.	Crataegus pinnatifida Bge. var. major N. E. Br.	Dry mature fruit	Multiple origins
24	Crataegi Folium	Rosaceae	Plant	Crataegus pinnatifida Bge. var. major N. E. Br.	Crataegus pinnatifida Bge. var. major N. E. Br.	Dry leaf	Multiple origins
25	Euphorbiae Semen	Euphorbiaceae	Plant	Euphorbia lathyris L.	Euphorbia lathyris L.	Dry mature seed	
26	Fritillariae Cirrhosae Bulbus	Liliaceae	Plant	Fritillaria unibracteata Hsiao et K. C. Hsia var. wabuensis (S. Y. Tang et S. C. Yue) Z. D. Liu, S. Wang et S. C. Chen	Fritillaria unibracteata Hsiao et K. C. Hsia var. wabuensis (S. Y. Tang et S. C. Yue) Z. D. Liu, S. Wang et S. C. Chen	Dry bulb	Multiple origins
27	Cyathulae Radix	Amaranthaceae	Plant	Cyathula officinalis Kuan	Cyathula officinalis Kuan	Dry root	
28	Aconiti Radix	Ranunculaceae	Plant	Aconitum carmichaelii Debx.	Aconitum carmichaelii Debx.	Dry maternal root	
29	Chuanxiong Rhizoma	Umbelliferae	Plant	Ligusticum chuanxiong Hort.	Ligusticum chuanxiong Hort.	Dry rhizome	

continued

No.	Name of TCM crude drugs	Family	Category	Name of the origin plant	Latin name of the origin plant	Medicinal part	Remark
30	Iridis Tectori Rhizoma	Iridaceae	Plant	*Iris tectorum* Maxim.	*Iris tectorum* Maxim.	Dry rhizome	
31	Toosendan Fructus	Meliaceae	Plant	*Melia toosendan* Sieb.et Zucc.	*Melia toosendan* Sieb.et Zucc.	Dry fruit	
32	Choerospondiatis Fructus	Anacardiaceae	Plant	*Choerospondias axillaris* (Roxb.) Burtt et Hill	*Choerospondias axillaris* (Roxb.) Burtt et Hill	Dry mature fruit	
33	Desmodii Styracifolii Herba	Leguminosae	Plant	*Desmodium styracifolium* (Osb.) Merr.	*Desmodium styracifolium* (Osb.) Merr.	Dry above—ground part	
34	Pogostemonis Herba	Lamiaceae	Plant	*Pogostemon cablin* (Blanco) Benth.	*Pogostemon cablin* (Blanco) Benth.	Dry above—ground part	
35	Ligustri Lucidi Fructus	Oleaceae	Plant	*Ligustrum lucidum* Ait.	*Ligustrum lucidum* Ait.	Dry mature fruit	
36	Foeniculi Fructus	Umbelliferae	Plant	*Foeniculum vulgare* Mill.	*Foeniculum vulgare* Mill.	Dry mature fruit	
37	Vaccariae Semen	Caryophyllaceae	Plant	*Vaccaria segetalis* (Neck.) Garcke	*Vaccaria segetalis* (Neck.) Garcke	Dry mature seed	
38	Asparagi Radix	Liliaceae	Plant	*Asparagus cochinchinensis* (Lour.) Merr.	*Asparagus cochinchinensis* (Lour.) Merr.	Dry root tuber	

continued

No.	Name of TCM crude drugs	Family	Category	Name of the origin plant	Latin name of the origin plant	Medicinal part	Remark
39	Trichosanthis Radix	Cucurbitaceae	Plant	*Trichosanthes kirilowii* Maxim. / *Trichosanthes rosthornii* Harms	*Trichosanthes kirilowii* Maxim. / *Trichosanthes rosthornii* Harms	Dry root	Multiple origins
40	Bambusae Concretio Silicea	Poaceae	Plant	*Schizostachyum chinense* Rendle / Bambusa textilis Mc Clure	*Schizostachyum chinense* Rendle / Bambusa textilis Mc Clure	Clumps formed after the secretion inside the stem dries up	Multiple origins
41	Gastrodiae Rhizoma	Orchidaceae	Plant	*Gastrodia elata* Bl.	*Gastrodia elata* Bl.	Dry tuber	
42	Borneolum	Lauraceae	Plant	*Cinnamomum camphora* (L.) Presl	*Cinnamomum camphora* (L.) Presl	Extraction of fresh twigs and leaves	
43	Chaenomelis Fructus	Rosaceae	Plant	*Chaenomeles speciosa* (Sweet) Nakai	*Chaenomeles speciosa* (Sweet) Nakai	Dry nearly mature fruit	
44	Hibisci Mutabilis Folium	Malvaceae	Plant	*Hibiscus mutabilis* L.	*Hibiscus mutabilis* L.	Dry leaf	
45	Aucklandiae Radix	Asteraceae	Plant	*Aucklandia lappa* Decne.	*Aucklandia lappa* Decne.	Dry root	
46	Gossampini Flos	Bombacaceae	Plant	*Gossampinus malabarica* (DC.) Merr.	*Gossampinus malabarica* (DC.) Merr.	Dry flower	
47	Schisandrae Chinensis Fructus	Magnoliaceae	Plant	*Schisandra chinensis* (Turcz.) Baill.	*Schisandra chinensis* (Turcz.) Baill.	Dry mature fruit	

continued

No.	Name of TCM crude drugs	Family	Category	Name of the origin plant	Latin name of the origin plant	Medicinal part	Remark
48	Pseudostellariae Radix	Caryophyllaceae	Plant	*Pseudostellaria heterophylla* (Miq.) Pax ex Pax et Hoffm.	*Pseudostellaria heterophylla* (Miq.) Pax ex Pax et Hoffm.	Dry root tuber	
49	Plantaginis Semen	Plantaginaceae	Plant	*Plantago asiatica* L.	*Plantago asiatica* L.	Dry mature seed	Multiple origins
50	Arctii Fructus	Asteraceae	Plant	*Arctium lappa* L.	*Arctium lappa* L.	Dry mature fruit	
51	Achyranthis Bidentatae Radix	Amaranthaceae	Plant	*Achyranthes bidentata* Bl.	*Achyranthes bidentata* Bl.	Dry root	
52	Wenyujin Rhizoma Concisum	Zingiberaceae	Plant	*Curcuma wenyujin* Y. H. Chen et C. Ling	*Curcuma wenyujin* Y. H. Chen et C. Ling	Dry rhizome	
53	Citri Grandis Exocarpium	Rutaceae	Plant	*Citrus grandis* 'Tomentosa' *Citrus grandis* (L.) Osbeck	*Citrus grandis* 'Tomentosa' *Citrus grandis* (L.) Osbeck	Immature and nearly mature dry outer pericarp	Multiple origins
54	Rosae Chinensis Flos	Rosaceae	Plant	*Rosa chinensis* Jacq.	*Rosa chinensis* Jacq.	Dry flower	
55	Salviae Miltiorrhizae Radix et Rhizoma	Lamiaceae	Plant	*Salvia miltiorrhiza* Bge.	*Salvia miltiorrhiza* Bge.	Dry root and rhizome	
56	Linderae Radix	Lauraceae	Plant	*Lindera aggregata* (Sims) Kosterm.	*Lindera aggregata* (Sims) Kos-term.	Dry root tuber	
57	Mume Fructus	Rosaceae	Plant	*Prunus mume* (Sieb.) Sieb. et Zucc.	*Prunus mume* (Sieb.) Sieb. et Zucc.	Dry nearly mature fruit	
58	Cannabis Fructus	Moraceae	Plant	*Cannabis sativa* L.	*Cannabis sativa* L.	Dry mature fruit	

continued

No.	Name of TCM crude drugs	Family	Category	Name of the origin plant	Latin name of the origin plant	Medicinal part	Remark
59	Crotonis Fructus	Euphorbiaceae	Plant	Croton tiglium L.	Croton tiglium L.	Dry mature fruit	
60	Morindae Officinalis Radix	Rubiaceae	Plant	Morinda officinalis How	Morinda officinalis How	Dry root	
61	Silybi Fructus	Asteraceae	Plant	Silybum marianum (L.) Gaertn.	Silybum marianum (L.) Gaertn.	Dry mature fruit	
62	Polygonati Odorati Rhizoma	Liliaceae	Plant	Polygonatum odoratum (Mill.) Druce	Polygonatum odoratum (Mill.) Druce	Dry rhizome	
63	Glycyrrhizae Radix et Rhizoma	Leguminosae	Plant	Glycyrrhiza uralensis Fisch.	Glycyrrhiza uralensis Fisch.	Dry root and rhizome	
64	Kansui Radix	Euphorbiaceae	Plant	Euphorbia kansui T. N. Liou ex T. P. Wang	Euphorbia kansui T. N. Liou ex T. P. Wang	Dry root tuber	
65	l–Borneolum	Asteraceae	Plant	Blumea balsamifera (L.) DC.	Blumea balsamifera (L.) DC.	Crystals produced from extraction and processing of fresh leaves	
66	Dendrobii Caulis	Orchidaceae	Plant	Dendrobium nobile Lindl. / Dendrobium devonianum Paxt	Dendrobium nobile Lindl. / Dendrobium devonianum Paxt	Fresh and dry stem	Multiple origins
67	Granati Pericarpium	Punicaceae	Plant	Punica granatum L.	Punica granatum L.	Dry pericarp	
68	Gentianae Radix et Rhizoma	Gentianaceae	Plant	Gentiana scabra Bge.	Gentiana scabra Bge.	Dry root and rhizome	Multiple origins

continued

No.	Name of TCM crude drugs	Family	Category	Name of the origin plant	Latin name of the origin plant	Medicinal part	Remark
69	Longan Arillus	Sapindaceae	Plant	*Dimocarpus longan* Lour.	*Dimocarpus longan* Lour.	Aril	
70	Fritillariae Ussuriensis Bulbus	Liliaceae	Plant	*Fritillaria ussuriensis* Maxim.	*Fritillaria ussuriensis* Maxim.	Dry bulb	
71	Glehniae Radix	Umbelliferae	Plant	*Glehnia littoralis* Fr. Schmidt ex Miq.	*Glehnia littoralis* Fr. Schmidt ex Miq.	Dry root	
72	Ilicis Chinensis Folium	Aquifoliaceae	Plant	*Ilex chinensis* Sims	*Ilex chinensis* Sims	Dry leaf	
73	Zingiberis Rhizoma Recens	Zingiberaceae	Plant	*Zingiber officinale* Rosc.	*Zingiber officinale* Rosc.	Fresh rhizome	
74	Bletillae Rhizoma	Orchidaceae	Plant	*Bletilla striata* (Thunb.) Reichb. f.	*Bletilla striata* (Thunb.) Reichb. f.	Dry tuber	
75	Atractylodis Macrocephalae Rhizoma	Asteraceae	Plant	*Atractylodes macrocephala* Koidz.	*Atractylodes macrocephala* Koidz.	Dry rhizome	
76	Paeoniae Radix Alba	Ranunculaceae	Plant	*Paeonia lactiflora* Pall.	*Paeonia lactiflora* Pall.	Dry root	
77	Angelicae Dahuricae Radix	Umbelliferae	Plant	*Angelica dahurica* (Fisch. ex Hoffm.) Benth. et Hook. f. / *Angelica dahurica* (Fisch. ex Hoffm.) Benth. et Hook. f. var. *formosana* (Boiss.) Shan et Yuan	*Angelica dahurica* (Fisch. ex Hoffm.) Benth. et Hook. f. / *Angelica dahurica* (Fisch. ex Hoffm.) Benth. et Hook. f. var. *formosana* (Boiss.) Shan et Yuan	Dry root	Multiple origins

continued

No.	Name of TCM crude drugs	Family	Category	Name of the origin plant	Latin name of the origin plant	Medicinal part	Remark
78	Typhonii Rhizoma	Araceae	Plant	*Typhonium giganteum* Engl.	*Typhonium giganteum* Engl.	Dry tuber	
79	Ginkgo Semen	Ginkgoaceae	Plant	*Ginkgo biloba* L.	*Ginkgo biloba* L.	Dry mature seed	
80	Lablab Semen Album	Leguminosae	Plant	*Dolichos lablab* L.	*Dolichos lablab* L.	Dry mature seed	
81	Trichosanthis Fructus	Cucurbitaceae	Plant	*Trichosanthes kirilowii* Maxim. / *Trichosanthes rosthornii* Harms	*Trichosanthes kirilowii* Maxim. / *Trichosanthes rosthornii* Harms	Dry mature fruit	Multiple origins
82	Trichosanthis Semen	Cucurbitaceae	Plant	*Trichosanthes kirilowii* Maxim. / *Trichosanthes rosthornii* Harms	*Trichosanthes kirilowii* Maxim. / *Trichosanthes rosthornii* Harms	Dry mature seed	Multiple origins
83	Trichosanthis Pericarpium	Cucurbitaceae	Plant	*Trichosanthes kirilowii* Maxim. / *Trichosanthes rosthornii* Harms	*Trichosanthes kirilowii* Maxim. / *Trichosanthes rosthornii* Harms	Dry mature pericarp	Multiple origins
84	Benincasae Exocarpium	Cucurbitaceae	Plant	*Benincasa hispida* (Thunb.) Cogn.	*Benincasa hispida* (Thunb.) Cogn.	Dry outer pericarp	
85	Rabdosiae Rubescentis Herba	Lamiaceae	Plant	*Rabdosia rubescens* (Hemsl.) Hara	*Rabdosia rubescens* (Hemsl.) Hara	Dry above—ground part	
86	Malvae Fructus	Malvaceae	Plant	*Malva verticillata* L.	*Malva verticillata* L.	Dry mature fruit	

continued

No.	Name of TCM crude drugs	Family	Category	Name of the origin plant	Latin name of the origin plant	Medicinal part	Remark
87	Scrophulariae Radix	Scrophulariaceae	Plant	*Scrophularia ningpoensis* Hemsl.	*Scrophularia ningpoensis* Hemsl.	Dry root	
88	Scutellariae Barbatae Herba	Lamiaceae	Plant	*Scutellaria barbata* D. Don	*Scutellaria barbata* D. Don	Dry whole herb	
89	Pinelliae Rhizoma	Araceae	Plant	*Pinellia ternata* (Thunb.) Breit.	*Pinellia ternata* (Thunb.) Breit.	Dry tuber	
90	Luffae Fructus Retinervus	Cucurbitaceae	Plant	*Luffa cylindrica* (L.) Roem.	*Luffa cylindrica* (L.) Roem.	Vascular bundle of dry mature fruit	
91	Lycii Cortex	Solanaceae	Plant	*Lycium barbarum* L.	*Lycium barbarum* L.	Dry root bark	Multiple origins
92	Rehmanniae Radix	Scrophulariaceae	Plant	*Rehmannia glutinosa* Libosch.	*Rehmannia glutinosa* Libosch.	Fresh and dry root tuber	
93	Lini Semen	Linaceae	Plant	*Linum usitatissimum* L.	*Linum usitatissimum* L.	Dry mature seed	
94	Mirabilitum Praeparatum	Cucurbitaceae	Plant	*Citrullus lanatus* (Thunb.) Matsumu.et Nakai	*Citrullus lanatus* (Thunb.) Matsumu.et Nakai	Processed mature and fresh fruits with mirabilite	
95	Croci Stigma	Iridaceae	Plant	*Crocus sativus* L.	*Crocus sativus* L.	Dry stigma	
96	Panacis Quinquefolii Radix	Araliaceae	Plant	*Panax quinquefolium* L.	*Panax quinquefolium* L.	Dry root	
97	Lilii Bulbus	Liliaceae	Plant	*Lilium brownii* F. E. Brown var. *viridulum* Baker / *Lilium lancifolium* Thunb.	*Lilium brownii* F. E. Brown var. *viridulum* Baker / *Lilium lancifolium* Thunb.	Dry fleshly scale leaf	Multiple origins

continued

No.	Name of TCM crude drugs	Family	Category	Name of the origin plant	Latin name of the origin plant	Medicinal part	Remark
98	Angelicae Sinensis Radix	Umbelliferae	Plant	Angelica sinensis (Oliv.) Diels	Angelica sinensis (Oliv.) Diels	Dry root	
99	Cistanches Herba	Orobanchaceae	Plant	Cistanche deserticola Y. C. Ma Cistanche tubulosa (Schenk) Wight	Cistanche deserticola Y. C. Ma Cistanche tubulosa (Schenk) Wight	Dry succulent stem with scale leaves	Multiple origins
100	Cinnamomi Cortex	Lauraceae	Plant	Cinnamomum cassia Presl	Cinnamomum cassia Presl	Dry bark	
101	Panacis Japonici Rhizoma	Araliaceae	Plant	Panax japonicus C. A. Mey.	Panax japonicus C. A. Mey.	Dry rhizome	
102	Bambusae Caulis In Taenias	Poaceae	Plant	Sinocalamus beecheyanus (Munro) McClure var. pubescens P. F. Li Phyllostachys nigra (Lodd.) Munro var. henonis (Mitf.) Stapf ex Rendle Bambusa tuldoides Munro	Sinocalamus beecheyanus (Munro) McClure var. pubescens P. F. Li Phyllostachys nigra (Lodd.) Munro var. henonis (Mitf.) Stapf ex Rendle Bambusa tuldoides Munro	Dry middle layer of stem	Multiple origins
103	Corydalis Rhizoma	Papaveraceae	Plant	Corydalis yanhusuo W. T. Wang	Corydalis yanhusuo W. T. Wang	Dry tuber	
104	Fritillariae Pallidiflorae Bulbus	Liliaceae	Plant	Fritillaria pallidiflora Schrenk	Fritillaria pallidiflora Schrenk	Dry bulb	Multiple origins

continued

No.	Name of TCM crude drugs	Family	Category	Name of the origin plant	Latin name of the origin plant	Medicinal part	Remark
105	Albiziae Cortex	Leguminosae	Plant	*Albizia julibrissin* Durazz.	*Albizia julibrissin* Durazz.	Dry bark	
106	Albiziae Flos	Leguminosae	Plant	*Albizia julibrissin* Durazz.	*Albizia julibrissin* Durazz.	Dry inflorescence or flower bud	
107	Cassiae Semen	Leguminosae	Plant	*Cassia obtusifolia* L.	*Cassia obtusifolia* L.	Dry mature seed	Multiple origins
				Cassia tora L.	*Cassia tora* L.		
108	Junci Medulla	Juncaceae	Plant	*Juncus effusus* L.	*Juncus effusus* L.	Dry stem pith	
109	Erigerontis Herba	Asteraceae	Plant	*Erigeron breviscapus* (Vant.) Hand. –Mazz.	*Erigeron breviscapus* (Vant.) Hand. –Mazz.	Dry whole herb	
110	Saposhnikoviae Radix	Umbelliferae	Plant	*Saposhnikovia divaricata* (Turcz.) Schischk.	*Saposhnikovia divaricata* (Turcz.) Schischk.	Dry root	
111	Carthami Flos	Asteraceae	Plant	*Carthamus tinctorius* L.	*Carthamus tinctorius* L.	Dry flower	
112	Hedysari Radix	Leguminosae	Plant	*Hedysarum polybotrys* Hand. –Mazz.	*Hedysarum polybotrys* Hand. –Mazz.	Dry root	
113	Ginseng Radix et Rhizoma Rubra	Araliaceae	Plant	*Panax ginseng* C. A. Mey.	*Panax ginseng* C. A. Mey.	Dry root and rhizome after steaming	
114	Ophiopogonis Radix	Liliaceae	Plant	*Ophiopogon japonicus* (L. f) Ker–Gawl.	*Ophiopogon japonicus* (L. f) Ker–Gawl.	Dry root tuber	
115	Hordei Fructus Germinatus	Poaceae	Plant	*Hordeum vulgare* L.	*Hordeum vulgare* L.	Processed products from mature fruits that have sprouted and been dried	

continued

No.	Name of TCM crude drugs	Family	Category	Name of the origin plant	Latin name of the origin plant	Medicinal part	Remark
116	Polygalae Radix	Polygalaceae	Plant	Polygala tenuifolia Willd.	Polygala tenuifolia Willd.	Dry root	Multiple origins
117	Vignae Semen	Leguminosae	Plant	Vigna angularis Ohwi et Ohashi	Vigna angularis Ohwi et Ohashi	Dry mature seed	Multiple origins
				Vigna umbellata Ohwi et Ohashi	Vigna umbellata Ohwi et Ohashi		
118	Zanthoxyli Pericarpium	Rutaceae	Plant	Zanthoxylum bungeanum Maxim.	Zanthoxylum bungeanum Maxim.	Dry mature pericarp	Multiple origins
119	Sinapis Semen	Cruciferae	Plant	Sinapis alba L.	Sinapis alba L.	Dry mature seed	Multiple origins
				Brassica juncea (L.) Czern. et Coss.	Brassica juncea (L.) Czern. et Coss.		
120	Atractylodis Rhizoma	Asteraceae	Plant	Atractylodes lancea (Thunb.) DC.	Atractylodes lancea (Thunb.) DC.	Dry rhizome	Multiple origins
121	Euryales Semen	Nymphaeaceae	Plant	Euryale ferox Salisb.	Euryale ferox Salisb.	Dry mature kernel	
122	Aloe	Liliaceae	Plant	Aloe ferox Miller	Aloe ferox Miller	Desiccate from concentrated juice	Multiple origins
				Aloe barbadensis Miller	Aloe barbadensis Miller		
123	Eucommiae Cortex	Eucommiaceae	Plant	Eucommia ulmoides Oliv.	Eucommia ulmoides Oliv.	Dry bark	
124	Eucommiae Folium	Eucommiaceae	Plant	Eucommia ulmoides Oliv.	Eucommia ulmoides Oliv.	Dry leaf	

No.	Name of TCM crude drugs	Family	Category	Name of the origin plant	Latin name of the origin plant	Medicinal part	Remark
125	Euodiae Fructus	Rutaceae	Plant	*Euodia rutaecarpa* (Juss.) Benth.	*Euodia rutaecarpa* (Juss.) Benth.	Dry nearly mature fruit	Multiple origins
126	Moutan Cortex	Ranunculaceae	Plant	*Paeonia suffruticosa* Andr.	*Paeonia suffruticosa* Andr.	Dry root bark	
127	Polygoni Multiflori Radix	Polygonaceae	Plant	*Polygonum multiflorum* Thunb.	*Polygonum multiflorum* Thunb.	Dry root tuber	
128	Gleditsiae Spina	Leguminosae	Plant	*Gleditsia sinensis* Lam.	*Gleditsia sinensis* Lam.	Dry thorns	
129	Citri Sarcodactylis Fructus	Rutaceae	Plant	*Citrus medica* L. var. *sarcodactylis* Swingle	*Citrus medica* L. var. *sarcodactylis* Swingle	Dry fruit	
130	Phyllanthi Fructus	Euphorbiaceae	Plant	*Phyllanthus emblica* L.	*Phyllanthus emblica* L.	Dry mature fruit	
131	Setariae Fructus Germinatus	Poaceae	Plant	*Setaria italica* (L.) Beauv.	*Setaria italica* (L.) Beauv.	Processed products from mature fruits that have sprouted and been dried	
132	Magnoliae Flos	Magnoliaceae	Plant	*Magnolia biondii* Pamp. *Magnolia sprengeri* Pamp. *Magnolia denudata* Desr.	*Magnolia biondii* Pamp. *Magnolia sprengeri* Pamp. *Magnolia denudata* Desr.	Dry flower bud	Multiple origins
133	Astragali Complanati Semen	Leguminosae	Plant	*Astragalus complanatus* R. Br.	*Astragalus complanatus* R. Br.	Dry mature seed	

163

continued

No.	Name of TCM crude drugs	Family	Category	Name of the origin plant	Latin name of the origin plant	Medicinal part	Remark
134	Aquilariae Lignum Resinatum	Thymelaeaceae	Plant	Aquilaria sinensis (Lour.) Gilg	Aquilaria sinensis (Lour.) Gilg	Wood containing resin	
135	Psoraleae Fructus	Leguminosae	Plant	Psoralea corylifolia L.	Psoralea corylifolia L.	Dry mature fruit	
136	Ganoderma	Polyporaceae	Fungi	Ganoderma lucidum (Leyss. ex Fr.) Karst. / Ganoderma sinense Zhao, Xu et Zhang	Ganoderma lucidum (Leyss. ex Fr.) Karst. / Ganoderma sinense Zhao, Xu et Zhang	Dry fruiting body	Multiple origins
137	Citri Reticulatae Pericarpium	Rutaceae	Plant	Citrus reticulata Blanco	Citrus reticulata Blanco	Dry mature pericarp	
138	Aconiti Lateralis Radix Praeparata	Ranunculaceae	Plant	Aconitum carmichaelii Debx.	Aconitum carmichaelii Debx.	Processed product of roots	
139	Lonicerae Japonicae Caulis	Caprifoliaceae	Plant	Lonicera japonica Thunb.	Lonicera japonica Thunb.	Dry stems and branches	
140	Abri Herba	Leguminosae	Plant	Abrus cantoniensis Hance	Abrus cantoniensis Hance	Dry whole plant	
141	Celosiae Cristatae Flos	Amaranthaceae	Plant	Celosia cristata L.	Celosia cristata L.	Dry inflorescence	
142	Citri Reticulatae Pericarpium Viride	Rutaceae	Plant	Citrus reticulata Blanco	Citrus reticulata Blanco	Dry young fruit and pericarp of immature fruit	
143	Canarii Fructus	Burseraceae	Plant	Canarium album Raeusch.	Canarium album Raeusch.	Dry mature fruit	

continued

No.	Name of TCM crude drugs	Family	Category	Name of the origin plant	Latin name of the origin plant	Medicinal part	Remark
144	Artemisiae Annuae Herba	Asteraceae	Plant	*Artemisia annua* L.	*Artemisia annua* L.	Dry above-ground part	
145	Indigo Naturalis	Cruciferae	Plant	*Isatis indigotica* Fort.	*Isatis indigotica* Fort.	Dry powder, clumps or granules produced from processed leaves or stem leaves	Multiple origins
		Acanthaceae	Plant	*Baphicacanthus cusia* (Nees) Bremek.	*Baphicacanthus cusia* (Nees) Bremek.		
		Polygonaceae	Plant	*Polygonum tinctorium* Ait.	*Polygonum tinctorium* Ait.		
146	Rosae Rugosae Flos	Rosaceae	Plant	*Rosa rugosa* Thunb.	*Rosa rugosa* Thunb.	Dry flower bud	
147	Corydalis Bungeanae Herba	Papaveraceae	Plant	*Corydalis bungeana* Turcz.	*Corydalis bungeana* Turcz.	Dry whole herb	
148	Armeniacae Semen Amarum	Rosaceae	Plant	*Prunus armeniaca* L.	*Prunus armeniaca* L.	Dry mature seed	Multiple origins
149	Eriobotryae Folium	Rosaceae	Plant	*Eriobotrya japonica* (Thunb.) Lindl.	*Eriobotrya japonica* (Thunb.) Lindl.	Dry leaf	
150	Isatidis Radix	Cruciferae	Plant	*Isatis indigotica* Fort.	*Isatis indigotica* Fort.	Dry root	
151	Pimi Pollen	Pinaceae	Plant	*Pinus massoniana* Lamb.	*Pinus massoniana* Lamb.	Dry pollen	Multiple origins
				Pinus tabulieformis Carr.	*Pinus tabulieformis* Carr.		

165

continued

No.	Name of TCM crude drugs	Family	Category	Name of the origin plant	Latin name of the origin plant	Medicinal part	Remark
152	Curcumae Radix	Zingiberaceae	Plant	*Curcuma kwangsiensis* S. G. Lee et C. F. Liang	*Curcuma kwangsiensis* S. G. Lee et C. F. Liang	Dry root tuber	Multiple origins
				Curcuma wenyujin Y. H. Chen et C. Ling	*Curcuma wenyujin* Y. H. Chen et C. Ling		
				Curcuma phaeocaulis Val.	*Curcuma phaeocaulis* Val.		
				Curcuma longa L.	*Curcuma longa* L.		
153	Laminariae Thallus, Eckloniae Thallus	Laminariaceae	Plant	*Laminaria japonica* Aresch.	*Laminaria japonica* Aresch.	Dry thallus	Multiple origins
154	Changii Radix	Umbelliferae	Plant	*Changium smyrnioides* Wolff	*Changium smyrnioides* Wolff	Dry root	
155	Siraitiae Fructus	Cucurbitaceae	Plant	*Siraitia grosvenorii* (Swingle) C. Jeffrey ex A. M. Lu et Z. Y. Zhang	*Siraitia grosvenorii* (Swingle) C. Jeffrey ex A. M. Lu et Z. Y. Zhang	Dry fruit	
156	Anemarrhenae Rhizoma	Liliaceae	Plant	*Anemarrhena asphodeloides* Bge.	*Anemarrhena asphodeloides* Bge.	Dry rhizome	
157	Quisqualis Fructus	Combretaceae	Plant	*Quisqualis indica* L.	*Quisqualis indica* L.	Dry mature fruit	
158	Platycladi Cacumen	Cupressaceae	Plant	*Platycladus orientalis* (L.) Franco	*Platycladus orientalis* (L.) Franco	Dry tip of a branch and leaves	
159	Eupatorii Herba	Asteraceae	Plant	*Eupatorium fortunei* Turcz.	*Eupatorium fortunei* Turcz.	Dry above-ground part	

No.	Name of TCM crude drugs	Family	Category	Name of the origin plant	Latin name of the origin plant	Medicinal part	Remark
160	Lonicerae Japonicae Flos	Caprifoliaceae	Plant	*Lonicera japonica* Thunb.	*Lonicera japonica* Thunb.	Dry flower bud or flower to blossom	
161	Houttuyniae Herba	Saururaceae	Plant	*Houttuynia cordata* Thunb.	*Houttuynia cordata* Thunb.	Fresh whole plant or dry above—ground part	
162	Lycopi Herba	Lamiaceae	Plant	*Lycopus lucidus* Turcz. var. *hirtus* Regel	*Lycopus lucidus* Turcz. var. *hirtus* Regel	Dry above—ground part	
163	Pini Lignum Nodi	Pinaceae	Plant	*Pinus massoniana* Lamb. *Pinus tabulieformis* Carr.	*Pinus massoniana* Lamb. *Pinus tabulieformis* Carr.	Dry nodule—like nodes and branching nodes	Multiple origins
164	Alismatis Rhizoma	Alismataceae	Plant	*Alisma orientale* (Sam.) Juzep.	*Alisma orientale* (Sam.) Juzep.	Dry tuber	
165	Asari Radix et Rhizoma	Aristolochiaceae	Plant	*Asarum heterotropoides* Fr. Schmidt var. *mandshuricum* (Maxim.) Kitag.	*Asarum heterotropoides* Fr. Schmidt var. *mandshuricum* (Maxim.) Kitag.	Dry above—ground part	Multiple origins
166	Schizonepetae Herba	Lamiaceae	Plant	*Schizonepeta tenuifolia* Briq.	*Schizonepeta tenuifolia* Briq.	Dry above—ground part	
167	Schizonepetae Spica	Lamiaceae	Plant	*Schizonepeta tenuifolia* Briq.	*Schizonepeta tenuifolia* Briq.	Dry spica	
168	Tsaoko Fructus	Zingiberaceae	Plant	*Amomum tsao-ko* Crevost et Lemaire	*Amomum tsao-ko* Crevost et Lemaire	Dry mature fruit	
169	Poria	Polyporaceae	Fungi	*Poria cocos* (Schw.) Wolf	*Poria cocos* (Schw.) Wolf	Dry sclerotium	

continued

No.	Name of TCM crude drugs	Family	Category	Name of the origin plant	Latin name of the origin plant	Medicinal part	Remark
170	Poriae Cutis	Polyporaceae	Fungi	*Poria cocos* (Schw.) Wolf	*Poria cocos* (Schw.) Wolf	Dry outer peel of sclerotium	
171	Leonuri Fructus	Lamiaceae	Plant	*Leonurus japonicus* Houtt.	*Leonurus japonicus* Houtt.	Dry mature fruit	
172	Trigonellae Semen	Leguminosae	Plant	*Trigonella foenum-graecum* L.	*Trigonella foenum-graecum* L.	Dry mature seed	
173	Piperis Fructus	Piperaceae	Plant	*Piper nigrum* L.	*Piper nigrum* L.	Dry, almost mature or mature fruit	
174	Litchi Semen	Sapindaceae	Plant	*Litchi chinensis* Sonn.	*Litchi chinensis* Sonn.	Dry mature seed	
175	Baphicacanthis Cusiae Rhizoma et Radix	Acanthaceae	Plant	*Baphicacanthus cusia* (Nees) Bremek.	*Baphicacanthus cusia* (Nees) Bremek.	Dry rhizome and root	
176	Aurantii Fructus	Rutaceae	Plant	*Citrus aurantium* L.	*Citrus aurantium* L.	Dry immature fruit	
177	Aurantii Fructus Immaturus	Rutaceae	Plant	*Citrus aurantium* L. *Citrus sinensis* Osbeck	*Citrus aurantium* L. *Citrus sinensis* Osbeck	Dry young fruit	Multiple origins
178	Platycladi Semen	Cupressaceae	Plant	*Platycladus orientalis* (L.) Franco	*Platycladus orientalis* (L.) Franco	Dry mature kernel	
179	Gardeniae Fructus	Rubiaceae	Plant	*Gardenia jasminoides* Ellis	*Gardenia jasminoides* Ellis	Dry mature fruit	
180	Lycii Fructus	Solanaceae	Plant	*Lycium barbarum* L.	*Lycium barbarum* L.	Dry mature fruit	
181	Kaki Calyx	Ebenaceae	Plant	*Diospyros kaki* Thunb.	*Diospyros kaki* Thunb.	Dry persistent calyx	

continued

No.	Name of TCM crude drugs	Family	Category	Name of the origin plant	Latin name of the origin plant	Medicinal part	Remark
182	Magnoliae Officinalis Cortex	Magnoliaceae	Plant	*Magnolia officinalis* Rehd. et Wils. var. *biloba* Rehd. et Wils.	*Magnolia officinalis* Rehd. et Wils. var. *biloba* Rehd. et Wils.	Dry stem bark, root bark and branch bark	Multiple origins
				Magnolia officinalis Rehd. et Wils.	*Magnolia officinalis* Rehd. et Wils.		
183	Magnoliae Officinalis Flos	Magnoliaceae	Plant	*Magnolia officinalis* Rehd. et Wils. var. *biloba* Rehd. et Wils.	*Magnolia officinalis* Rehd. et Wils. var. *biloba* Rehd. et Wils.	Dry flower bud	Multiple origins
				Magnolia officinalis Rehd. et Wils.	*Magnolia officinalis* Rehd. et Wils.		
184	Amomi Fructus	Zingiberaceae	Plant	*Amomum villosum* Lour.	*Amomum villosum* Lour.	Dry mature fruit	Multiple origins
				Amomum longiligulare T.L.Wu	*Amomum longiligulare* T.L.Wu		
185	Bruceae Fructus	Simaroubaceae	Plant	*Brucea javanica* (L.) Merr.	*Brucea javanica* (L.) Merr.	Dry mature fruit	
186	Allii Tuberosi Semen	Liliaceae	Plant	*Allium tuberosum* Rottl. ex Spreng.	*Allium tuberosum* Rottl. ex Spreng.	Dry mature seed	
187	Citri Fructus	Rutaceae	Plant	*Citrus medica* L.	*Citrus medica* L.	Dry mature fruit	Multiple origins
				Citrus wilsonii Tanaka	*Citrus wilsonii* Tanaka		
188	Moslae Herba	Lamiaceae	Plant	*Mosla chinensis* 'Jiangxiangru'	*Mosla chinensis* 'Jiangxiangru'	Dry above-ground part	Multiple origins

continued

No.	Name of TCM crude drugs	Family	Category	Name of the origin plant	Latin name of the origin plant	Medicinal part	Remark
189	Angelicae Pubescentis Radix	Umbelliferae	Plant	*Angelica pubescens* Maxim. f. *biserrata* Shan et Yuan	*Angelica pubescens* Maxim. f. *biserrata* Shan et Yuan	Dry root	
190	Impatientis Semen	Balsaminaceae	Plant	*Impatiens balsamina* L.	*Impatiens balsamina* L.	Dry mature seed	
191	Curcumae Longae Rhizoma	Zingiberaceae	Plant	*Curcuma longa* L.	*Curcuma longa* L.	Dry rhizome	
192	Peucedani Radix	Umbelliferae	Plant	*Peucedanum praeruptorum* Dunn	*Peucedanum praeruptorum* Dunn	Dry root	
193	Polygoni Multiflori Caulis	Polygonaceae	Plant	*Polygonum multiflorum* Thunb.	*Polygonum multiflorum* Thunb.	Dry rattan stems	
194	Andrographis Herba	Acanthaceae	Plant	*Andrographis paniculata* (Burm.f.) Nees	*Andrographis paniculata* (Burm.f.) Nees	Dry above—ground part	
195	Gentianae Macrophyllae Radix	Gentianaceae	Plant	*Gentiana macrophylla* Pall.	*Gentiana macrophylla* Pall.	Dry root	Multiple origins
196	Raphani Semen	Cruciferae	Plant	*Raphanus sativus* L.	*Raphanus sativus* L.	Dry mature seed	
197	Nelumbinis Semen	Nymphaeaceae	Plant	*Nelumbo nucifera* Gaertn.	*Nelumbo nucifera* Gaertn.	Dry mature seed	
198	Nelumbinis Plumula	Nymphaeaceae	Plant	*Nelumbo nucifera* Gaertn.	*Nelumbo nucifera* Gaertn.	Dry spire and radicle in mature seeds	
199	Nelumbinis Receptaculum	Nymphaeaceae	Plant	*Nelumbo nucifera* Gaertn.	*Nelumbo nucifera* Gaertn.	Dry receptacle	

continued

No.	Name of TCM crude drugs	Family	Category	Name of the origin plant	Latin name of the origin plant	Medicinal part	Remark
200	Nelumbinis Stamen	Nymphaeaceae	Plant	*Nelumbo nucifera* Gaertn.	*Nelumbo nucifera* Gaertn.	Dry stamen	
201	Curcumae Rhizoma	Zingiberaceae	Plant	*Curcuma kwangsiensis* S. G. Lee et C. F. Liang	*Curcuma kwangsiensis* S. G. Lee et C. F. Liang	Dry rhizome	Multiple origins
				Curcuma wenyujin Y. H. Chen et C. Ling	*Curcuma wenyujin* Y. H. Chen et C. Ling		
				Curcuma phaeocaulis Val.	*Curcuma phaeocaulis* Val.		
202	Nelumbinis Folium	Nymphaeaceae	Plant	*Nelumbo nucifera* Gaertn.	*Nelumbo nucifera* Gaertn.	Dry leaf	
203	Cinnamomi Ramulus	Lauraceae	Plant	*Cinnamomum cassia* Presl	*Cinnamomum cassia* Presl	Dry twig	
204	Platycodonis Radix	Campanulaceae	Plant	*Platycodon grandiflorum* (Jacq.) A. DC.	*Platycodon grandiflorum* (Jacq.) A. DC.	Dry root	
205	Persicae Semen	Rosaceae	Plant	*Prunus persica* (L.) Batsch	*Prunus persica* (L.) Batsch	Dry mature seed	Multiple origins
206	Persicae Ramulus	Rosaceae	Plant	*Prunus persica* (L.) Batsch	*Prunus persica* (L.) Batsch	Dry branches	
207	Juglandis Semen	Juglandaceae	Plant	*Juglans regia* L.	*Juglans regia* L.	Dry mature seed	
208	Prunellae Spica	Lamiaceae	Plant	*Prunella vulgaris* L.	*Prunella vulgaris* L.	Dry cluster	
209	Bupleuri Radix	Umbelliferae	Plant	*Bupleurum chinense* DC.	*Bupleurum chinense* DC.	Dry root	Multiple origins

continued

No.	Name of TCM crude drugs	Family	Category	Name of the origin plant	Latin name of the origin plant	Medicinal part	Remark
210	Codonopsis Radix	Campanulaceae	Plant	*Codonopsis tangshen* Oliv.	*Codonopsis tangshen* Oliv.	Dry root	Multiple origins
				Codonopsis pilosula (Franch.) Nannf.	*Codonopsis pilosula* (Franch.) Nannf.		
				Codonopsis pilosula Nannf. var. *modesta* (Nannf.) L. T. Shen	*Codonopsis pilosula* Nannf. var. *modesta* (Nannf.) L. T. Shen		
211	Dendrobii Officinalis Caulis	Orchidaceae	Plant	*Dendrobium officinale* Kimura et Migo	*Dendrobium officinale* Kimura et Migo	Dry stem	
212	Belamcandae Rhizoma	Iridaceae	Plant	*Belamcanda chinensis* (L.) DC.	*Belamcanda chinensis* (L.) DC.	Dry rhizome	
213	Cynanchi Paniculati Radix Et Rhizoma	Asclepiadaceae	Plant	*Cynanchum paniculatum* (Bge.) Kitag.	*Cynanchum paniculatum* (Bge.) Kitag.	Dry root and rhizome	
214	Campsis Flos	Bignoniaceae	Plant	*Campsis grandiflora* (Thunb.) K. Schum.	*Campsis grandiflora* (Thunb.) K. Schum.	Dry flower	Multiple origins
				Campsis radicans (L.) Seem.	*Campsis radicans* (L.) Seem.		
215	Alpiniae Officinarum Rhizoma	Zingiberaceae	Plant	*Alpinia officinarum* Hance	*Alpinia officinarum* Hance	Dry rhizome	
216	Puerariae Thomsonii Radix	Leguminosae	Plant	*Pueraria thomsonii* Benth.	*Pueraria thomsonii* Benth.	Dry root	

continued

No.	Name of TCM crude drugs	Family	Category	Name of the origin plant	Latin name of the origin plant	Medicinal part	Remark
217	Leonuri Herba	Lamiaceae	Plant	*Leonurus japonicus* Houtt.	*Leonurus japonicus* Houtt.	Fresh or dry above-ground part	
218	Alpiniae Oxyphyllae Fructus	Zingiberaceae	Plant	*Alpinia oxyphylla* Miq.	*Alpinia oxyphylla* Miq.	Dry mature fruit	
219	Fritillariae Thunbergii Bulbus	Liliaceae	Plant	*Fritillaria thunbergii* Miq.	*Fritillaria thunbergii* Miq.	Dry bulb	
220	Mori Folium	Moraceae	Plant	*Morus alba* L.	*Morus alba* L.	Dry leaf	
221	Mori Cortex	Moraceae	Plant	*Morus alba* L.	*Morus alba* L.	Dry root bark	
222	Mori Ramulus	Moraceae	Plant	*Morus alba* L.	*Morus alba* L.	Dry twig	
223	Mori Fructus	Moraceae	Plant	*Morus alba* L.	*Morus alba* L.	Dry cluster	
224	Scutellariae Radix	Lamiaceae	Plant	*Scutellaria baicalensis* Georgi	*Scutellaria baicalensis* Georgi	Dry root	
225	Astragali Radix	Leguminosae	Plant	*Astragalus membranaceus* (Fisch.) Bge. var. *mongholicus* (Bge.) Hsiao / *Astragalus membranaceus* (Fisch.) Bge.	*Astragalus membranaceus* (Fisch.) Bge. var. *mongholicus* (Bge.) Hsiao / *Astragalus membranaceus* (Fisch.) Bge.	Dry root	Multiple origins
226	Coptidis Rhizoma	Ranunculaceae	Plant	*Coptis chinensis* Franch.	*Coptis chinensis* Franch.	Dry rhizome	Multiple origins
227	Phellodendri Chinensis Cortex	Rutaceae	Plant	*Phellodendron chinense* Schneid.	*Phellodendron chinense* Schneid.	Dry bark	

continued

No.	Name of TCM crude drugs	Family	Category	Name of the origin plant	Latin name of the origin plant	Medicinal part	Remark
228	Abelmoschi Corolla	Malvaceae	Plant	*Abelmoschus manihot* (L.) Medic.	*Abelmoschus manihot* (L.) Medic.	Dry corolla	
229	Cuscutae Semen	Convolvulaceae	Plant	*Cuscuta chinensis* Lam.	*Cuscuta chinensis* Lam.	Dry mature seed	Multiple origins
230	Cichorii Herba, Cichorii Radix	Asteraceae	Plant	*Cichorium intybus* L. *Cichorium glandulosum* Boiss. et Huet	*Cichorium intybus* L. *Cichorium glandulosum* Boiss. et Huet	Dry above-ground part and root	Multiple origins
231	Chrysanthemi Flos	Asteraceae	Plant	*Chrysanthemum morifolium* Ramat.	*Chrysanthemum morifolium* Ramat.	Dry capitulum	
232	Mume Flos	Rosaceae	Plant	*Prunus mume* (Sieb.) Sieb. et Zucc.	*Prunus mume* (Sieb.) Sieb. et Zucc.	Dry flower bud	
233	Ginkgo Folium	Ginkgoaceae	Plant	*Ginkgo biloba* L.	*Ginkgo biloba* L.	Dry leaf	
234	Stellariae Radix	Caryophyllaceae	Plant	*Stellaria dichotoma* L. var. *lanceolata* Bge.	*Stellaria dichotoma* L. var. *lanceolata* Bge.	Dry root	
235	Melo Semen	Cucurbitaceae	Plant	*Cucumis melo* L.	*Cucumis melo* L.	Dry mature seed	
236	Gleditsiae Fructus Abnormalis	Leguminosae	Plant	*Gleditsia sinensis* Lam.	*Gleditsia sinensis* Lam.	Dry sterile fruit	
237	Polyporus	Polyporaceae	Fungi	*Polyporus umbellatus* (Pers.) Fries	*Polyporus umbellatus* (Pers.) Fries	Dry sclerotium	
238	Sojae Semen Praeparatum	Leguminosae	Plant	*Glycine max* (L.) Merr.	*Glycine max* (L.) Merr.	Fermented processed products of mature seeds	

continued

No.	Name of TCM crude drugs	Family	Category	Name of the origin plant	Latin name of the origin plant	Medicinal part	Remark
239	Dipsaci Radix	Dipsacaceae	Plant	*Dipsacus asper* Wall. ex Henry	*Dipsacus asper* Wall. ex Henry	Dry root	
240	Farfarae Flos	Asteraceae	Plant	*Tussilago farfara* L.	*Tussilago farfara* L.	Dry flower bud	
241	Trachycarpi Petiolus	Arecaceae	Plant	*Trachycarpus fortunei* (Hook. f.) H. Wendl.	*Trachycarpus fortunei* (Hook. f.) H. Wendl.	Dry petiole	
242	Perillae Fructus	Lamiaceae	Plant	*Perilla frutescens* (L.) Britt.	*Perilla frutescens* (L.) Britt.	Dry mature fruit	
243	Perillae Folium	Lamiaceae	Plant	*Perilla frutescens* (L.) Britt.	*Perilla frutescens* (L.) Britt.	Dry leaves (with twigs)	
244	Perillae Caulis	Lamiaceae	Plant	*Perilla frutescens* (L.) Britt.	*Perilla frutescens* (L.) Britt.	Dry stem	
245	Asteris Radix et Rhizoma	Asteraceae	Plant	*Aster tataricus* L. f.	*Aster tataricus* L. f.	Dry root and rhizome	
246	Sesami Semen Nigrum	Pedaliaceae	Plant	*Sesamum indicum* L.	*Sesamum indicum* L.	Dry mature seed	
247	Sojae Semen Nigrum	Leguminosae	Plant	*Glycine max* (L.) Merr.	*Glycine max* (L.) Merr.	Dry mature seed	
248	Nigellae Semen	Ranunculaceae	Plant	*Nigella glandulifera* Freyn et Sint.	*Nigella glandulifera* Freyn et Sint.	Dry mature seed	Multiple origins
249	Fritillariae Hupehensis Bulbus	Liliaceae	Plant	*Fritillaria hupehensis* Hsiao et K. C. Hsia	*Fritillaria hupehensis* Hsiao et K. C. Hsia	Dry bulb	

continued

No.	Name of TCM crude drugs	Family	Category	Name of the origin plant	Latin name of the origin plant	Medicinal part	Remark
250	Ricini Semen	Euphorbiaceae	Plant	*Ricinus communis* L.	*Ricinus communis* L.	Dry mature seed	
251	Taraxaci Herba	Asteraceae	Plant	*Taraxacum mongolicum* Hand. –Mazz.	*Taraxacum mongolicum* Hand. –Mazz.	Dry whole herb	Multiple origins
252	Ailanthi Cortex	Simaroubaceae	Plant	*Ailanthus altissima* (Mill.) Swingle	*Ailanthus altissima* (Mill.) Swingle	Dry root bark and dry bark	
253	Sophorae Flos	Leguminosae	Plant	*Sophora japonica* L.	*Sophora japonica* L.	Dry flower and flower bud	
254	Sophorae Fructus	Leguminosae	Plant	*Sophora japonica* L.	*Sophora japonica* L.	Dry mature fruit	
255	Liquidambaris Fructus	Hamamelidaceae	Plant	*Liquidambar formosana* Hance	*Liquidambar formosana* Hance	Dry and mature infructescence	
256	Physalis Calyx seu Fructus	Solanaceae	Plant	*Physalis alkekengi* L. var. *franchetii* (Mast.) Makino	*Physalis alkekengi* L. var. *franchetii* (Mast.) Makino	Dry persistent calyx, calyx with fruit	
257	Polygoni Tinctorii Folium	Polygonaceae	Plant	*Polygonum tinctorium* Ait.	*Polygonum tinctorium* Ait.	Dry leaf	
258	Torreyae Semen	Taxaceae	Plant	*Torreya grandis* Fort.	*Torreya grandis* Fort.	Dry mature seed	
259	Arecae Semen	Arecaceae	Plant	*Areca catechu* L.	*Areca catechu* L.	Dry mature seed	
260	Papaveris Pericarpium	Papaveraceae	Plant	*Papaver somniferum* L.	*Papaver somniferum* L.	Dry mature fruit shell	
261	Capsici Fructus	Solanaceae	Plant	*Capsicum annuum* L.	*Capsicum annuum* L.	Dry mature fruit	

continued

No.	Name of TCM crude drugs	Family	Category	Name of the origin plant	Latin name of the origin plant	Medicinal part	Remark
262	Oryzae Fructus Germinatus	Poaceae	Plant	Oryza sativa L.	Oryza sativa L.	Processed products from mature fruits that have sprouted and been dried	
263	Allii Macrostemonis Bulbus	Liliaceae	Plant	Allium chinense G. Don	Allium chinense G. Don	Dry bulb	Multiple origins
264	Coicis Semen	Poaceae	Plant	Coix lacryma-jobi L. var. ma-yuen (Roman.) Stapf	Coix lacryma-jobi L. var. ma-yuen (Roman.) Stapf	Dry mature kernel	
265	Menthae Haplocalycis Herba	Lamiaceae	Plant	Mentha haplocalyx Briq.	Mentha haplocalyx Briq.	Dry above—ground part	
266	Belladonnae Herba	Solanaceae	Plant	Atropa belladonna L.	Atropa belladonna L.	Dry whole herb	
267	Citri Exocarpium Rubrum	Rutaceae	Plant	Citrus reticulata Blanco	Citrus reticulata Blanco	Dry outer pericarp	
268	Citri reticulatae Semen	Rutaceae	Plant	Citrus reticulata Blanco	Citrus reticulata Blanco	Dry mature seed	
269	Ligustici Rhizoma et Radix	Umbelliferae	Plant	Ligusticum jeholense Nakai et Kitag.	Ligusticum jeholense Nakai et Kitag.	Dry rhizome and root	Multiple origins
270	Santali Albi Lignum	Santalaceae	Plant	Santalum album L.	Santalum album L.	Dry heartwood of the tree trunk	

continued

No.	Name of TCM crude drugs	Family	Category	Name of the origin plant	Latin name of the origin plant	Medicinal part	Remark
271	Nelumbinis Rhizomatis Nodus	Nymphaeaceae	Plant	*Nelumbo nucifera* Gaertn.	*Nelumbo nucifera* Gaertn.	Dry rhizome node	
272	Dianthi Herba	Caryophyllaceae	Plant	*Dianthus chinensis* L.	*Dianthus chinensis* L.	Dry above–ground part	Multiple origins

Notes: 1. Type and source of TCM crude drugs: TCM crude drugs of which origins are plants (including fungi, the same below) in the *Pharmacopoeia of the People's Republic of China* (2015 Edition). Processed products are not listed separately (e.g., of zingiberis rhizoma and zingiberis rhizoma praeparatum, only zingiberis rhizoma is listed, while rhizoma zingiberis praeparatum is not), and TCM crude drugs for which different parts are used as ingredients (e.g., perillae fructus, perillae folium, and perillae caulis) are recorded separately according to the *Pharmacopoeia of the People's Republic of China*. A total of 272 TCM crude drugs from 255 plant origins are artificially cultivated.

2. Standard for "artificial cultivation" : Large–scale artificial cultivation has been achieved in production, the cultivation technology is mature or relatively mature, and artificially cultivated TCM crude drugs have become the mainstream of the market. For TCM crude drugs of multiple origins, only those plants of "artificially cultivated" origins are listed. For example, for TCM crude drugs of the origin glycyrrhiza uralensis fisch., only *Glycyrrhiza uralensis* that has been artificially cultivated on a large scale is listed. *G. glabra* and *G. inflata* are mainly wild and will not be included. In addition, it is noted in the "Remark" column that the TCM crude drug is of "multiple origins" . The TCM crude drug of which the cultivation technology has been basically successful, but the scale is small, and the cultivated products have not yet become the main source of commercially available and clinical medicines (e.g., Rhodiolae Crenulatae Radix et Rhizoma, Lobeliae Chinensis Herba, Notopterygii Rhizoma Et Radix, Polygonati Rhizoma, and Paridis Rhizoma, etc.), those which are mainly imported, and those not cultivated in a large scale in China (e.g., Caryophylli Flos, Myristicae Semen, and Sterculiae Lychnophorae Semen, etc.) have not been included.

3. Sorting method: Consistent with the *Pharmacopoeia of the People's Republic of China*, sorted by the number of strokes in the first Chinese character of TCM crude drugs.

中药资源评估技术指导原则

一、概述

为了保护中药资源，实现中药资源可持续利用，保障中药资源的稳定供给和中药产品的质量可控，依据《中华人民共和国药品管理法》《药品注册管理办法》等有关规定，制定本指导原则。

本技术指导原则所述中药资源是指：专用于中成药、中药饮片等生产的植物、动物及矿物资源。本原则所述中药资源评估是指：药品上市许可持有人或中药生产企业对未来 5 年内中药资源的预计消耗量与预计可获得量之间的比较，以及对中药产品生产对中药资源可持续利用可能造成的影响进行科学评估的过程。

二、基本原则

（一）坚持资源保护与产业发展相结合

中药资源评估工作应与"坚持节约资源和保护环境的基本国策"相符，在加强中药资源保护的同时，积极推动中药资源可持续利用。

（二）药材资源的供给与消耗平衡原则

使用药材资源的药品上市许可持有人或生产企业应提供评估资料证明预计药材年消耗量与可获得药材资源量之间平衡。如使用野生药材，应保证药材年消耗量低于相应药品上市许可持有人或生产企业可获得的规定产地药材的年增长量。应强化质量优先意识，在保证质量符合产品要求的前提下评估可持续的产量，从质量和供应两方面进行综合评估。

（三）坚持动态评估原则

中药产品在其立项、研制、上市后等阶段均应开展药材资源评估。根据中药资源预计消耗量和预计可获得量的变化及时更新评估报告。

已上市中药产品原则上每 5 年对中药资源重新评估一次。中成药再注册时，如处方中含有濒危野生药材，其生产有可能导致相应药材资源枯竭的，药品上市许可持有人或生产企业应在再注册前开展中药资源评估。

三、中药资源评估内容

中药资源评估主要包括预计消耗量、潜在风险和可持续利用措施三个方面。对于复方中成药，其处方中所含的每一药味均应当单独进行资源评估。

（一）背景资料

用于中药资源评估的背景资料包括以下内容：

1. 市场规模分析：中成药从产品适应症定位、目标人群、所治疗疾病的发病率、达到治疗效果的每个患者平均所需药品量和生物量、产品潜在的市场规模等方面论述。中药饮片从销售目标市场覆盖范围论述。

2. 处方及实际投料：列出每一药味的名称及其处方量；明确每一药味的实际投料量。

3. 中药资源基本信息：明确药品上市许可持有人或生产企业所用中药资源基原物种及其生物学特性，所使用中药资源的药用部位和产地初加工信息，野生或种植养殖的来源情况。

4. 产地基本信息：中药材产地地理位置（野生提供来源区域）、种植养殖基地面积、生产和组织方式。进口中药材应当提供原产地证明及进口商相关信息。

5. 中药材质量信息：选择中药资源物种、基地位置或来源区域的主要依据；对中药材质量进行的相关研究。

（二）预计消耗量

中药资源预计消耗量是指在评估年限内产品预计消耗掉的中药材总数量。

1. 中成药

中成药根据处方和预计年销售量计算被评估产品预计消耗量，计算公式为：

预计消耗量（吨）＝每个最小包装单位消耗中药材量（克）× 预计年销售最小包装总数 × 百万分之一

其中：①每个最小包装单位消耗中药材克数，以背景资料2提供的资料为依据计算。②预计年销售最小包装总数可以参考同类上市产品近5年的年销售量，或根据产品自身既往销售情况估算，此部分资料主要从背景资料1获得。

2. 中药饮片

每个产品可根据其每年所有销售终端（医院、药房等）的累计销售量或参考同类产品市场销售量估算。此部分资料主要从背景资料1和2获得。

（三）预计可获得量

重点描述中药生产企业能够获得特定药材资源的途径及可获得量。

对来源于人工种植养殖的中药材品种，应当说明基地的范围、基地年产量；对来源于野生的中药材品种，应当说明野生中药材的来源区域范围、可获得量等。

（四）潜在风险

中药资源潜在风险可从中药材再生能力、中药材成药周期、分布区域、濒危等级、特殊价值等方面分析，相关内容可来源于背景资料3、4。

1. 再生能力

应当说明所使用中药材是否为可再生资源以及再生的限制条件，包括人工繁殖是否存在障碍、特殊生境需求等。

2. 中药材成药周期

应当说明中药资源从幼苗生长到繁殖器官成熟所需要的时间和生产符合药品标准的中药材所需要的时间，可以引用文献数据或实测数据。

3. 分布区域

应当说明所使用中药资源分布范围，重点从中药资源道地性和品质变异的角度说明，可以引用文献数据或实测数据。

4. 濒危等级

应当关注国家、地方或国际珍稀濒危保护名录的更新情况，并说明所使用中药资源是否被列为保护对象，以及是否收录在相关保护名录中。

5. 特殊价值

应当说明所使用中药资源在生态系统和生物多样性中的特殊作用和价值。例如，甘草、麻黄对防风固沙具有重要生态价值，过度采挖可能导致土壤沙化。

6. 风险特别提示

所使用中药资源含有以下任何一种情形时，需要在中药资源评估报告结论部分对该资源含有的风险进行特别提示：

①不可进行人工繁育：该类中药材生长条件或繁育机制尚不清楚，不能进行人工种植养殖，中药材可持续供给存在障碍。

②中药材成药周期在5年以上（含5年）：该类中药材从繁殖体种植养殖开始计算，生长成为达到药用标准中药材的时间超过5年，生产周期长导致产量波动大，供需动态匹配困难。

③对生境有特殊需求，分布较窄：该类中药材仅分布在特定区域，产量难以扩大，过度采挖极易导致物种濒危。

④为野生珍稀濒危资源：该类药材已经出现资源问题，已收入野生珍稀濒危资源名录，国内外法律法规对该种资源的使用具有限制措施。

⑤质量不稳定：该类中药材不同区域质量变异较大或品种容易混杂，容易出现质量问题。

⑥存在严重连作障碍：该类中药材由于病虫害、营养等因素，无法在同一地块反复种植，需要不断更换种植地，质量管理有难度。

⑦其他可能造成资源量或质量问题的风险：如进口药材、产地变迁、气候变化、环境污染等。

（五）可持续利用和稳定质量措施

中药资源可持续利用措施的评估需着重说明以下情形：

1. 可持续获得性

对来源于人工种植养殖的中药材品种，应当提供基地发展5年规划；对来源于野生的中药材品种，应当明确年产量，说明5年自然更新、野生抚育和野生变家种家养等情况。

2. 稳定质量措施

应当明确并固定中药材基原、来源区域、采收时间、产地初加工方法等。来源于人工种植养殖的，还应当说明种植养殖符合中药材生产质量管理规范要求的措施。

四、中药资源评估决策和动态调整

分析可持续利用措施是否能够有效防范潜在风险，根据预计消耗量与预计可获得量的匹配情况，可作出中药资源评估决策。

可持续利用措施能够有效防范潜在风险，预计消耗量与预计可获得量相匹配的，说明中药产品对中药资源可持续利用带来的风险较低。

可持续利用措施无法有效防范潜在风险，预计消耗量与预计可获得量不相匹配的，说明中药产品对中药资源可持续利用带来的风险较高，则应慎重考虑产品的研发或上市，并需要调整预计消耗量或可持续利用措施。

经过调整，仍无法有效防范潜在风险，预计消耗量与预计可获得量不相匹配的，说明中药产品的生产有可能导致相关中药资源的枯竭。

附：1. 中药资源评估报告格式要求

2. 种植中药材参考名录（植物类）

附 1

中药资源评估报告格式要求

一个完整的中药产品资源评估报告由概述和产品涉及的每一味中药材的资源评估分报告组成。

1 概述

概述包括：封面、声明、产品简介、评估过程介绍、主要评估结论、涉及商业秘密的说明。

1.1 封面

封面应包括：题目（产品名称 + 所用药材名称 + 资源评估报告）、上市许可持有人或生产企业名称、评估日期等。

1.2 声明

本产品的中药资源评估报告资料真实完整、来源合法、未侵犯他人的权益。如有不实之处，我们承担由此导致的一切法律后果。

1.3 产品简介

介绍产品所涉及中药材品种，以及产品所处注册申报阶段或上市后生产销售情况。

（1）研发过程摘要：简述产品研发背景、目的；产品研发过程概述。

（2）市场规模分析：可从中药产品适用人群、所治疗疾病的发病率、分析达到治疗效果的每个患者平均所需药品量以及同类产品市场信息等方面进行综合分析。

中药饮片生产企业从销售目标市场覆盖范围分析中药饮片的市场规模。

1.4 评估过程综述

综述产品资源评估的组织实施过程。

1.5 主要评估结论

概述所涉及的每一味中药材资源的评估结论。

1.6 涉及商业秘密的说明

说明所涉及商业秘密的内容、范围。

2 中药资源评估分报告

中药资源评估分报告由封面、说明、分报告和相关附件等 4 部分内容组成，并按此顺序排列。

2.1 封面

封面应含有报告题目、评估单位、评估主要负责人和评估时间等信息。

2.2 说明

2.2.1 评估所需数据的来源及其可靠性、完整性和真实性

2.2.2 评估人信息

包括主要参与评估人员的姓名、单位、职称、职务、专业背景等。

2.3 分报告

2.3.1 标题

药材名（中药产品所用）+ 资源评估分报告，例如：山茱萸（六味地黄丸所用）资源评估分报告。

2.3.2 摘要

简明扼要地概括评估所用数据的来源、评估方法、评估结果、评估结论等。

2.3.3 一般背景资料

（1）最小包装所需药材量。

（2）中药资源基本信息：包括药品上市许可持有人或生产企业所用中药资源基原物种信息，所使用中药资源的药用部位和产地初加工信息，来源于野生或种植养殖情况。

（3）产地信息：药品上市许可持有人或生产企业所用中药资源产地、位置（野生药材提供来源区域）、面积、生产和组织方式。进口中药材需要提供原产国及进口商相关信息。

（4）质量信息：包括选择中药资源物种、基地位置或来源区域的主要依据，对中药材质量进行的相关研究，所采用质量标准及标准编制依据。

2.3.4 预计消耗量评估

（1）预计消耗量的计算过程。

（2）各项数据来源的说明。

2.3.5 预计可获得量评估

说明预计可获得量计算过程，以及数据来源。

2.3.6 潜在风险评估

（1）再生能力。

（2）中药材成药周期。

（3）分布区域。

（4）濒危等级。

（5）特殊价值。

（6）风险特别提示。

2.3.7 中药资源可持续利用和稳定质量措施

（1）可持续获得性的措施。

（2）稳定质量的措施。

（3）措施有效性评估。

2.3.8 最终结论

根据评估结果，言简意赅地表述评估结论。

2.3.9 不确定性分析

任何材料和数据方面的不确定性（如：知识的不足、数据限制、有争议问题等）都要在该节进行充分的讨论，并就各种不确定性对结果可靠性的影响程度进行详细说明。

2.3.10 参考资料

若评估报告中引用了文献和文件，在评估报告的最后要提供引用文献和文件的出处。

2.4 相关附件

2.4.1 中药材种植养殖基地相关证明文件

如：土地证或土地租赁合同、合作协议等复印件。

2.4.2 规范化种植养殖技术规程

2.4.3 符合中药产品特性的中药材质量研究资料

2.4.4 其他与本报告有关的证明文件

如：供销合同、相关检查报告等。

2.4.5 数据汇总表

数据汇总表

产品名称	（中成药或中药饮片名称）		
药材名	（参看注1）		
基原	（参看注2）	拉丁学名	（参看注2）
药用部位	□植物（□根　□果实和种子　□全草　□根及根茎　□花　□皮　□叶　□茎木　□树脂　□生理或病理产物） □动物（□全体　□器官　□生理或病理产物　□组织　□角骨　□贝壳） □矿物 □菌　□藻　□地衣　□其他：_____		

续表

	年份	每个最小包装单位消耗中药材量 *（克）	预计年销售最小包装总数 *	预计年消耗量（吨）
预计消耗的资源量	年			
	年			
	年			
	年			
	合计			
风险特征评估	人工繁育	□不可　　□不成熟　　□成熟		
	分布区域	□1-2省　□3-6省　□6省以上		
	中药材成药周期（参看注3）	成药年限	□1-2年　□3-5年　□5年以上 □其他：_____	
		采收周期	□1-2年　□3-5年　□5年以上 □其他：_____	
	中国特有种	□是　　□否		
	野生珍稀濒危	□是　　□否（参看注4） 备注：_____		
	具有特殊价值	□是　　□否（参看注4） 备注：_____		
	需要提示风险			

续表

		产地位置	地区（精确到县） 道地产区（□是　□否　□其他：＿＿＿＿＿＿＿＿）		
可持续利用措施	种植中药材	面积	亩		
		基地位置	经度：	纬度：	地区：
		生产组织方式	□公司自建　□合作基地 □其他：＿＿＿＿＿＿＿＿＿＿＿＿		
		是否规范化种植	□是（GAP 基地　□是　□否） □否 其他：＿＿＿＿＿＿＿＿＿＿＿＿		
		产地初加工方式			
		预计可获得量	年份	可用面积（亩）	亩产量（千克/亩）	预计可获得量（吨）
			年			
			年			
			年			
			年			
			年			
			合计			
	养殖中药材	基地位置	经度：	纬度：	地区：
		生产组织方式	□公司自建　□合作基地 □其他：＿＿＿＿＿＿＿＿＿＿＿＿		
		是否规范化养殖	□是（GAP 基地　□是　□否） □否 其他：＿＿＿＿＿＿＿＿＿＿＿＿		
		产地初加工方式			
		预计可获得量	年份	养殖数量	预计可获得量（吨）
			年		
			年		
			年		
			年		
			年		
			合计		

续表

		基地位置	经度：		纬度：	地区：
可持续利用措施	野生中药材	面积	亩			
		获取途径	□自采　　□收购　□其他：＿＿＿＿＿＿			
		限制措施	□有围栏　　□无　　□其他：＿＿＿＿＿＿			
		采收时间	XX 月—XX 月			
		产地初加工方式				
		预计可获得量	年份		可用区域	预计可获得量（吨）
			年			
			年			
			年			
			年			
			年			
			合计			
	其他措施					
评估结论	资源量		预计可获得量≥预计消耗量　□确认			
	资源质量		质量稳定□确认			

注：1. 为了科学和完整地获取中药资源评估的相关数据，申请人应按照以上表格汇总数据。每个中药材单独填写一张数据汇总表。

2. 中药资源基原物种信息以《中国药典》为主，《中国药典》未收载的以《中国植物志》《中国动物志》以及具有同等效力的分类学专著的名称为准，名称有更新的以最新名称为准，拉丁学名应遵循双名法。具有种下分类单元或栽培品种或品系的应进一步详述。

3. 成药年限（以植物药材为例）是指从幼苗生长到符合药用要求首次采收所需要的时间。采收周期（以植物药材为例）是指从上次采收到下次采收中药材所需要的时间。

4. 野生药材相关保护名录：《濒危野生动植物物种国际贸易公约》（CITES）附录1、2，《国家重点保护野生动物名录》，《国家重点保护野生植物名录（第1批）》，《国家重点保护野生药材物种名录》等及地方保护名录。

5. 标 * 部分，中药饮片无需填写。

附 2

种植中药材参考名录（植物类）

序号	药材名	科	类别	基原植物名称	基原植物拉丁学名	部位	备注
1	八角茴香	木兰科	植物	八角茴香	*Illicium verum* Hook. f.	干燥成熟果实	
2	人参	五加科	植物	人参	*Panax ginseng* C. A. Mey.	干燥根和根茎	
3	人参叶	五加科	植物	人参	*Panax ginseng* C. A. Mey.	干燥叶	
4	刀豆	豆科	植物	刀豆	*Canavalia gladiata* (Jacq.) DC.	干燥成熟种子	
5	三七	五加科	植物	三七	*Panax notoginseng* (Burk.) F. H. Chen	干燥根和根茎	
6	三棱	黑三棱科	植物	黑三棱	*Sparganium stoloniferum* Buch. –Ham.	干燥块茎	
7	干姜	姜科	植物	姜	*Zingiber officinale* Rosc.	干燥根茎	
8	土木香	菊科	植物	土木香	*Inula helenium* L.	干燥根	
9	土贝母	葫芦科	植物	土贝母	*Bolbostemma paniculatum* (Maxim.) Franquet	干燥块茎	
10	土荆皮	松科	植物	金钱松	*Pseudolarix amabilis* (Nelson) Rehd.	干燥根皮或近根树皮	
11	大豆黄卷	豆科	植物	大豆	*Glycine max* (L.) Merr.	成熟种子经发芽干燥的炮制加工品	
12	大皂角	豆科	植物	皂荚	*Gleditsia sinensis* Lam.	干燥成熟果实	
13	大青叶	十字花科	植物	菘蓝	*Isatis indigotica* Fort.	干燥叶	

续表

序号	药材名	科	类别	基原植物名称	基原植物拉丁学名	部位	备注
14	大枣	鼠李科	植物	枣	*Ziziphus jujuba* Mill.	干燥成熟果实	
15	大黄	蓼科	植物	药用大黄	*Rheum officinale* Baill.	干燥根和根茎	多基原
				掌叶大黄	*Rheum palmatum* L.		
16	大蒜	百合科	植物	大蒜	*Allium sativum* L.	鳞茎	
17	大腹皮	棕榈科	植物	槟榔	*Areca catechu* L.	干燥果皮	
18	山麦冬	百合科	植物	湖北麦冬	*Liriope spicata*（Thunb.）Lour. var. *prolifera* Y. T. Ma	干燥块根	多基原
19	山茱萸	山茱萸科	植物	山茱萸	*Cornus officinalis* Sieb. et Zucc.	干燥成熟果肉	
20	山药	薯蓣科	植物	薯蓣	*Dioscorea opposita* Thunb.	干燥根茎	
21	山柰	姜科	植物	山柰	*Kaempferia galanga* L.	干燥根茎	
22	山银花	忍冬科	植物	黄褐毛忍冬	*Lonicera fulvotomentosa* Hsu et S. C. Cheng	干燥花蕾、带初开的花	多基原
				灰毡毛忍冬	*Lonicera macranthoides* Hand.–Mazz.		
23	山楂	蔷薇科	植物	山里红	*Crataegus pinnatifida* Bge. var. *major* N. E. Br.	干燥成熟果实	多基原
24	山楂叶	蔷薇科	植物	山里红	*Crataegus pinnatifida* Bge. var. *major* N. E. Br.	干燥叶	多基原
25	千金子	大戟科	植物	续随子	*Euphorbia lathyris* L.	干燥成熟种子	
26	川贝母	百合科	植物	瓦布贝母	*Fritillaria unibracteata* Hsiao et K. C. Hsia var. *wabuensis*（S. Y. Tang et S. C. Yue）Z. D. Liu, S. Wang et S. C. Chen	干燥鳞茎	多基原

续表

序号	药材名	科	类别	基原植物名称	基原植物拉丁学名	部位	备注
27	川牛膝	苋科	植物	川牛膝	*Cyathula officinalis* Kuan	干燥根	
28	川乌	毛茛科	植物	乌头	*Aconitum carmichaelii* Debx.	干燥母根	
29	川芎	伞形科	植物	川芎	*Ligusticum chuanxiong* Hort.	干燥根茎	
30	川射干	鸢尾科	植物	鸢尾	*Iris tectorum* Maxim.	干燥根茎	
31	川楝子	楝科	植物	川楝	*Melia toosendan* Sieb. et Zucc.	干燥果实	
32	广枣	漆树科	植物	南酸枣	*Choerospondias axillaris* (Roxb.) Burtt et Hill	干燥成熟果实	
33	广金钱草	豆科	植物	广金钱草	*Desmodium styracifolium* (Osb.) Merr.	干燥地上部分	
34	广藿香	唇形科	植物	广藿香	*Pogostemon cablin* (Blanco) Benth.	干燥地上部分	
35	女贞子	木犀科	植物	女贞	*Ligustrum lucidum* Ait.	干燥成熟果实	
36	小茴香	伞形科	植物	茴香	*Foeniculum vulgare* Mill.	干燥成熟果实	
37	王不留行	石竹科	植物	麦蓝菜	*Vaccaria segetalis* (Neck.) Garcke	干燥成熟种子	
38	天冬	百合科	植物	天冬	*Asparagus cochinchinensis* (Lour.) Merr.	干燥块根	
39	天花粉	葫芦科	植物	栝楼	*Trichosanthes kirilowii* Maxim.	干燥根	多基原
				双边栝楼	*Trichosanthes rosthornii* Harms		
40	天竺黄	禾本科	植物	华思劳竹	*Schizostachyum chinense* Rendle	秆内的分泌液干燥后、块状物	多基原
				青皮竹	*Bambusa textilis* McClure		

续表

序号	药材名	科	类别	基原植物名称	基原植物拉丁学名	部位	备注
41	天麻	兰科	植物	天麻	*Gastrodia elata* Bl.	干燥块茎	
42	天然冰片（右旋龙脑）	樟科	植物	樟	*Cinnamomum camphora*（L.）Presl	新鲜枝、叶经提取加工制成	
43	木瓜	蔷薇科	植物	贴梗海棠	*Chaenomeles speciosa*（Sweet）Nakai	干燥近成熟果实	
44	木芙蓉叶	锦葵科	植物	木芙蓉	*Hibiscus mutabilis* L.	干燥叶	
45	木香	菊科	植物	木香	*Aucklandia lappa* Decne.	干燥根	
46	木棉花	木棉科	植物	木棉	*Gossampinus malabarica*（DC.）Merr.	干燥花	
47	五味子	木兰科	植物	五味子	*Schisandra chinensis*（Turcz.）Baill.	干燥成熟果实	
48	太子参	石竹科	植物	孩儿参	*Pseudostellaria heterophylla*（Miq.）Pax ex Pax et Hoffm.	干燥块根	
49	车前子	车前科	植物	车前	*Plantago asiatica* L.	干燥成熟种子	多基原
50	牛蒡子	菊科	植物	牛蒡	*Arctium lappa* L.	干燥成熟果实	
51	牛膝	苋科	植物	牛膝	*Achyranthes bidentata* Bl.	干燥根	
52	片姜黄	姜科	植物	温郁金	*Curcuma wenyujin* Y. H. Chen et C. Ling	干燥根茎	
53	化橘红	芸香科	植物	化州柚	*Citrus grandis* 'Tomentosa'	未成熟、近成熟的干燥外层果皮	多基原
				柚	*Citrus grandis*（L.）Osbeck		
54	月季花	蔷薇科	植物	月季	*Rosa chinensis* Jacq.	干燥花	
55	丹参	唇形科	植物	丹参	*Salvia miltiorrhiza* Bge.	干燥根和根茎	
56	乌药	樟科	植物	乌药	*Lindera aggregata*（Sims）Kosterm.	干燥块根	

续表

序号	药材名	科	类别	基原植物名称	基原植物拉丁学名	部位	备注
57	乌梅	蔷薇科	植物	梅	*Prunus mume*(Sieb.) Sieb. et Zucc.	干燥近成熟果实	
58	火麻仁	桑科	植物	大麻	*Cannabis sativa* L.	干燥成熟果实	
59	巴豆	大戟科	植物	巴豆	*Croton tiglium* L.	干燥成熟果实	
60	巴戟天	茜草科	植物	巴戟天	*Morinda officinalis* How	干燥根	
61	水飞蓟	菊科	植物	水飞蓟	*Silybum marianum*(L.) Gaertn.	干燥成熟果实	
62	玉竹	百合科	植物	玉竹	*Polygonatum odoratum*(Mill.) Druce	干燥根茎	
63	甘草	豆科	植物	甘草	*Glycyrrhiza uralensis* Fisch.	干燥根和根茎	
64	甘遂	大戟科	植物	甘遂	*Euphorbia kansui* T. N. Liou ex T. P. Wang	干燥块根	
65	艾片（左旋龙脑）	菊科	植物	艾纳香	*Blumea balsamifera*(L.)DC.	新鲜叶经提取加工制成的结晶	
66	石斛	兰科	植物	金钗石斛	*Dendrobium nobile* Lindl.	新鲜或干燥茎	多基原
				齿瓣石斛	*Dendrobium devonianum* Paxt		
67	石榴皮	石榴科	植物	石榴	*Punica granatum* L.	干燥果皮	
68	龙胆	龙胆科	植物	龙胆	*Gentiana scabra* Bge.	干燥根和根茎	多基原
69	龙眼肉	无患子科	植物	龙眼	*Dimocarpus longan* Lour.	假种皮	
70	平贝母	百合科	植物	平贝母	*Fritillaria ussuriensis* Maxim.	干燥鳞茎	
71	北沙参	伞形科	植物	珊瑚菜	*Glehnia littoralis* Fr. Schmidt ex Miq.	干燥根	
72	四季青	冬青科	植物	冬青	*Ilex chinensis* Sims	干燥叶	
73	生姜	兰科	植物	姜	*Zingiber officinale* Rosc.	新鲜根茎	

193

续表

序号	药材名	科	类别	基原植物名称	基原植物拉丁学名	部位	备注
74	白及	姜科	植物	白及	*Bletilla striata*（Thunb.）Reichb. f.	干燥块茎	
75	白术	菊科	植物	白术	*Atractylodes macrocephala* Koidz.	干燥根茎	
76	白芍	毛茛科	植物	芍药	*Paeonia lactiflora* Pall.	干燥根	
77	白芷	伞形科	植物	白芷	*Angelica dahurica*（Fisch. ex Hoffm.）Benth. et Hook. f.	干燥根	多基原
				杭白芷	*Angelica dahurica*（Fisch. ex Hoffm.）Benth. et Hook. f. var. *formosana*（Boiss.）Shan et Yuan		
78	白附子	天南星科	植物	独角莲	*Typhonium giganteum* Engl.	干燥块茎	
79	白果	银杏科	植物	银杏	*Ginkgo biloba* L.	干燥成熟种子	
80	白扁豆	豆科	植物	扁豆	*Dolichos lablab* L.	干燥成熟种子	
81	瓜蒌	葫芦科	植物	栝楼	*Trichosanthes kirilowii* Maxim.	干燥成熟果实	多基原
				双边栝楼	*Trichosanthes rosthornii* Harms		
82	瓜蒌子	葫芦科	植物	栝楼	*Trichosanthes kirilowii* Maxim.	干燥成熟种子	多基原
				双边栝楼	*Trichosanthes rosthornii* Harms		
83	瓜蒌皮	葫芦科	植物	栝楼	*Trichosanthes kirilowii* Maxim.	干燥成熟果皮	多基原
				双边栝楼	*Trichosanthes rosthornii* Harms		

续表

序号	药材名	科	类别	基原植物名称	基原植物拉丁学名	部位	备注
84	冬瓜皮	葫芦科	植物	冬瓜	*Benincasa hispida*（Thunb.）Cogn.	干燥外层果皮	
85	冬凌草	唇形科	植物	碎米桠	*Rabdosia rubescens*（Hemsl.）Hara	干燥地上部分	
86	冬葵果	锦葵科	植物	冬葵	*Malva verticillata* L.	干燥成熟果实	
87	玄参	玄参科	植物	玄参	*Scrophularia ningpoensis* Hemsl.	干燥根	
88	半枝莲	唇形科	植物	半枝莲	*Scutellaria barbata* D. Don	干燥全草	
89	半夏	天南星科	植物	半夏	*Pinellia ternata*（Thunb.）Breit.	干燥块茎	
90	丝瓜络	葫芦科	植物	丝瓜	*Luffa cylindrica*（L.）Roem.	干燥成熟果实的维管束	
91	地骨皮	茄科	植物	宁夏枸杞	*Lycium barbarum* L.	干燥根皮	多基原
92	地黄	玄参科	植物	地黄	*Rehmannia glutinosa* Libosch.	新鲜、干燥块根	
93	亚麻子	亚麻科	植物	亚麻	*Linum usitatissimum* L.	干燥成熟种子	
94	西瓜霜	葫芦科	植物	西瓜	*Citrullus lanatus*（Thunb.）Matsumu. et Nakai	成熟新鲜果实与皮硝经加工制成	
95	西红花	鸢尾科	植物	番红花	*Crocus sativus* L.	干燥柱头	
96	西洋参	五加科	植物	西洋参	*Panax quinquefolium* L.	干燥根	
97	百合	百合科	植物	百合	*Lilium brownii* F. E. Brown var. *viridulum* Baker	干燥肉质鳞叶	多基原
				卷丹	*Lilium lancifolium* Thunb.		
98	当归	伞形科	植物	当归	*Angelica sinensis*（Oliv.）Diels	干燥根	

续表

序号	药材名	科	类别	基原植物名称	基原植物拉丁学名	部位	备注
99	肉苁蓉	列当科	植物	肉苁蓉	*Cistanche deserticola* Y. C. Ma	干燥带鳞叶的肉质茎	多基原
				管花肉苁蓉	*Cistanche tubulosa* (Schenk) Wight		
100	肉桂	樟科	植物	肉桂	*Cinnamomum cassia* Presl	干燥树皮	
101	竹节参	五加科	植物	竹节参	*Panax japonicus* C. A. Mey.	干燥根茎	
102	竹茹	禾本科	植物	大头典竹	*Sinocalamus beecheyanus* (Munro) McClure var. *pubescens* P. F. Li	茎秆的干燥中间层	多基原
				淡竹	*Phyllostachys nigra* (Lodd.) Munro var. *henonis* (Mitf.) Stapf ex Rendle		
				青秆竹	*Bambusa tuldoides* Munro		
103	延胡索（元胡）	罂粟科	植物	延胡索	*Corydalis yanhusuo* W. T. Wang	干燥块茎	
104	伊贝母	百合科	植物	伊犁贝母	*Fritillaria pallidiflora* Schrenk	干燥鳞茎	多基原
105	合欢皮	豆科	植物	合欢	*Albizia julibrissin* Durazz.	干燥树皮	
106	合欢花	豆科	植物	合欢	*Albizia julibrissin* Durazz.	干燥花序或花蕾	
107	决明子	豆科	植物	决明	*Cassia obtusifolia* L.	干燥成熟种子	多基原
				小决明	*Cassia tora* L.		
108	灯心草	灯心草科	植物	灯心草	*Juncus effusus* L.	干燥茎髓	
109	灯盏细辛（灯盏花）	菊科	植物	短葶飞蓬	*Erigeron breviscapus* (Vant.) Hand. –Mazz.	干燥全草	

续表

序号	药材名	科	类别	基原植物名称	基原植物拉丁学名	部位	备注
110	防风	伞形科	植物	防风	*Saposhnikovia divaricata*（Turcz.）Schischk.	干燥根	
111	红花	菊科	植物	红花	*Carthamus tinctorius* L.	干燥花	
112	红芪	豆科	植物	多序岩黄芪	*Hedysarum polybotrys* Hand. –Mazz.	干燥根	
113	红参	五加科	植物	人参栽培品	*Panax ginseng* C. A. Mey.	蒸制后的干燥根和根茎	
114	麦冬	百合科	植物	麦冬	*Ophiopogon japonicus*（L. f）Ker–Gawl.	干燥块根	
115	麦芽	禾本科	植物	大麦	*Hordeum vulgare* L.	成熟果实经发芽干燥的炮制加工品	
116	远志	远志科	植物	远志	*Polygala tenuifolia* Willd.	干燥根	多基原
117	赤小豆	豆科	植物	赤豆	*Vigna angularis* Ohwi et Ohashi	干燥成熟种子	多基原
				赤小豆	*Vigna umbellata* Ohwi et Ohashi		多基原
118	花椒	芸香科	植物	花椒	*Zanthoxylum bungeanum* Maxim.	干燥成熟果皮	多基原
119	芥子	十字花科	植物	白芥	*Sinapis alba* L.	干燥成熟种子	多基原
				芥	*Brassica juncea*（L.）Czern. et Coss.		
120	苍术	菊科	植物	茅苍术	*Atractylodes lancea*（Thunb.）DC.	干燥根茎	多基原
121	芡实	睡莲科	植物	芡	*Euryale ferox* Salisb.	干燥成熟种仁	

197

续表

序号	药材名	科	类别	基原植物名称	基原植物拉丁学名	部位	备注
122	芦荟	百合科	植物	好望角芦荟	*Aloe ferox* Miller	汁液浓缩干燥物	多基原
				库拉索芦荟	*Aloe barbadensis* Miller		
123	杜仲	杜仲科	植物	杜仲	*Eucommia ulmoides* Oliv.	干燥树皮	
124	杜仲叶	杜仲科	植物	杜仲	*Eucommia ulmoides* Oliv.	干燥叶	
125	吴茱萸	芸香科	植物	吴茱萸	*Euodia rutaecarpa*（Juss.）Benth.	干燥近成熟果实	多基原
126	牡丹皮	毛茛科	植物	牡丹	*Paeonia suffruticosa* Andr.	干燥根皮	
127	何首乌	蓼科	植物	何首乌	*Polygonum multiflorum* Thunb.	干燥块根	
128	皂角刺	豆科	植物	皂荚	*Gleditsia sinensis* Lam.	干燥棘刺	
129	佛手	芸香科	植物	佛手	*Citrus medica* L. var. *sarcodactylis* Swingle	干燥果实	
130	余甘子	大戟科	植物	余甘子	*Phyllanthus emblica* L.	干燥成熟果实	
131	谷芽	禾本科	植物	粟	*Setaria italica*（L.）Beauv.	成熟果实经发芽干燥的炮制加工品	
132	辛夷	木兰科	植物	望春花	*Magnolia biondii* Pamp.	干燥花蕾	多基原
				武当玉兰	*Magnolia sprengeri* Pamp.		
				玉兰	*Magnolia denudata* Desr.		
133	沙苑子	豆科	植物	扁茎黄芪	*Astragalus complanatus* R. Br.	干燥成熟种子	
134	沉香	瑞香科	植物	白木香	*Aquilaria sinensis*（Lour.）Gilg	含有树脂的木材	
135	补骨脂	豆科	植物	补骨脂	*Psoralea corylifolia* L.	干燥成熟果实	

续表

序号	药材名	科	类别	基原植物名称	基原植物拉丁学名	部位	备注
136	灵芝	多孔菌科	真菌	赤芝	*Ganoderma lucidum*（Leyss. ex Fr.）Karst.	干燥子实体	多基原
				紫芝	*Ganoderma sinense* Zhao，Xu et Zhang		
137	陈皮	芸香科	植物	橘及其栽培变种	*Citrus reticulata* Blanco	干燥成熟果皮	
138	附子	毛茛科	植物	乌头	*Aconitum carmichaelii* Debx.	子根的加工品	
139	忍冬藤	忍冬科	植物	忍冬	*Lonicera japonica* Thunb.	干燥茎枝	
140	鸡骨草	豆科	植物	广州相思子	*Abrus cantoniensis* Hance	干燥全株	
141	鸡冠花	苋科	植物	鸡冠花	*Celosia cristata* L.	干燥花序	
142	青皮	芸香科	植物	橘及其栽培变种	*Citrus reticulata* Blanco	干燥幼果、未成熟果实的果皮	
143	青果	橄榄科	植物	橄榄	*Canarium album* Raeusch.	干燥成熟果实	
144	青蒿	菊科	植物	黄花蒿	*Artemisia annua* L.	干燥地上部分	
145	青黛	十字花科	植物	菘蓝	*Isatis indigotica* Fort.	叶或茎叶经加工制得的干燥粉末、团块或颗粒	多基原
		爵床科	植物	马蓝	*Baphicacanthus cusia*（Nees）Bremek.		
		蓼科	植物	蓼蓝	*Polygonum tinctorium* Ait.		
146	玫瑰花	蔷薇科	植物	玫瑰	*Rosa rugosa* Thunb.	干燥花蕾	
147	苦地丁	罂粟科	植物	紫堇	*Corydalis bungeana* Turcz.	干燥全草	
148	苦杏仁	蔷薇科	植物	杏	*Prunus armeniaca* L.	干燥成熟种子	多基原

续表

序号	药材名	科	类别	基原植物名称	基原植物拉丁学名	部位	备注
149	枇杷叶	蔷薇科	植物	枇杷	*Eriobotrya japonica* (Thunb.)Lindl.	干燥叶	
150	板蓝根	十字花科	植物	菘蓝	*Isatis indigotica* Fort.	干燥根	
151	松花粉	松科	植物	马尾松	*Pinus massoniana* Lamb.	干燥花粉	多基原
				油松	*Pinus tabulieformis* Carr.		
152	郁金	姜科	植物	广西莪术	*Curcuma kwangsiensis* S. G. Lee et C. F. Liang	干燥块根	多基原
				温郁金	*Curcuma wenyujin* Y. H. Chen et C. Ling		
				蓬莪术	*Curcuma phaeocaulis* Val.		
				姜黄	*Curcuma longa* L.		
153	昆布	海带科	植物	海带	*Laminaria japonica* Aresch.	干燥叶状体	多基原
154	明党参	伞形科	植物	明党参	*Changium smyrnioides* Wolff	干燥根	
155	罗汉果	葫芦科	植物	罗汉果	*Siraitia grosvenorii* (Swingle)C. Jeffrey ex A. M. Lu et Z. Y. Zhang	干燥果实	
156	知母	百合科	植物	知母	*Anemarrhena asphodeloides* Bge.	干燥根茎	
157	使君子	使君子科	植物	使君子	*Quisqualis indica* L.	干燥成熟果实	
158	侧柏叶	柏科	植物	侧柏	*Platycladus orientalis* (L.)Franco	干燥枝梢和叶	
159	佩兰	菊科	植物	佩兰	*Eupatorium fortunei* Turcz.	干燥地上部分	
160	金银花	忍冬科	植物	忍冬	*Lonicera japonica* Thunb.	干燥花蕾、带初开的花	

序号	药材名	科	类别	基原植物名称	基原植物拉丁学名	部位	备注
161	鱼腥草	截菜科	植物	截菜	*Houttuynia cordata* Thunb.	新鲜全草或干燥地上部分	
162	泽兰	唇形科	植物	地瓜儿苗	*Lycopus lucidus* Turcz. *var. hirtus* Regel	干燥地上部分	
163	油松节	松科	植物	马尾松	*Pinus massoniana* Lamb.	干燥瘤状节、分枝节	多基原
				油松	*Pinus tabulieformis* Carr.		
164	泽泻	泽泻科	植物	泽泻	*Alisma orientale*（Sam.）Juzep.	干燥块茎	
165	细辛	马兜铃科	植物	北细辛	*Asarum heterotropoides* Fr. Schmidt var. *mandshuricum*（Maxim.）Kitag.	干燥地上部分	多基原
166	荆芥	唇形科	植物	荆芥	*Schizonepeta tenuifolia* Briq.	干燥地上部分	
167	荆芥穗	唇形科	植物	荆芥	*Schizonepeta tenuifolia* Briq.	干燥花穗	
168	草果	姜科	植物	草果	*Amomum tsao-ko* Crevost et Lemaire	干燥成熟果实	
169	茯苓	多孔菌科	真菌	茯苓	*Poria cocos*（Schw.）Wolf	干燥菌核	
170	茯苓皮	多孔菌科	真菌	茯苓	*Poria cocos*（Schw.）Wolf	菌核干燥外皮	
171	茺蔚子	唇形科	植物	益母草	*Leonurus japonicus* Houtt.	干燥成熟果实	
172	胡芦巴	豆科	植物	胡芦巴	*Trigonella foenum-graecum* L.	干燥成熟种子	
173	胡椒	胡椒科	植物	胡椒	*Piper nigrum* L.	干燥近成熟、成熟果实	
174	荔枝核	无患子科	植物	荔枝	*Litchi chinensis* Sonn.	干燥成熟种子	
175	南板蓝根	爵床科	植物	马蓝	*Baphicacanthus cusia*（Nees）Bremek.	干燥根茎和根	

序号	药材名	科	类别	基原植物名称	基原植物拉丁学名	部位	备注
176	枳壳	芸香科	植物	酸橙及其栽培变种	*Citrus aurantium* L.	干燥未成熟果实	
177	枳实	芸香科	植物	酸橙及其栽培变种	*Citrus aurantium* L.	干燥幼果	多基原
				甜橙及其栽培变种	*Citrus sinensis* Osbeck		
178	柏子仁	柏科	植物	侧柏	*Platycladus orientalis*（L.）Franco	干燥成熟种仁	
179	栀子	茜草科	植物	栀子	*Gardenia jasminoides* Ellis	干燥成熟果实	
180	枸杞子	茄科	植物	宁夏枸杞	*Lycium barbarum* L.	干燥成熟果实	
181	柿蒂	柿树科	植物	柿	*Diospyros kaki* Thunb.	干燥宿萼	
182	厚朴	木兰科	植物	凹叶厚朴	*Magnolia officinalis* Rehd. et Wils. var. *biloba* Rehd. et Wils.	干燥干皮、根皮及枝皮	多基原
				厚朴	*Magnolia officinalis* Rehd. et Wils.		
183	厚朴花	木兰科	植物	凹叶厚朴	*Magnolia officinalis* Rehd. et Wils. var. *biloba* Rehd. et Wils.	干燥花蕾	多基原
				厚朴	*Magnolia officinalis* Rehd. et Wils.		
184	砂仁	姜科	植物	阳春砂	*Amomum villosum* Lour.	干燥成熟果实	多基原
				海南砂仁	*Amomum longiligulare* T. L. Wu		
185	鸦胆子	苦木科	植物	鸦胆子	*Brucea javanica*（L.）Merr.	干燥成熟果实	
186	韭菜子	百合科	植物	韭菜	*Allium tuberosum* Rottl. ex Spreng.	干燥成熟种子	

序号	药材名	科	类别	基原植物名称	基原植物拉丁学名	部位	备注
187	香橼	芸香科	植物	枸橼	*Citrus medica* L.	干燥成熟果实	多基原
				香圆	*Citrus wilsonii* Tanaka		
188	香薷	唇形科	植物	江香薷	*Mosla chinensis* 'Jiangxiangru'	干燥地上部分	多基原
189	独活	伞形科	植物	重齿毛当归	*Angelica pubescens* Maxim. f. *biserrata* Shan et Yuan	干燥根	
190	急性子	凤仙花科	植物	凤仙花	*Impatiens balsamina* L.	干燥成熟种子	
191	姜黄	姜科	植物	姜黄	*Curcuma longa* L.	干燥根茎	
192	前胡	伞形科	植物	白花前胡	*Peucedanum praeruptorum* Dunn	干燥根	
193	首乌藤	蓼科	植物	何首乌	*Polygonum multiflorum* Thunb.	干燥藤茎	
194	穿心莲	爵床科	植物	穿心莲	*Andrographis paniculata* (Burm. f.) Nees	干燥地上部分	
195	秦艽	龙胆科	植物	秦艽	*Gentiana macrophylla* Pall.	干燥根	多基原
196	莱菔子	十字花科	植物	萝卜	*Raphanus sativus* L.	干燥成熟种子	
197	莲子	睡莲科	植物	莲	*Nelumbo nucifera* Gaertn.	干燥成熟种子	
198	莲子心	睡莲科	植物	莲	*Nelumbo nucifera* Gaertn.	成熟种子中的干燥幼叶及胚根	
199	莲房	睡莲科	植物	莲	*Nelumbo nucifera* Gaertn.	干燥花托	
200	莲须	睡莲科	植物	莲	*Nelumbo nucifera* Gaertn.	干燥雄蕊	
201	莪术	姜科	植物	广西莪术	*Curcuma kwangsiensis* S. G. Lee et C. F. Liang	干燥根茎	多基原
				温郁金	*Curcuma wenyujin* Y. H. Chen et C. Ling		
				蓬莪术	*Curcuma phaeocaulis* Val.		

序号	药材名	科	类别	基原植物名称	基原植物拉丁学名	部位	备注
202	荷叶	睡莲科	植物	莲	*Nelumbo nucifera* Gaertn.	干燥叶	
203	桂枝	樟科	植物	肉桂	*Cinnamomum cassia* Presl	干燥嫩枝	
204	桔梗	桔梗科	植物	桔梗	*Platycodon grandiflorum* (Jacq.) A. DC.	干燥根	
205	桃仁	蔷薇科	植物	桃	*Prunus persica* (L.) Batsch	干燥成熟种子	多基原
206	桃枝	蔷薇科	植物	桃	*Prunus persica* (L.) Batsch	干燥枝条	
207	核桃仁	胡桃科	植物	胡桃	*Juglans regia* L.	干燥成熟种子	
208	夏枯草	唇形科	植物	夏枯草	*Prunella vulgaris* L.	干燥果穗	
209	柴胡	伞形科	植物	柴胡	*Bupleurum chinense* DC.	干燥根	多基原
210	党参	桔梗科	植物	川党参	*Codonopsis tangshen* Oliv.	干燥根	多基原
				党参	*Codonopsis pilosula* (Franch.) Nannf.		
				素花党参	*Codonopsis pilosula* Nannf. var. *modesta* (Nannf.) L. T. Shen		
211	铁皮石斛	兰科	植物	铁皮石斛	*Dendrobium officinale* Kimura et Migo	干燥茎	
212	射干	鸢尾科	植物	射干	*Belamcanda chinensis* (L.) DC.	干燥根茎	
213	徐长卿	萝藦科	植物	徐长卿	*Cynanchum paniculatum* (Bge.) Kitag.	干燥根和根茎	
214	凌霄花	紫葳科	植物	凌霄	*Campsis grandiflora* (Thunb.) K. Schum.	干燥花	多基原
				美洲凌霄	*Campsis radicans* (L.) Seem.		

续表

序号	药材名	科	类别	基原植物名称	基原植物拉丁学名	部位	备注
215	高良姜	姜科	植物	高良姜	*Alpinia officinarum* Hance	干燥根茎	
216	粉葛	豆科	植物	甘葛藤	*Pueraria thomsonii* Benth.	干燥根	
217	益母草	唇形科	植物	益母草	*Leonurus japonicus* Houtt.	新鲜或干燥地上部分	
218	益智	姜科	植物	益智	*Alpinia oxyphylla* Miq.	干燥成熟果实	
219	浙贝母	百合科	植物	浙贝母	*Fritillaria thunbergii* Miq.	干燥鳞茎	
220	桑叶	桑科	植物	桑	*Morus alba* L.	干燥叶	
221	桑白皮	桑科	植物	桑	*Morus alba* L.	干燥根皮	
222	桑枝	桑科	植物	桑	*Morus alba* L.	干燥嫩枝	
223	桑葚	桑科	植物	桑	*Morus alba* L.	干燥果穗	
224	黄芩	唇形科	植物	黄芩	*Scutellaria baicalensis* Georgi	干燥根	
225	黄芪	豆科	植物	蒙古黄芪	*Astragalus membranaceus* (Fisch.) Bge. var. *mongholicus* (Bge.) Hsiao	干燥根	多基原
				膜荚黄芪	*Astragalus membranaceus* (Fisch.) Bge.		
226	黄连	毛茛科	植物	黄连	*Coptis chinensis* Franch.	干燥根茎	多基原
227	黄柏	芸香科	植物	黄皮树	*Phellodendron chinense* Schneid.	干燥树皮	
228	黄蜀葵花	锦葵科	植物	黄蜀葵	*Abelmoschus manihot* (L.) Medic.	干燥花冠	
229	菟丝子	旋花科	植物	菟丝子	*Cuscuta chinensis* Lam.	干燥成熟种子	多基原
230	菊苣	菊科	植物	菊苣	*Cichorium intybus* L.	干燥地上部分、根	多基原
				毛菊苣	*Cichorium glandulosum* Boiss. et Huet		

续表

序号	药材名	科	类别	基原植物名称	基原植物拉丁学名	部位	备注
231	菊花	菊科	植物	菊	*Chrysanthemum morifolium* Ramat.	干燥头状花序	
232	梅花	蔷薇科	植物	梅	*Prunus mume*（Sieb.）Sieb. et Zucc.	干燥花蕾	
233	银杏叶	银杏科	植物	银杏	*Ginkgo biloba* L.	干燥叶	
234	银柴胡	石竹科	植物	银柴胡	*Stellaria dichotoma* L. var. *lanceolata* Bge.	干燥根	
235	甜瓜子	葫芦科	植物	甜瓜	*Cucumis melo* L.	干燥成熟种子	
236	猪牙皂	豆科	植物	皂荚	*Gleditsia sinensis* Lam.	干燥不育果实	
237	猪苓	多孔菌科	真菌	猪苓	*Polyporus umbellatus*（Pers.）Fries	干燥菌核	
238	淡豆豉	豆科	植物	大豆	*Glycine max*（L.）Merr.	成熟种子的发酵加工品	
239	续断	川续断科	植物	川续断	*Dipsacus asper* Wall. ex Henry	干燥根	
240	款冬花	菊科	植物	款冬	*Tussilago farfara* L.	干燥花蕾	
241	棕榈	棕榈科	植物	棕榈	*Trachycarpus fortunei*（Hook. f.）H. Wendl.	干燥叶柄	
242	紫苏子	唇形科	植物	紫苏	*Perilla frutescens*（L.）Britt.	干燥成熟果实	
243	紫苏叶	唇形科	植物	紫苏	*Perilla frutescens*（L.）Britt.	干燥叶（带嫩枝）	
244	紫苏梗	唇形科	植物	紫苏	*Perilla frutescens*（L.）Britt.	干燥茎	
245	紫菀	菊科	植物	紫菀	*Aster tataricus* L. f.	干燥根和根茎	
246	黑芝麻	脂麻科	植物	脂麻	*Sesamum indicum* L.	干燥成熟种子	
247	黑豆	豆科	植物	大豆	*Glycine max*（L.）Merr.	干燥成熟种子	

续表

序号	药材名	科	类别	基原植物名称	基原植物拉丁学名	部位	备注
248	黑种草子	毛茛科	植物	腺毛黑种草	*Nigella glandulifera* Freyn et Sint.	干燥成熟种子	多基原
249	湖北贝母	百合科	植物	湖北贝母	*Fritillaria hupehensis* Hsiao et K. C. Hsia	干燥鳞茎	
250	蓖麻子	大戟科	植物	蓖麻	*Ricinus communis* L.	干燥成熟种子	
251	蒲公英	菊科	植物	药用蒲公英	*Taraxacum officinale* F. H. Wigg.	干燥全草	多基原
252	椿皮	苦木科	植物	臭椿	*Ailanthus altissima* (Mill.) Swingle	干燥根皮、干皮	
253	槐花	豆科	植物	槐	*Sophora japonica* L.	干燥花及花蕾	
254	槐角	豆科	植物	槐	*Sophora japonica* L.	干燥成熟果实	
255	路路通	金缕梅科	植物	枫香树	*Liquidambar formosana* Hance	干燥成熟果序	
256	锦灯笼	茄科	植物	酸浆	*Physalis alkekengi* L. var. *franchetii* (Mast.) Makino	干燥宿萼、带果实的宿萼	
257	蓼大青叶	蓼科	植物	蓼蓝	*Polygonum tinctorium* Ait.	干燥叶	
258	榧子	红豆杉科	植物	榧	*Torreya grandis* Fort.	干燥成熟种子	
259	槟榔	棕榈科	植物	槟榔	*Areca catechu* L.	干燥成熟种子	
260	罂粟壳	罂粟科	植物	罂粟	*Papaver somniferum* L.	干燥成熟果壳	
261	辣椒	茄科	植物	辣椒或其栽培变种	*Capsicum annuum* L.	干燥成熟果实	
262	稻芽	禾本科	植物	稻	*Oryza sativa* L.	成熟果实经发芽干燥的炮制加工品	
263	薤白	百合科	植物	薤	*Allium chinense* G. Don	干燥鳞茎	多基原

续表

序号	药材名	科	类别	基原植物名称	基原植物拉丁学名	部位	备注
264	薏苡仁	禾本科	植物	薏苡	*Coix lacryma-jobi* L. var. *ma-yuen* (Roman.)Stapf	干燥成熟种仁	
265	薄荷	唇形科	植物	薄荷	*Mentha haplocalyx* Briq.	干燥地上部分	
266	颠茄草	茄科	植物	颠茄	*Atropa belladonna* L.	干燥全草	
267	橘红	芸香科	植物	橘及其栽培变种	*Citrus reticulata* Blanco	干燥外层果皮	
268	橘核	芸香科	植物	橘及其栽培变种	*Citrus reticulata* Blanco	干燥成熟种子	
269	藁本	伞形科	植物	辽藁本	*Ligusticum jeholense* Nakai et Kitag.	干燥根茎和根	多基原
270	檀香	檀香科	植物	檀香	*Santalum album* L.	树干的干燥心材	
271	藕节	睡莲科	植物	莲	*Nelumbo nucifera* Gaertn.	干燥根茎节部	
272	瞿麦	石竹科	植物	石竹	*Dianthus chinensis* L.	干燥地上部分	多基原

注：1. 药材种类来源：来自于2015年版《中国药典》中，基原为植物（含菌类，下同）的中药材。炮制品未单列（如干姜、炮姜只列出了干姜，炮姜未列出），不同部位入药的药材单列（如紫苏子、紫苏叶、紫苏梗），按药典单独收录。共有来自255种植物基原的272种药材属于人工栽培。

2. "人工栽培"标准：在生产上已实现大规模人工种植，栽培技术成熟或较成熟，人工种植药材已占市场主流。对于多基原药材，只列出属于"人工栽培"的基原植物，如甘草药材的基原植物，只列出已有大规模人工种植的甘草*Glycyrrhiza uralensis*，而光果甘草*G.glabra*和胀果甘草*G.inflata*主要来自野生，未收录，并在备注栏提示该药材来自"多基原"。对于栽培技术已基本成功，但种植规模小，栽培品尚未成为市场和临床用药主要来源（如红景天、半边莲、羌活、黄精、重楼等），以及主要来自进口，在国内暂无大规模栽培的药材（如丁香、肉豆蔻、胖大海等）未收录。

3. 排序方式：与《中国药典》一致，按药材首字笔画排序。

Guideline on Processing Study of Prepared Slices/ Decoction pieces for New Traditional Chinese Medicines (TCMs) (Trial)

I. Overview

The processing of decoction pieces for new TCMs is closely associated with the quality control and therapeutic effects of preparations of new TCMs. It is necessary to comply with TCM theories during the R&D of new TCMs, and conduct studies based on the characteristics of new TCMs and study design needs. This guideline will provide technical guidance on the processing of decoction pieces for new TCMs, so as to provide safe and effective decoction pieces with stable quality for the production of TCM preparations.

This guideline mainly includes the processing technology, adjuvants used for processing, standards for decoction pieces, packaging and storage, etc., and are intended to provide a reference for studies on the processing of decoction pieces for new TCMs.

II. General Principles

(I) Following TCM theories

The study of decoction pieces processing should follow the theory of traditional Chinese medicine, inherit traditional processing experience and technology, and uphold the principle of preserving traditions while pursuing innovation. The processing methods, process parameters, degree of processing, storage conditions, and maintenance management of decoction pieces should respect the traditional processing experience and techniques. It is encouraged to conduct studies on the processing of decoction pieces by integrating traditional experience and modern science and technology.

(II) Meeting the needs of study design for new TCMs

Studies on the processing of decoction pieces should meet the needs of study design for new TCMs. Processing parameters and quality requirements should be determined based on the studies on critical quality attributes of TCM crude drugs and the manufacturing equipment capacity, etc. For decoction pieces of new TCMs, if other processing methods are necessary, sufficient studies should be conducted. The specifications of decoction pieces for new TCMs may be different from those for clinical dispensing. Appropriate specifications of and quality requirements for decoction pieces should be determined based on the characteristics of TCM crude drugs, production scale of preparations, extraction process characteristics, and quality control requirements in the context of following the traditional processing methods. The processing of decoction pieces should comply with the requirements of *Good Manufacturing Practice*.

(III) Establishing and improving quality standards

Corresponding standards for decoction pieces should be established and improved according to the needs of study design for new TCMs and the study results of correlation among quality standards for TCM crude drugs, decoction pieces and TCM preparations. Test items should be determined by taking into account their correlation with safety and efficacy. TCM crude drugs and adjuvants for processing should meet relevant standards. Corresponding standards should be established for those decoction pieces and adjuvants without standards. Standards that have been established but cannot meet the quality control requirements should be improved.

(IV) Strengthening quality control throughout the process

Whole quality control should be implemented throughout the processing of decoction pieces. Study and control should be strengthened for critical parts and risk control points that may cause fluctuations in the quality of TCM preparations during processing. Documentation for the processing of decoction pieces should be standardized. In addition, it is encouraged to establish a traceability system for decoction pieces using modern information technologies for tracing the source and destination.

III. Basic Contents

(I) Processing technology

On the basis of inheriting traditional technologies, studies should be conducted on specific processing technologies such as cleansing, cutting, and roasting and broiling to determine process parameters and manufacturing equipment, etc. by considering TCM theories, clinical medication, and the needs of study design for new TCMs. In addition, the processes should be validated. The manufacturing equipment used in processing should be appropriate to the processing technologies, production scale and quality requirements for decoction pieces.

1. Cleansing

Common methods include picking, winnowing, purifying by water, sifting, cutting, scraping, peeling, eliminating, brushing, wiping, grinding, and bumping, etc. Cleansing should be performed depending on TCM crude drugs and production requirements of TCM preparations. Appropriate cleansing methods should be selected through studies to meet the specified purity requirements.

While decoction pieces are directly used in oral preparations as raw powder after being pulverized, studies should be conducted on the types and levels of microbial contamination in TCM crude drugs (decoction pieces) during the cleansing process, such as washing. Suitable measures such as methods, equipment, and conditions should be adopted to effectively reduce the microbial contamination level in the context of ensuring the quality of decoction pieces.

2. Cutting

Except for a few TCM crude drugs that are cut in the fresh or dry condition, most TCM crude drugs need to be softened to facilitate cutting. Common softening methods include spraying, elutriating, soaking, flushing, and moistening, etc. Appropriate softening methods should be selected through studies to avoid losing or damaging active components. Process parameters such as specific method, equipment, water absorption, temperature, and time for softening should be defined.

It is encouraged to carry out studies on new cutting techniques in the context of respecting traditional processing experience, ensuring the quality of decoction pieces, and complying with the relevant requirements of *Good Manufacturing Practice*, and process parameters and quality standards should be studied and established. If freshly sliced varieties from the places of growth are not recorded in national drug standards or standards of provinces, autonomous regions and municipalities directly under the Central Government for TCM crude drugs (decoction pieces) or in the specifications for processing, sufficient comparative studies with traditional methods should be conducted. While TCM crude drugs are processed into decoction pieces suitable for extraction by smashing or other techniques, the rationality of the method should be studied and explained, and appropriate methods and parameters should be selected based on characteristics of TCM crude drugs to ensure that the size distribution of the decoction pieces after smashing falls into a suitable range.

3. Roasting and broiling

Common methods include stir-frying, stir-frying with liquid adjuvants, calcining, steaming, boiling, multi-step processing, and roasting, etc. The critical process parameters should be studied and determined by fully considering the impact of temperature, time, types and amounts of adjuvant materials used on the quality of decoction pieces, as well as the characteristics and specifications of the decoction pieces, production equipment, and scale, etc. For example, if stir-frying is used, the equipment (e.g., model, working principle, and critical technical parameters), specifications of decoction pieces, feeding amount, stir-frying temperature (determine the test point of stir-frying temperature based on the equipment), rotational speed, and stir-frying time should be determined. If adjuvants are needed, the type, amount, and adding way should be determined. It is encouraged to adopt methods that combine traditional experience with modern technology for judgment. For example, intelligent recognition, image comparison, and other methods can be used to assess the processing degree of medicinal slices based on their characteristics, and a rational range should be defined to ensure the stability of the quality between batches.

For special roasting and broiling methods such as fermentation, germination, water-grinding, and frost-like powder making, the traditional processing technologies should be fully respected, and critical process parameters and manufacturing equipment should be determined.

4. Drying

The decoction pieces needing drying during processing should be treated timely to avoid microbial contamination, deterioration, and spoilage caused by delayed drying. Common drying methods include drying under sunshine, drying in the shade, and drying in a stove or oven. Appropriate drying methods and conditions should be selected by taking into account the properties of decoction pieces. Studies should be conducted on the drying equipment, temperature, duration, and thickness of decoction pieces, and the method and process parameters should be defined. Effective strategies should be taken during the drying process to prevent contamination and cross-contamination of decoction pieces, and novel low-temperature drying technologies are encouraged to be used.

(II) Adjuvants used for processing

1. Preparation of adjuvants used for processing

If the adjuvants used for processing are outsourced, those prepared with traditional technologies should be selected. For example, vinegar should be brewed from rice, wheat, and sorghum, etc., without adding coloring agents or flavor agents, etc.

If adjuvants used during processing procedures are self-prepared, such adjuvants should be prepared using the methods recorded in the specifications for processing of decoction pieces and standards for TCM crude drugs and prepared slices/decoction pieces. In-process control should be strengthened to ensure stable quality of the adjuvants used during processing procedures. If necessary, preparation methods should be studied to confirm the preparation methods and process parameters. For example, licorice juice and ginger juice that are prepared right before use should be prepared using the methods specified in the specifications for processing, and the process parameters should be studied and detailed (e.g., amount of water added, number of times of extraction, and decoction duration).

If the preparation method of adjuvants is not recorded in the national drug standards or standards of provinces, autonomous regions and municipalities directly under the Central Government for TCM crude drugs and prepared slices/ decoction pieces or in the specifications for processing, appropriate preparation methods and process parameters should be determined through studies on the basis of respecting traditional experience.

For adjuvants derived from animals, inactivation study and verification should be performed on pathogenic microorganisms that may cause zoonoses.

2. Standards for adjuvants used for processing

If the adjuvants used for processing already have pharmaceutical standards or edible standards , the original standards can still be used. If necessary, the standards can be improved based on traditional experience and processing requirements. If there are no such standards, a quality standard meeting pharmaceutical requirements should be studied and established based on quality characteristics of the adjuvants.

Targeted studies should be strengthened on adjuvants of special origins. Heavy metals and harmful elements should be studied for those adjuvants originated from minerals. Where necessary, corresponding test items should be established in the standards for adjuvants. The use of adjuvants derived from animals should be evaluated for pathogens, and if necessary, corresponding test methods should be established.

The substances for preparing adjuvants used for processing should also meet the quality requirements of related products.

3. Packaging and storage of adjuvants used for processing

Appropriate packaging materials/containers should be selected according to the characteristics of adjuvants. If necessary, studies on the compatibility between adjuvants and packaging materials/containers should be performed. In addition, storage conditions of the adjuvants used for processing should be determined on the basis of the results from stability studies.

(Ⅲ) Standards for decoction pieces

The standards for decoction pieces should highlight the processing characteristics of TCMs, summarize traditional processing experience, reflect quality characteristics, demonstrate the correlation among quality standards for TCM crude drugs, decoction pieces and TCM preparations, and address the requirements for overall quality management of the complex TCM system. Developing reasonable standards for decoction pieces and implementing quality control throughout processing are beneficial for ensuring stable quality of the decoction pieces. For decoction pieces subject to special processing or those characterized by "different functions between unprocessed and processed ones", specific quality control methods should be established to distinguish from those non- processing ones.

The standards for decoction pieces should generally include: name, origin, place of origin, processing, appearance, identification, tests, extractive, assay, property and flavor and meridian tropism, functions and indications, usage and dosage, precautions, and storage, etc. In addition, it is encouraged to conduct studies on characteristics and common problems such as coloring, weight gain, adulteration, and likeliness to mildew and decay of the decoction pieces. According to the needs of risk management, it may be necessary to add specific test items according to the relevant national supplementary test methods or studies, establish corresponding test methods, and include them into standards, when necessary.

The main study contents and general requirements of some items in the standards for decoction pieces are briefly described below:

[Processing] To clarify the requirements for the processing method, critical process parameters, types and amounts of adjuvants, and degree of processing of decoction pieces.

[Appearance] To describe the shape, size, color, taste, flavor, and texture according to characteristics of the decoction pieces for actual production. Colored pictures of the decoction pieces should be attached, if necessary.

[Identification] To establish a specific identification method for decoction pieces by adopting methods such as traditional experience-based methods, microscopic identification, chemical reactions, chromatography, and spectroscopy, etc.

Especially for counterfeit or easily-confused decoction pieces, a comprehensive comparative study should be conducted to demonstrate the specificity of the method. In the process of studying identification methods, it is encouraged to improve the specificity of identification methods using reference TCM crude drugs (decoction pieces), reference extracts, and standard spectrum, etc. In order to improve the specificity of the thin layer chromatography identification method, descriptions of the number, color, and location of identification spots should be improved according to study results.

[Test] Water content, total ash, acid-insoluble ash, and sulfur dioxide residues in decoction pieces should be studied and if necessary, included in specifications, and reasonable limits should be established. Safety test items such as heavy metals and harmful elements, pesticide residues, and mycotoxin should be studied in conjunction with the source of TCM crude drugs and manufacturing and preparation process and if necessary, included in standards. For toxic decoction pieces or decoction pieces considered toxic upon modern studies, the test item for the limit of toxic components should be established in the standards. For directly-crushed decoction pieces, microbial test items should be added to the quality standards based on the manufacturing processes of TCM preparations. Specific test items should be established for decoction pieces originated from animals, minerals, and resins or fermented techniques according to their characteristics.

[Extractive] Select appropriate solvents to establish the test method for extractives according to components contained in the decoction pieces and the extraction process of TCM preparations. In addition, the correlation with TCM crude drugs and TCM preparations should be studied, and rational limits should be established.

[Assay] A method for assay of active makers, analytical makers or major chemical classes related to safety and efficacy should be studied and established based on quality characteristics of the decoction pieces and TCM preparations. The correlation with TCM crude drugs and TCM preparations should be studied, and reasonable limits should be defined. For the toxic components that are also active components in the decoction pieces, a method for their assay should be established, and reasonable limits should be defined.

If the quality control items in the quality standard for a TCM preparation are related to the quality of decoction pieces, corresponding quality control items should be established in the standards for decoction pieces and rational quality requirements should be determined according to study results.

(IV) Packaging and storage

The packaging and storage of decoction pieces should facilitate their preservation and use. Appropriate packaging materials (containers) and storage conditions should be determined according to characteristics of decoction pieces, the actual production and processing experience.

1. Packaging

Appropriate packaging materials (containers) and package specifications should be selected according to characteristics of decoction pieces and their storage and use requirements, in conjunction with the actual production experience. The packaging of decoction pieces should not affect their quality, and should facilitate their storage, transportation and use. Packaging materials and containers in direct contact with decoction pieces should comply with national drug and food package quality standards. Attention should be paid to the packaging of special decoction pieces that are prone to volatilization, contamination, dampness and deterioration. The packages of decoction pieces should have obvious packaging marks and comply with relevant national regulations.

2. Storage

Combining traditional experience and the characteristics of decoction pieces, Appropriate storage conditions and suitable maintenance techniques should be determined based on the stability test results of the decoction pieces. Necessary maintenance and management should be carried out during the storage period. If insect and moth proofing is required, the methods and parameters used should be studied. Maintenance should not affect the quality of decoction pieces, and detailed records should be maintained.

IV. Main References

1. China Food and Drug Administration. *Technical Guidelines for Pretreatment of TCM crude drugs for Traditional Chinese Medicines and Natural Medicines*. 2005.

2. Ministry of Health. *Good Manufacturing Practice (2010 Revision)*. 2011.

中药新药用饮片炮制研究技术指导原则（试行）

一、概述

中药新药用饮片炮制与新药制剂的质量控制和临床疗效密切相关，需要在新药研制阶段遵循中医药理论，围绕新药特点和研究设计需要开展研究。为指导中药新药用饮片炮制研究，为中药制剂生产提供安全、有效和质量稳定的饮片，制定本指导原则。

本指导原则主要包括炮制工艺、炮制用辅料、饮片标准、包装与贮藏等内容，旨在为中药新药用饮片炮制的研究提供参考。

二、一般原则

（一）遵循中医药理论

饮片炮制研究应遵循中医药理论，继承传统炮制经验和技术，守正创新。饮片炮制方法、工艺参数、炮制程度、贮藏条件及养护管理等应尊重传统炮制经验和技术。鼓励采用传统经验与现代科学技术相结合的方式开展饮片炮制研究。

（二）满足中药新药研究设计的需要

饮片炮制研究应满足中药新药研究设计的需要，根据药材的关键质量属性、生产设备能力等研究确定炮制工艺参数及质量要求。中药新药用饮片，如确需采用其他炮制方法的，应进行充分的研究。中药新药用饮片与临床调剂用饮片的规格可不同，应在遵循传统炮制方法基础上，根据药材特点及制剂生产规模、提取工艺特点、质量控制要求等确定合适的饮片规格和质量要求。饮片炮制应符合药品生产质量管理规范的要求。

（三）建立完善质量标准

根据中药新药研究设计的需要，药材、饮片及中药制剂质量标准关联性的研究结果，建立完善相应的饮片标准，其检测项目的设立应关注与安全性、有效性的关联。炮制用药材及辅料均应符合相关标准。无标准的饮片、炮制用辅料，应研究建立相应的标准。已有标准但尚不能满足质量控制需要的，应研究完善相应的标准。

（四）加强全过程质量控制

饮片炮制应进行全过程质量控制，对炮制过程中导致中药制剂质量波动的关键环节和风险控制点加强研究和控制，规范饮片炮制的文件管理。鼓励运用现代信息技术建立饮片追溯体系，实现来源可查、去向可追。

三、基本内容

（一）炮制工艺

根据中医药理论、临床用药及中药新药研究设计需要，在继承传统工艺的基础上，对药材进行净制、切制、炮炙等炮制具体工艺研究，确定工艺参数、生产设备等，并进行工艺验证。炮制所用的生产设备应与炮制工艺、生产规模及饮片质量要求相适应。

1. 净制

常用的方法有挑选、风选、水选、筛选、剪切、刮、削、剔除、刷、擦、碾、撞等。应根据药材情况及中药制剂生产要求进行净制，通过研究选择合适的净制方法，达到规定的净度要求。

饮片粉碎后以药粉直接入药的口服制剂，应在水洗等净制环节对药材（饮片）中微生物污染种类及污染水平进行研究，在保证饮片质量的前提下，采用合理的方法、设备、条件等，有效降低微生物污染水平。

2. 切制

除少数药材鲜切、干切外，一般需经过软化处理，使药材利于切制。常用的软化方法包括喷淋、淘洗、泡、漂、润等，应研究选择合适的软化方法，避免有效成份损失或破坏，明确软化的具体方法、设备、吸水量、温度、时间等工艺参数。

鼓励开展新型切制技术研究，应以尊重传统加工炮制经验和保证饮片质量为前提，并符合药品生产质量管理规范的有关要求，研究制定工艺参数和质量标准。产地趁鲜切制品种未收载于国家药品标准或省、自治区、直辖市的药材（饮片）标准或炮制规范的，应与传统方法进行充分的对比研究。药材采用破碎等技术加工成适合提取的饮片形式的，应研究说明方法的合理性，并根据药材特性选择合适的方法及参数，使破碎后饮片的大小分布在合适的范围内。

3. 炮炙

常用的方法有炒、炙、煅、蒸、煮、复制、煨等。炮炙应充分考虑温度、时间、所用辅料的种类和用量等对饮片质量的影响，结合饮片特点及规格、生产设备及规模等，研究确定炮炙关键工艺参数。如炒制，一般应明确炒药设备（如型号、工作原理及关键技术参数等）、饮片规格、投料量、炒制温度（应结合设备情况明确炒制温度的测试点）、转速、炒制时间等工艺参数。如需加辅料，应明确辅料种类、用量、加入方式等内容。炮炙程度（即终点控制）鼓励采用传统经验与现代技术相结合的方法进行判断，如可采用智能识别、图像对比等方法，根据性状对饮片炮炙程度进行判断，规定合理范围，保证批间质量的稳定。

对于发酵法、发芽法、水飞法、制霜法等特殊炮炙方法，应充分尊重传统炮制工艺，明确关键工艺参数、生产设备等。

4. 干燥

炮制过程中需干燥的饮片应及时处理，避免因干燥不及时而引起微生物污染及变质、腐败等。常用的干燥方法包括晒干或阴干、烘干等。应根据具体饮片性质选择适宜的干燥方法和条件，应对干燥设备、温度、时间、物料厚度等进行研究，明确方法及工艺参数。在干燥过程中应采取有效措施防止饮片被污染和交叉污染，鼓励采用新型低温干燥技术。

（二）炮制用辅料

1. 炮制用辅料制备

炮制用辅料需外购的，一般应选用以传统工艺制备的产品。如醋，应为米、麦、高粱等酿制而成，不得添加着色剂、调味剂等。

炮制用辅料需自行制备的，一般应按饮片炮制规范、药材／饮片标准收载的制备方法制备，加强过程控制，保证炮制用辅料质量稳定，必要时应进行制备方法的研究，明确制备方法及工艺参数。如甘草汁、姜汁等临用前配制的，应按炮制规范规定的方法制备，并研究细化工艺参数（如加水量、提取次数、煎煮时间等）。

辅料制备方法未收载于国家药品标准或省、自治区、直辖市的药材／饮片标准或炮制规范的，应尊重传统经验，进行制备方法研究，明确适宜的制备方法及工艺参数。

来源于动物的辅料，应对可能引发人畜共患病的病原微生物进行灭活研究和验证。

2. 炮制用辅料标准

炮制用辅料已有药用或食用标准的，一般可沿用原标准，必要时根据传统经验及炮制要求进行完善。无标准的，应结合其质量特点，研究建立符合药用要求的质量标准。

特殊来源的辅料，应加强针对性研究。如来源于矿物的辅料，应对重金属及有害元素等进行研究，必要时在辅料标准中建立相应检测项；来源于动物的辅料，应对可能引发人畜共患病的病原微生物等进行研究，必要时建立相应检测方法。

制备炮制用辅料所用原材料也应符合相关产品的质量要求。

3.炮制用辅料的包装及贮藏

应根据辅料特点选择合适的包装材料/容器，必要时应进行辅料与包材的相容性研究。根据稳定性研究结果确定炮制用辅料的贮藏条件。

（三）饮片标准

饮片标准应突出中药炮制特色，注重对传统炮制经验进行总结，反映饮片的质量特点，体现饮片与药材、中药制剂质量标准的关联性，体现中药复杂体系整体质量控制的要求。制定合理的饮片标准，并对饮片炮制进行全过程质量控制，有利于保证饮片质量的稳定。采用特殊方法炮制或具有"生熟异治"特点的饮片应建立区别于对应生品的专属性质控方法。

饮片标准的内容一般包括：名称、基原、产地、炮制、性状、鉴别、检查、浸出物、含量测定、性味与归经、功能与主治、用法与用量、注意、贮藏等。另外，鼓励针对饮片特点和染色、增重、掺杂使假、易霉烂变质等常见问题加强研究，根据风险管理的需要，参照国家相关补充检验方法或研究增加针对性的检测项目，建立相应的检测方法，必要时列入标准。

以下就饮片标准中部分项目的主要研究内容及一般要求进行简要说明：

【炮制】明确饮片的炮制方法、关键工艺参数、辅料种类及用量、炮制程度的要求等。

【性状】根据实际生产用饮片的特点描述其形状、大小、色泽、味道、气味、质地等；必要时附饮片彩色图片。

【鉴别】采用传统经验方法、显微鉴别法、化学反应法、色谱法、光谱法等手段建立饮片的专属性鉴别方法，尤其是存在伪品、易混淆品的饮片，应进行充分的对比研究说明其专属性。在鉴别方法的研究过程中，鼓励采用对照药材（饮片）、对照提取物、标准图谱等为对照，提高鉴别方法的专属性。为提高薄层色谱鉴别方法的专属性，应根据研究结果完善鉴别斑点个数、颜色、位置等内容的描述。

【检查】应对饮片中水分、总灰分、酸不溶性灰分、二氧化硫残留量等项目进行研究，必要时列入标准，并制定合理的限度。对于重金属及有害元素、农药残留、真菌毒素等安全性检查项目，应结合药材来源、生产加工过程等研究，必要时列入标准。毒性饮片或现代研究公认有毒性的饮片，标准中应建立毒性成份的限量检查项。饮片直接粉碎入药的，应根据中药制剂工艺情况，在质量标准中增加微生物检查项。动物类、矿物类、发酵类、树脂类等饮片，应根据其特点建立针对性的检查项。

【浸出物】应结合饮片中成份、中药制剂提取工艺等因素，选择合适的溶剂建立浸出物检测方法，并考察与药材、中药制剂的相关性，制定合理的限度。

【含量测定】根据饮片及中药制剂的质量特点，研究建立与安全性、有效性相关联的有效成份、指标成份或大类成份等的含量测定方法，考察与药材、中药制剂的相关性，并规定合理的含量限度。饮片中既是毒性成份又是有效成份的，应建立其含量测定方法，并规定合理的含量限度。

中药制剂质量标准中建立的质控项目与饮片质量相关的，应在饮片标准中建立相应质控项目，并根据研究结果确定合理的质量要求。

（四）包装与贮藏

饮片的包装、贮藏应便于保存和使用，根据饮片的特性，结合实际生产加工经验，确定合适的包装材料（容器）和贮藏条件。

1. 包装

应根据饮片特点、保存及使用要求，结合实际生产经验，选择合适的包装材料（容器）及包装规格。饮片的包装应不影响饮片的质量，且方便储存、运输、使用。直接接触饮片的包装材料和容器应符合国家药品、食品包装质量标准。关注易挥发、易污染、受潮易变质等特殊饮片的包装。饮片包装上应有明显的包装标识，并应符合国家相关规定。

2. 贮藏

结合传统经验及饮片特点，根据饮片的稳定性考察结果确定合适的贮藏条件和适宜的养护技术。贮藏期间需进行必要的养护管理，如需采取防虫防蛀等处理的，应对所用方法、参数等进行研究，养护处理应不影响饮片质量，并详细记录。

四、主要参考文献

1. 国家食品药品监督管理局.《中药、天然药物原料的前处理技术指导原则》. 2005 年.

2. 卫生部.《药品生产质量管理规范（2010 年修订）》. 2011 年.

Guideline for Homogenization Studies of Traditional Chinese Medicines (TCMs) (Trial)

I. Overview

The ingredients of TCM preparations are originated from TCM crude drugs. In the production process of TCM preparations, quality differences of TCM crude drugs may influence that of ingredients, intermediates and finished products, directly affecting the batch-to-batch quality stability of TCM preparations. This Guideline is developed to reduce quality fluctuations for these reasons, improve the batch-to-batch quality consistency of TCM preparations, and promote high-quality development of the TCM industry.

The term "homogenization" mentioned in the Guideline refers to appropriate measures in the feeding process of qualified ingredients with certain quality fluctuations across different batches, without changing the feeding amount, so as to reduce batch-to-batch quality fluctuations of TCM preparations and achieve the expected quality objectives.

The Guideline is intended to provide a reference for homogenization studies of TCM preparations. The methods should be determined according to specific study situations. Homogenization is not a necessary measure for the production of TCM preparations.

II. Basic Principles

(I) Aim for the batch-to-batch quality stability of preparations

Batch-to-batch quality stability of TCM preparations is the basis for ensuring their clinical safety and efficacy, and it is also the goal of homogenization studies. Evaluation indicators that can reflect safety, efficacy, and overall quality of medicines should be selected as much as possible for the homogenization studies. Reasonable homogenization requirements should be determined based on the quality objectives, safety and efficacy study data of TCM preparations, relevant knowledge gained from the R&D and production of medicines, and in conjunction with the characteristics of specific products and process study data, so as to ensure the batch-to-batch quality stability of TCM preparations.

(II) Comply with the requirements of the *Good Manufacturing Practice*

The homogenization process should comply with the requirements of the *Good Manufacturing Practice*. If homogenization is adopted, it should be included in the quality management system. The homogenization method should be thoroughly studied and validated, and quality risk management be strengthened. Potential quality risks should be proactively identified, scientifically evaluated and effectively controlled. A standardized operating procedure should be established to effectively prevent potential risks such as contamination and errors during the homogenization process. Homogenization operations should have complete records, and the contents should be true, accurate and reliable. The source, destination, and quality information of TCM crude drugs, prepared slices/decoction pieces, intermediates, and corresponding preparations should be traced according to these records.

(III) Carry out targeted studies based on the characteristics of the product

Different feeding forms for ingredients such as decoction pieces and extracts, different quality differences, so homongenization studies should be conducted based on the characteristics of different products of TCM preparations. For formulas containing ingredients originated from toxic TCM crude drugs, special attention should be paid to safety requirements.

III. Main Contents

(I) Object of homongenization

Considering the characteristics of ingredients and the manufacturing process of TCM preparations, the object of homongenization is an ingredient under [Formula] of quality standards for TCM preparations, including decoction pieces and extracts.

(II) Preparation before homongenization

1. Quality qualification. The ingredients for homongenization should meet the requirements of national drug standards or drug registration standards as well as the requirements of internal control quality standards. If ingredients contain decoction pieces and extracts that do not have national drug standards or drug registration standards, quality standards for such ingredients should be established separately and attached to quality standards for preparations. The quality standards for extracts should include their preparation processes.

2. Correlation study of TCM crude drugs. It is required to strengthen the study on the quality correlation between the object of homongenization and TCM crude drugs. It is encouraged to establish TCM crude drugs bases, set up a quality traceability system for TCM crude drugs, and ensure relatively stable quality and sources of TCM crude drugs.

3. Representativeness of samples. Reasonable sampling methods should be used to ensure that the test data can better reflect the actual quality situation of the object of homongenization.

4. Timeliness of data. Attention should be paid to the timeliness of quality test data of the object of homongenization. A rational deadline for using relevant test data should be determined in conjunction with the stability study results. Re-test should be performed before homongenization, if necessary.

(III) Selection of homongenization indicators

Adequate studies should be carried out based on the characteristics of the object of homongenization, and homongenization indicators that meet the quality objectives and risk management requirements of preparations should be selected. Homongenization indicators are mainly those associated with critical quality attributes of TCM preparations, such as the content of active components, markers, and major chemical classes; extractives content; fingerprint chromatogram; and bioassay, etc. It is encouraged to use the method that can test multiple markers at the same time and to use new techniques and methods that can reflect the quality of medicines.

(IV) Quality requirements for homongenization

The batch-to-batch quality stability of preparations produced after homongenization should be considered as the objective. Targeted studies should be conducted based on the characteristics of the product to determine reasonable homongenization requirements (i.e., the limit and range of homongenization indicators or the design space composed of multiple indicators) to improve the limit and range of preparation indicators. With the accumulation of the data on R&D, production and application, the design space can be continuously optimized.

General considerations for determining homongenization requirements include:

1. The test data of multiple batches of samples used for drug clinical trials (mainly including the samples used for phase II, III, and IV clinical trials, bioequivalence studies, and real-world studies) have an important value in determining limits and ranges.

2. In the context of insufficient clinical study data, study data of non-clinical pharmacodynamics, toxicology, and pharmacokinetics, etc. also have certain reference value.

3. Transfer rules of chemical components among ingredients, intermediates, and preparations, as well as quality objectives of corresponding preparations.

4. Relevant knowledge obtained from the R&D, technology transfer, and commercial-scale production of medicines, including statistical analysis results of process study and production data of multiple batches.

(V) Calculation method of homongenization

Homongenization calculation is intended to calculate the number of batches and proportion of the object of homongenization to meet homongenization requirements based on the quality test data of different batches of the object of homongenization. Homongenization should not change the feeding amount. In principle, any calculation method that can meet homongenization requirements may be used. It is suggested to pay attention to whether the relevant data has additivity. For example, similarity should not be directly calculated during fingerprint data calculating, while peak area per unit (A/W) can be used instead.

(VI) Others

1. One or more ingredients with greater batch-to-batch quality differences may require honogenization, or all ingredients can be subject to be homongenized depending on the products.

2. If an ingredient is originated from TCM crude drugs and prepared slices/decoction pieces of different origins, the origins should be fixed. If it is difficult to fix the origins, the feeding proportion of the decoction pieces of different origins should be determined, and then the decoction pieces of the same origin be homongenized.

3. Where the quality of samples before and after homongenization is evaluated by fingerprint chromatograms, in addition to similarity, it is recommended to add the range of fluctuation of the peak area of principal chromatographic peaks, the number of common peaks, the number of non-common peaks, the sum of peak areas, and the peak characteristics of fingerprint chromatograms (e.g., the size ranking of the peak area of principal chromatographic peaks or the proportion of the peak area of principal chromatographic peaks) depending on circumstances.

中药均一化研究技术指导原则（试行）

一、概述

中药制剂的处方药味源自中药材。在中药制剂的生产过程中，中药材的质量差异会传递至处方药味、中间体及成品，直接影响中药制剂批间质量的稳定。为减少此类原因导致的质量波动，提高中药制剂批间质量一致性，推动中药产业高质量发展，制定本指导原则。

本指导原则中的"均一化"是指：为减少中药制剂批间质量波动并达到预期质量目标，在不改变投料量的前提下，对不同批次的具有一定质量波动的合格处方药味，采用适当方法投料的措施。

本指导原则旨在为中药制剂的均一化研究提供参考，其方法应根据具体情况研究确定。均一化不是中药制剂生产必须采用的措施。

二、基本原则

（一）以制剂批间质量稳定为目标

中药制剂批间质量稳定是保证其临床用药安全有效的基础，也是均一化研究的目标。均一化研究应尽可能选择反映药品安全性、有效性及整体质量状况的评价指标。根据中药制剂的质量目标、安全性及有效性研究数据、药品研发及生产获得的相关知识，结合具体产品的特点和工艺研究数据，确定合理的均一化要求，保证中药制剂批间质量相对稳定。

（二）符合药品生产质量管理规范要求

均一化过程应符合药品生产质量管理规范的要求。采用均一化处理的，应将均一化纳入质量管理体系。均一化方法应经充分研究及验证，加强质量风险管理，主动识别、科学评估和有效控制潜在的质量风险。应建立均一化操作规程，有效防止均一化过程中可能的污染、差错等风险。均一化操作应有完整记录，内容真实、准确、可靠。根据记录可追溯药材、饮片、中间体及相关制剂的来源、去向及质量信息。

（三）根据品种特点开展针对性研究

饮片、提取物等处方药味的投料形式不同，质量差异有别，应根据中药制剂品种的特点开展均一化研究。对于处方含有源自毒性药材的处方药味，应特别关注安全性方面的要求。

三、主要内容

（一）均一化对象

从中药制剂处方药味及生产工艺的特点考虑，均一化对象为中药制剂质量标准【处方】项下的药味，包括饮片、提取物等。

（二）均一化前的准备

1. 质量合格。均一化用处方药味应符合国家药品标准或药品注册标准的要求，同时也需符合内控质量标准的要求。如处方药味含有无国家药品标准且不具有药品注册标准的中药饮片、提取物，应单独建立该药味的质量标准，并附于制剂标准中，提取物的质量标准应包括其制备工艺。

2. 药材相关研究。应加强均一化对象与药材之间的质量相关性研究。鼓励建立药材基地，建立药材质量追溯体系，保证药材质量及来源的相对稳定。

3. 取样的代表性。应采用合理的取样方法，使检验数据较好反映均一化对象的实际质量状况。

4. 数据的时效性。应关注均一化对象质量检验数据的时效性，结合稳定性考察结果，确定相关检验数据合理使用的期限，必要时在均一化前重新检验。

（三）均一化指标选择

应根据均一化对象的特点开展充分研究，选择满足制剂质量目标及风险管理要求的均一化指标。均一化指标主要是与中药制剂关键质量属性相关的指标，如有效成份、指标成份、大类成份的含量；浸出物量；指纹图谱；生物活性等。鼓励采用同时测定多个成份的方法及反映药品质量的新技术、新方法。

（四）均一化质量要求

应以均一化后制成的制剂批间质量稳定为目标，根据品种特点开展针对性研究，合理确定均一化要求（如均一化指标的限度范围或多个指标构成的设计空间），以完善制剂指标的限度范围。随着研发、生产和使用数据的积累，该设计空间可不断优化。

确定均一化要求的一般考虑：

1. 药品临床试验用多批次样品（主要包括Ⅱ、Ⅲ、Ⅳ期临床试验、生物等效性试验及真实世界研究等所用样品）的检验数据，对于确定限度范围具有重要价值。

2. 在临床研究数据不足的情况下，非临床药效学、毒理学和药代动力学研究数据等也具有一定参考价值。

3.处方药味、中间体、制剂之间的化学成份转移规律，以及相应制剂的质量目标。

4.药品研发、技术转移、商业规模生产等环节获得的相关知识，包括对多批工艺研究和生产数据的统计分析结果。

（五）均一化计算方法

均一化计算是根据不同批次均一化对象的质量检验数据，计算出达到均一化要求所需的均一化对象的批次及比例。均一化不应改变投料量。原则上，能够满足均一化要求的计算方法都可以使用。建议关注相关数据是否具加和性，如在指纹图谱数据计算时，不宜直接对相似度进行计算，可改用单位质量峰面积（A/W）等为指标。

（六）其他

1.可根据需要对一个或多个批间质量差异较大的处方药味等进行均一化处理，也可根据品种情况对全部药味进行均一化处理。

2.如处方药味来源于不同基原的药材/饮片，应固定基原。如难以固定为一个基原，应确定不同基原的饮片投料比例，再分别对同基原的饮片进行均一化处理。

3.用指纹图谱对均一化前后样品质量进行评价的，除相似度外，建议根据情况增加主要色谱峰峰面积的波动范围、共有峰个数、非共有峰个数及峰面积和、指纹图谱峰形特征（如主要色谱峰的峰面积大小排序或主要色谱峰的峰面积比例）等指标。

Guideline for Study on Manufacturing Process of Compound Preparations of Traditional Chinese Medicines (TCMs) (Trial)

I. Overview

This guideline is mainly used to instruct the applicant to carry out studies on manufacturing process of compound preparations of TCMs with prepared slices/ decoction pieces. The applicant should carry out necessary studies under guidance of TCM theories, based on clinical medication needs, formula composition, drug properties and characteristics of dosage form, showing respect for traditional medication experience, and in combination with modern technology and production practices, to specify process route and process parameters, so as to achieve reasonable and feasible manufacturing process, and consistent, stable and controllable product quality, thus to guarantee the safety and efficacy of TCMs.

This guideline covers the following contents: pre-treatment study, extraction, purification, concentration and drying study, preparation study, packaging study, pilot-scale study, commercial manufacturing study, and process validation, etc.

Compound preparations of TCMs are characterized with complex compositions, multiple chemical components and targets etc; different formulas are of different ingredients, and for the same ingredient, different processing may be applied for varied indications and clinical requirements; with the many existing preparation processes, technologies and methods, new technologies and new methods emerge constantly; and the key points that ought to be considered for different preparation processes, methods and technologies, those difficult points that ought to be studied, and the technical parameters that ought to be determined may all be different. Therefore, the study on manufacturing process of compound preparations of TCMs should not only follow TCM theories and show respect for traditional medication experience, but also follow the general laws of pharmaceutical investigation; based on modern research outcomes and the relationship between formula compositions and ingredients, the physiochemical properties and pharmacological action of the components contained in ingredients, considering the preparation process and manufacturing practice, environmental protection and energy-saving requirements, studies should be conducted using associated disciplinary knowledge, reasonable study design and evaluation indicators. It is encouraged to apply new technologies, new methods and new excipients conforming to product characteristics.

II. Basic Principles and Requirements

(I) Abiding by the traditional medication experience

Study on compound preparations of TCMs is based on knowledge of TCM in life, health and disease, and also based on records in ancient books and modern literature, as well as study, exploration and data accumulation from practical clinical application. Study on manufacturing process of compound preparations of TCMs should abide by TCM theories, and show respect for traditional medication experience. Therefore, the more systematic and deeper literature study in the preliminary phase and the more sufficient data accumulated in clinical application, the better the study core and key points can be grasped.

(II) Quality by design

Study on compound preparations of TCMs should be based on the concept of "Quality by design". In the preliminary phase of manufacturing process study of compound preparations of TCMs, the process route and dosage form of TCMs should be designed as oriented by clinical value and on the basis of understanding formula compatibility, clinical application and other conditions, and tests and studies should be carried out to understand key quality attributes and quantitative and qualitative transfer of the product, and determine the key process parameters. In addition, design space that can meet product quality design requirements and has stable manufacturing process should be established in accordance with material properties and process conditions, etc., such as determining the control range of process parameters. Quality risk management should be carried out, and quality control strategy and drug quality standard system should be established in accordance with the design space.

(III) Holistic quality evaluation

Evaluation during the study on manufacturing process of compound preparations of TCMs should embody overall quality characteristics of compound preparations. Appropriate evaluation indicators should be selected in combination with characteristics of compound preparations of TCMs from aspects such as clinical application conditions, formula compatibility, chemical components contained, pharmacological and pharmaceutical effects, etc. Attention should be paid to the relevance to the safety and efficacy of drugs.

Indicators selected for study on manufacturing process should be comprehensive, scientific and objective, and should be quantifiable as much as possible. Such indicators should be able to reflect changes in relevant manufacturing processes, and also reflect integrity and consistency of drug quality as well as transfer law of active components, to guarantee controllability of the manufacturing process. Evaluation indicators and judgment criteria for intermediates/intermediate products and dynamic process control should be established. Environment-friendly and cost-effective manufacturing process should be established to serve as the quality evaluation indicators.

Manufacturing process and manufacturing equipment are closely related to each other. Therefore, the concept that manufacturing equipment serves the drug quality should be established, and the selection of manufacturing equipment should conform to the requirements for manufacturing process.

(IV) Constant improvement of manufacturing process

In order to guarantee homogeneity and stability of the product quality, it is of great significance to constantly improve the manufacturing process of compound preparations of TCMs. The processes and process parameters determined in various study phases may have certain limitations due to process conditions, batch sizes and other factors. Therefore, scale-up validation and improvement are g conducted, and validation of manufacturing conditions at commercial scale should be performed before marketing to determine the manufacturing process and process parameters.

In the study on manufacturing process of new compound preparations of TCMs, under the condition of unchanged process route and key process parameters, study on optimization of manufacturing process can be carried out before confirmatory clinical trial. Studies in various pre-market phases and post-market studies on improvement of manufacturing process may be carried out in reference to relevant guidelines.

III. Main Contents

(I) Pre-treatment study

Pre-treatment methods of TCM crude drugs include cleansing, cutting, roasting and broiling, pulverization, and sterilization, etc. Study on processing of decoction pieces should show respect for processing technology of decoction pieces applied in clinical practices, conform to the needs for study design of compound preparations of TCMs, and conform to relevant technical requirements. In accordance with characteristics of specific medicines, requirements for dosage form and preparation design etc., , if pre-treatment such as pulverization and sterilization is required for decoction pieces, appropriate method, equipment, process conditions and parameters should be selected, and relevant quality control requirements should be determined.

(II) Study on extraction, purification, concentration and drying

Compound preparations of TCMs have complex ingredients, and therefore, in order to retain the active components as much as possible, reduce the dosage and facilitate the preparations, etc., extraction and purification are generally required. Reasonable and correct use of extraction and purification technologies has a direct relation to the performance of pharmaceutical effect and utilization of TCM crude drugs resources. Study on extraction, purification, concentration and drying of compound preparations of TCMs should center on the efficacy and safety of the medicines, lay emphasis on TCMs formula compatibility theory and traditional clinical application experience (e.g., combined decoction, separated decoction, decoct first, decoct later, etc.), pay attention to the interaction of ingredients, and quantitative and qualitative transfer of decoction pieces, intermediates/intermediate products and preparations, and also take feasibility, safety, energy saving, consumption reduction, environmental protection and other requirements for scale manufacturing into consideration.

1. Process route

Different extraction, purification, concentration and drying methods have their own characteristics and usages. Therefore, appropriate process route, method and evaluation indicators should be selected in accordance with the process design purpose, and in combination with physiochemical properties, pharmaceutical effect and safety study results of the components related to the therapeutic activity and safety, as well as existing literature reports.

Study on screening of process route should pay attention to:

Study on screening of process route related to efficacy. For compound preparations of TCMs originated from clinically effective formulas, the following aspects (including but not limited to) may be taken into consideration: 1) Clinical medication experience. Differences and similarities between the process route used and that of clinical medication (e.g., preparations of medical institutions, etc.) should be taken into consideration. If manufacturing process different from that of clinical medication is used, it is generally suitable to compare with the manufacturing process of clinical medication. 2) Pharmacodynamic test or literature references. In pharmacodynamic test, comparison study of process route can be carried out by selecting appropriate pharmacodynamic model and main pharmacodynamic indicators with clinical medication (e.g., decoction), etc. as the control. 3) Comparison of active components. For example, compare active components etc. when contrasting with clinical medication (e.g., decoction).

Study on screening of process route related to safety. Safety of the medicines should be studied when screening the efficacy. Consideration should be made from the following aspects (including but not limited to): adverse reactions and literature reports from preliminary clinical medication, comparison of animal safety indicators of different process routes with pharmacodynamics tests, toxic and harmful ingredients and single dose toxicity.

Rationality of manufacturing process is the basic work of study on manufacturing process of compound preparations of TCMs, and the more evidence supporting rationality of the process route, the more guarantee there is for study in later period. Attention should be paid to R&D risks that might be caused by irrational manufacturing process.

1.1 Extraction and purification process

Extraction of compound preparations of TCMs should be conducted on the basis of making full understanding of the traditional application mode, taking characteristics of decoction pieces, properties of active ingredients and requirements for dosage form into consideration, and paying attention to active ingredients, toxic ingredients and properties of extracts as well as quantitative and qualitative transfer of other quality attributes. Class I and Class II organic solvents should be avoided as the extraction solvent as much as possible.

For purification of compound preparations of TCMs, scientific, reasonable, stable and feasible manufacturing process can be designed in accordance with traditional TCM medication experience, or based on the existence state, polarity and solubleness, etc. of some active ingredients confirmed in the medicines. However, due to complexity of the ingredients in compound preparations of TCMs, the necessity and appropriateness of purification should be taken into consideration.

1.2 Concentration and drying process

In accordance with physiochemical properties of the materials, requirements for preparations, and factors influencing the concentration and drying effect, corresponding manufacturing process should be selected to enable the products obtained to reach required relative density and water content, etc., thus facilitating preparation of the final products. The main manufacturing process steps and process conditions as well as study factors need to be determined. The main ingredients should be studied, and attention should be paid to unstable ingredients.

2. Process conditions

Upon preliminary determination of the process route, scientific and reasonable test design and optimization should be performed for the process technologies and methods applied. Accurate, simple, representative and quantifiable comprehensive evaluation indicators and reasonable methods should be applied to optimize the manufacturing process, and multiple-factor and multi-level study should be performed based on pre-test. It is encouraged to apply new technologies and new methods, but for newly established methods, the rationality and feasibility study should be carried out.

Appropriate manufacturing process and equipment should be selected in accordance with specific product, and manufacturing process flow and the equipment used should be fixed.

Study on process conditions should pay attention to the relation between material properties, process parameters and the product quality, and key process parameters and their ranges should be determined.

2.1 Optimization of extraction and purification process conditions

Different extraction methods would have different factors influencing the extraction effect. Therefore, the selection of influence factors and determination of extraction parameters should be performed in accordance with the extraction method and equipment applied. Generally, it is required to select influence factors including solvent, extraction times and extraction duration etc., manufacturing equipment and process conditions, in order to optimize the extraction process. In addition, mature and well-recognized optimal selection method should be adopted, and the applicability of new method (if applied) should be taken into consideration.

The purification process should be selected in accordance with the purification purpose, principle of the method to be used and the influence factors. Generally, it is required to consider physiochemical properties of the active components to be reserved and the substances to be removed, the requirements of the dosage form to be made and the preparation process, as well as the bridging with manufacturing conditions.

Process parameters should be determined with references to tests, describing the test method, study indicators, and validation investigations etc. Determination of the ranges of process parameters should be supported by relevant study data.

2.2 Optimization of concentration and drying process conditions

The methods and degree of concentration and drying, equipment, process parameters and other factors have a direct influence on the stability of ingredients in the materials. Therefore, the process conditions should be studied and optimized in combination with the requirements of preparations.

The concentration and drying methods as well as main process parameters should be studied, and the determination of ranges of process parameters should be supported by relevant study data.

(III) Preparation study

During the preparation study compound preparations of TCMs, according to the properties and amount of medicinal substances for preparation process, and in combination with medication experience and indications, etc., appropriate dosage form, excipients, manufacturing process, and equipment should be selected.

For the optimization of preparation process, main changes of process study (including batch size, equipment and process parameters, etc.) and relevant supporting validation study should be described.

1. Selection of dosage forms

Different dosage forms of the medicines may result in different pharmaceutical effects, thus affecting clinical efficacy and adverse reactions of the medicines.

Selection of dosage forms should reference the early medication experience to meet clinical medical needs based on the comprehensive analysis of physiochemical and biological properties, and dosage form characteristics, etc. of the medicines. The convictive references and experimental data should be provided to adequately elucidate the scientificity, rationality and necessity of the selection of dosage form.

The following aspects should be primarily considered for the selection of dosage forms:

1.1 Clinical needs and medication objects

It should be considered that different dosage forms may be applicable to different clinical symptoms, as well as the compliance and physiological conditions, etc. of medication objects.

1.2 Properties and amount of medicinal substances used for preparation process

Active ingredients of TCMs are complex, and the solubleness and stability of various ingredients are different during absorption, distribution, metabolism and excretion process *in vivo*. Therefore, appropriate dosage forms should be selected in accordance with the properties of medicines.

The formula amount, amount and properties of medicinal substances used for preparation process, clinical medication dosage, and loading quantity of different dosage forms, etc. should be considered for the selection of dosage forms.

1.3 Safety

The safety of medicines should be fully considered when the dosage forms are selected. Attention should be paid to possible safety hazards (including toxicity and side effects) caused by dosage form and administration route.

In addition, the study before formula design of medicinal preparations needs to be emphasized. Relevant studies should be carried out on the basis of understanding the basic properties, dosage form characteristics and preparation requirements of medicines. The theories, methods and technologies of relevant disciplines should be referenced during the selection and design of the dosage form.

2. Study on formulas of preparations

Study on formulas of preparations is a process for screening appropriate excipients and determining formulas of preparations based on the properties of medicinal substances used for preparation process, dosage form characteristics and clinical medication requirements, etc. Study on formulas of preparations is an important content of preparation study.

2.1 Pre-formula study of preparations

Pre-formula study of preparations is the basis of the study on preparation process, for the purpose of enabling the preparation formula and preparation process to adapt to requirements for industrialized manufacturing, and guaranteeing the rationality, feasibility and inter-batch consistency of manufacturing.

In the pre-formula study of compound preparations of TCMs, the properties of medicinal substances used for preparation process should be studied. For example, for solid preparations, dissolution characteristics, moisture absorption, fluidity, stability and compressibility, etc. of the medicinal substance for preparation process should be mainly studied; and for oral liquid preparations, dissolution characteristics, acid-base property, stability, smell, and odor, etc. of the medicinal substance for preparation process should be mainly studied.

2.2 Selection of excipients

In the study of preparation process, of excipients should be selected. The excipients used should conform to the medicinal requirements, and new excipients should also conform to the relevant requirements.

Selection of excipients should generally take the following principles into consideration: meet the requirements of preparation process, stability and action characteristics of final products, have no adverse interaction with active components, and avoid the influence on drug testing. Considering the characteristics of compound preparations of TCMs, reducing the administration dosage and improving the medication compliance, the preparation formula should be able to obtain good preparations with as little amount of excipients as possible.

2.3 Study on screening of formulas of preparations

Study on screening of formulas of preparations should take the following factors into consideration: requirements for clinical medication, properties of the medicinal substances and excipients used for preparation process, and dosage form characteristics, etc. Through the study on formula screening, the formula composition of preparations is preliminary determined, and the types, models, specifications and amounts, etc. of the excipients used are clarified.

3. Study on preparation process

Through the study on preparation process, the formula design can be further improved, and the preparation formula, process and equipment are finally confirmed. In addition, it is required to pay attention to the stability of preparations.

3.1 Requirements for preparation process

Study on preparation process should generally take selection of preparation process and preparation technology into consideration, pay attention to bridging between the laboratory conditions and the pilot scale and manufacturing, and consider the feasibility and adaptability of commercial manufacturing equipment.

Unit operation or key process should be studied to guarantee the stability of quality. The technical conditions of each process should be studied to determine the detailed preparation process. During the preparation process, special attention should be paid to the homogeneity of toxic ingredients and medicines with small dosage but strong activity.

3.2 Preparation technology and preparation equipment

During the study of preparations, specific preparation technology and equipment may always have a great influence on the preparation process as well as the category and amount of the excipients used, so they should be correctly selected.

During the study of preparations, influences of equipment type and process parameters on key quality attributes of preparations should be emphatically studied. The diversified mathematical modeling methods can be used to carry out correlation studies among the properties of medicinal substances used for preparation process, process parameters, and evaluation indicators of key quality attributes, establish the design space for key material attributes, key process parameters and key evaluation indicators of medicinal substances used for preparation process, and explore corresponding process control technology, to reduce the inter-batch quality difference, guarantee the stability of drug quality, and then guarantee the safety and efficacy of drugs. Advanced preparation technology and corresponding preparation equipment are important aspects for improving the preparation level and product quality, which should also be paid attention.

(IV) Study on selection of package

Study on selection of package of compound preparations of TCMs mainly refers to the study on selection of packaging materials (containers) in direct contact with finished preparations and intermediates/intermediate products (if applicable), and also includes the study on selection of secondary packaging materials (containers).

Packaging materials (containers) in direct contact with drugs should be selected in accordance with influence factors and the stability study results of the product. Selection of packaging materials (containers) in direct contact with drugs should conform to relevant requirements of packaging materials (containers) in direct contact with drugs, drug packaging and label management, etc.

Under some special conditions or conditions with insufficient literature materials, the study on compatibility between drugs and packaging materials (containers) in direct contact with drugs should be strengthened. Especially for liquid preparations or semi-solid preparations containing organic solvents, on the one hand, it is possible to study whether ingredients in the packaging materials (especially additive ingredients in the packaging materials) will seep into the drugs to cause changes of product quality in accordance with the migration experimental results; and on the other hand, it is possible to study whether the adsorption/exudation of packaging materials could cause changes in drug concentration and precipitation, etc., thus leading to safety concerns in accordance with the adsorption test results. For new packaging materials (containers) in direct contact with drugs or packaging materials (containers) of specific dosage forms, not only the stability test should be carried out, but also appropriate study items should be added.

(V) Pilot-scale study

Pilot-scale study is the validation and improvement of rationality of laboratory process, and is an inevitable procedure for guaranteeing that the process can reach manufacturing stability and operability. After completing a series of studies on manufacturing process of compound preparations of TCMs, scale-up study should be carried out under the conditions which are basically consistent with the manufacturing conditions, to provide a basis for realizing the validation of manufacturing process at commercial scale. Pilot-scale study should take bridging with manufacturing at commercial scale into consideration. During the pilot-scale study process, the specific process procedures should be formulated, and proper records should be kept.

Through the pilot-scale study, the key steps, control range of key process parameters and yield range of intermediates/intermediate products (e.g., extracts, etc.) are explored, and the problems existing in process feasibility, labor protection, environmental protection and manufacturing cost, etc. are discovered, so as to provide a basis for manufacturing at commercial scale.

The pilot-scale study equipment should generally have consistent working principle with the manufacturing equipment, and the main technical parameters should be basically consistent. Pilot-scale study samples, if used in clinical trials, should be prepared in workshops conforming to conditions in the *Good Manufacturing Practice* (GMP).

Since for different dosage forms of drugs, the manufacturing process, equipment, workshop conditions, excipients and packaging, etc. differ greatly, the dosage form should be considered in pilot-scale study, and in particular, how to carry out work by adapting to manufacturing characteristics should be taken into consideration.

Feeding amount of pilot-scale study should take bridging with study on manufacturing at commercial scale into consideration, to provide a basis for manufacturing at commercial scale. Feeding amount, yield rate of intermediates/intermediate product and rate of finished products are important indicators for measuring the feasibility and stability of pilot-scale study. Feeding amount of pilot-scale study should meet the purpose of pilot-scale study. Yield rate of intermediates/intermediate product and rate of finished products should be stable relatively.

Generally pilot-scale study involves multiple batches to reach the purpose of stable process.

(VI) Study on manufacturing at commercial scale

Study on manufacturing at commercial scale mainly involves the homogeneity and stability of product quality under large-scale condition, especially the consistency of quality of samples used in clinical trials, which also covers comparison and evaluation. Through the study, all process steps and control ranges of process parameters applicable to manufacturing at commercial scale are specified, the decoction pieces, intermediates/intermediate product, and quality risk points are clarified, and the stability, environmental protection and economy of manufacturing process are guaranteed.

Manufacturing at commercial scale should pay attention to its match with the equipment, as well as fluency and convenience of various manufacturing procedures. Homogeneity and stability of product quality and manufacturing efficiency are important indicators for measuring large-scale manufacturing.

Stability of manufacturing at commercial scale generally should be performed through multiple batches. During the test, the process parameters and quality attribute relationship should be noticed, and the fluctuation of quality should be concerned. Relevant records should be improved, standardized and traceable.

(Ⅶ) Process validation

Validation of key processes and key process parameters should be completed before carrying out clinical trials, and complete process validation should be performed before applying for marketing authorization. Manufacturing environment for process validation should conform to the requirements of *Good Manufacturing Practice* (GMP), and the manufacturing equipment should match with the proposed manufacturing scale.

The process validation should be performed according to the designed protocol, and a process validation report should be formed afterwards. For the pilot-scale process or manufacturing at commercial scale, appropriate indicators should be selected, the process validation protocol should be designed, and the influence of personnel, equipment, materials, manufacturing environment, management and control measures, etc. on product quality are studied under proposed manufacturing scale, process conditions and parameters. If the design space or range of process parameters has been proposed, the extreme value of the proposed design space or the range of process parameters should be studied in the process validation, to validate the feasibility of manufacturing process and the consistency of product quality.

中药复方制剂生产工艺研究
技术指导原则（试行）

一、概述

本指导原则主要用于指导申请人开展以中药饮片为原料的中药复方制剂生产工艺研究。申请人应在中医药理论指导下，根据临床用药需求、处方组成、药物性质及剂型特点，尊重传统用药经验，结合现代技术与生产实际进行必要的研究，以明确工艺路线和具体工艺参数，做到工艺合理、可行、药品质量均一稳定可控，保障药品的安全、有效。

本指导原则涉及以下内容：前处理研究、提取纯化与浓缩干燥研究、成型研究、包装选择研究、中试研究、商业规模生产研究、工艺验证等。

由于中药复方组成复杂、化学成份众多以及存在多靶点作用等特点；不同处方药味组成不同，相同的药味针对不同的适应症和临床需求，可能需要采用不同的处理工艺；制剂制备工艺、技术与方法繁多，新技术与新方法不断涌现；不同的制备工艺、方法与技术所应考虑的重点，需进行研究的难点，要确定的技术参数，均有可能不同。因此中药复方制剂生产工艺的研究既要遵循中医药理论，尊重传统用药经验，又要遵循药品研究的一般规律，利用现代研究成果，在分析处方组成和各药味之间的关系、各药味所含成份的理化性质和药理作用的基础上，结合制剂工艺和生产实际、环保节能等要求，综合应用相关学科的知识，采用合理的试验设计和评价指标，开展相关研究。鼓励采用符合产品特点的新技术、新方法、新辅料。

二、基本原则及要求

（一）尊重传统用药经验

中药复方制剂的研究是基于中医药对生命、健康、疾病的认识，是以既往古籍及现代文献记载以及实际临床应用过程中的研究探索和数据积累为基础的。中药复方制剂工艺研究应遵循中医药理论，尊重传统用药经验。因此前期的文献研究工作越系统、深入，临床应用中积累的数据越充分，越能更好地把握研究的核心和重点。

（二）质量源于设计

中药复方制剂研究应基于"质量源于设计"的理念。中药复方制剂工艺研究初期就应以临床价值为导向，在了解药物配伍、临床应用等情况的基础上，设计工艺路线和药物剂型，通过试验研究，理解产品的关键质量属性和量质传递，确定关键工艺参数；根据物料性质、工艺条件等，建立能满足产品质量设计要求且工艺稳健的设计空间，如确定工艺参数控制范围等，并根据设计空间，开展质量风险管理，确立质量控制策略和药品质量标准体系。

（三）整体质量评价

中药复方制剂生产工艺研究中的评价应体现复方整体质量特性。应结合复方中药的特点，从临床应用情况、组方配伍、所含的化学成份、药理药效等方面选择适宜的评价指标。关注与药品安全性及有效性的相关性。

工艺研究选择的指标应该是全面、科学、客观，并尽可能是可量化的，能够客观反映相关工艺过程的变化，能够反映药物质量的整体性、一致性和药效物质的转移规律，保证工艺过程可控。应建立中间体/中间产物和工艺动态过程控制评价指标及判断标准。应建立环境友好、成本适宜的生产工艺，并作为质量评价指标。

生产工艺与生产设备密切相关，应树立生产设备是为药品质量服务的理念，生产设备的选择应符合生产工艺的要求。

（四）工艺持续改进

为保证产品质量的均一稳定，中药复方制剂工艺持续改进具有重要意义。各研究阶段确定的工艺路线和工艺参数，由于工艺条件、批量规模等因素的影响，会有一定的局限性。因此一般需要通过扩大生产规模进行验证和改进，上市前应进行商业规模的生产条件验证，确定生产工艺和工艺参数。

中药复方制剂新药生产工艺研究中，工艺路线、关键工艺参数不变的前提下，工艺优化研究工作可在确证性临床试验前进行。上市前各研究阶段及上市后的工艺改进研究，可参照相关指导原则。

三、主要内容

（一）前处理研究

药材前处理方法包括：净制、切制、炮炙、粉碎、灭菌等。饮片炮制研究应尊重临床应用的饮片炮制工艺，符合中药复方制剂研究设计的需要，符合相关技术要求。根据具体药物特点、剂型和制剂设计等要求，如需对饮片进行粉碎、灭菌等前处理，应选择合适的方法、设备、工艺条件和参数，确定相关质量控制要求。

（二）提取纯化、浓缩干燥研究

中药复方制剂成份复杂，为尽可能保留药效物质、降低服用量、便于制剂等，一般需要经过提取、纯化处理。提取、纯化技术的合理、正确运用与否直接关系到药物疗效的发挥和药材资源的利用。中药复方制剂提取纯化、浓缩干燥研究过程中应围绕药物有效性和安全性，注重中医组方配伍理论和临床传统应用经验（如合煎、分煎、先煎、后下等），关注组方药味相互作用以及饮片、中间体/中间产物和制剂的量质传递，并考虑规模化生产的可行性，安全、节能、降耗、环保等要求。

1. 工艺路线

不同的提取纯化、浓缩干燥方法均有其特点与使用范围，应根据工艺设计目的，并结合与治疗作用及安全性相关的药物成份的理化性质，药效、安全性研究结果，已有的文献报道，选择适宜工艺路线、方法和评价指标。

工艺路线筛选研究需要关注：

与有效性相关的工艺路线筛选研究。对来源于临床有效方剂的中药复方，一般可以但不限于从以下方面考虑：1）临床用药经验。应考虑采用的工艺路线与临床用药（如医疗机构制剂等）工艺路线的异同，如采用与临床用药不同的生产工艺，一般宜与临床用药的工艺进行比较。2）药效学试验依据或文献依据。药效学试验可以以临床用药形式（如汤剂）等为对照，选择适宜的药效模型和主要药效学指标，进行工艺路线的对比研究。3）药效物质基础的比较。如与临床用药形式（如汤剂）对照，从物质基础等方面进行比较。

与安全性相关的工艺路线筛选研究。应在有效性筛选的同时考察药物的安全性。一般可以但不限于以下方面考虑：前期临床用药时产生的不良反应、文献报道，采用药效试验对比不同工艺路线时动物的安全性指标，有毒、有害成份，单次给药毒性试验结果。

工艺合理性研究是中药复方制剂工艺研究的基础性工作，支持工艺路线合理性的证据越多，为后期研究提供更多保障。应注意工艺不合理可能引发的研发风险。

1.1 提取与纯化工艺

中药复方制剂的提取应在充分理解传统应用方式的基础上，考虑饮片特点、有效成份性质以及剂型的要求，关注有效成份、有毒成份、浸出物的性质和其他质量属性的量质传递。提取溶剂应尽量避免选择使用一、二类有机溶剂。

中药复方制剂的纯化可依据中药传统用药经验或根据药物中已确认的一些有效成份的存在状态、极性、溶解性等设计科学、合理、稳定、可行的工艺。但由于中药复方制剂中成份的复杂性，应考虑纯化的必要性和适宜性。

1.2 浓缩与干燥工艺

依据物料的理化性质、制剂的要求，影响浓缩、干燥效果的因素，选择相应工艺，使所得产物达到要求的相对密度、含水量等，以便于制剂成型。需确定主要工艺环节及工艺条件与考察因素。应考察主要成份，关注不稳定成份。

2. 工艺条件

工艺路线初步确定后，对采用的工艺技术与方法，应进行科学、合理的试验设计和优化。工艺的优选应采用准确、简便、具有代表性、可量化的综合性评价指标与合理的方法，在预试验的基础上对多因素、多水平进行考察。鼓励新技术新方法的应用，但对于新建立的方法，应进行方法的合理性、可行性研究。

应根据具体品种的情况选择适宜的工艺及设备，固定工艺流程及其所用设备。

工艺条件研究中应关注物料性质、工艺参数与产品质量的关系，确定关键工艺参数及范围。

2.1 提取与纯化工艺条件的优化

采用的提取方法不同，影响提取效果的因素有别，因此应根据所采用的提取方法与设备，考虑影响因素的选择和提取参数的确定。一般需对溶媒、提取次数、提取时间等影响因素及生产设备、工艺条件进行选择，优化提取工艺。通常采用成熟公认的优选方法，如果使用新方法应考虑其适用性。

应根据纯化的目的、拟采用方法的原理和影响因素选择纯化工艺。一般应考虑拟保留的药效物质与去除物质的理化性质、拟制成的剂型与成型工艺的需要以及与生产条件的桥接。

工艺参数的确定应有试验依据，说明试验方法、考察指标、验证试验等。工艺参数范围的确定也应有相关研究数据支持。

2.2 浓缩与干燥工艺条件的优化

浓缩与干燥的方法和程度、设备和工艺参数等因素都直接影响物料中成份的稳定，应结合制剂的要求对工艺条件进行研究和优化。

应研究浓缩干燥工艺方法、主要工艺参数，工艺参数范围的确定应有相关研究数据支持。

（三）成型研究

中药复方制剂成型研究应根据制剂成型所用原料的性质和用量，结合用药经验、适应症等，选择适宜的剂型、辅料、生产工艺及设备。

成型工艺的优化，应重点描述工艺研究的主要变化（包括批量、设备、工艺参数等）及相关的支持性验证研究。

1. 剂型选择

药物剂型的不同，可能导致药物作用效果的差异，从而关系到药物的临床疗效及不良反应。

剂型选择应借鉴前期用药经验，以满足临床医疗需要为宗旨，在对药物理化性质、生物学特性、剂型特点等方面综合分析的基础上进行。应提供具有说服力的文献依据、试验资料，充分阐述剂型选择的科学性、合理性、必要性。

剂型的选择应主要考虑以下方面：

1.1 临床需要及用药对象

应考虑不同剂型可能适用于不同的临床病证需要，以及用药对象的顺应性和生理情况等。

1.2 制剂成型所用原料的性质和用量

中药有效成份复杂，各成份溶解性、稳定性，在体内的吸收、分布、代谢、排泄过程各不相同，应根据药物的性质选择适宜的剂型。

选择剂型时应考虑处方量、制剂成型所用原料的量及性质、临床用药剂量，以及不同剂型的载药量等。

1.3 安全性

选择剂型时需充分考虑药物安全性。应关注剂型因素和给药途径可能产生的安全隐患（包括毒性和副作用）。

另外，需要重视药物制剂处方设计前研究工作。在认识药物的基本性质、剂型特点以及制剂要求的基础上，进行相关研究。在剂型选择和设计中注意借鉴相关学科的理论、方法和技术。

2. 制剂处方研究

制剂处方研究是根据制剂成型所用原料性质、剂型特点、临床用药要求等，筛选适宜的辅料，确定制剂处方的过程。制剂处方研究是制剂研究的重要内容。

2.1 制剂处方前研究

制剂处方研究是制剂成型研究的基础，其目的是使制剂处方和制剂工艺适应工业化生产的要求，保证生产时的合理性、可行性及批间一致性。

中药复方制剂处方前研究中，应研究制剂成型所用原料的性质。例如，制备固体制剂应主要研究制剂成型所用原料的溶解特性、吸湿性、流动性、稳定性、可压性等；制备口服液体制剂应主要研究制剂成型所用原料的溶解特性、酸碱性、稳定性以及嗅、味等。

2.2 辅料的选择

制剂成型工艺的研究中，应对辅料的选用进行研究。所用辅料应符合药用要求，新辅料还应符合相关要求。

辅料选择一般应考虑以下原则：满足制剂成型、稳定、作用特点的要求，不与药物发生不良相互作用，避免影响药品的检测。考虑到中药复方制剂的特点，减少服用量及提高用药顺应性，制剂处方应能在尽可能少的辅料用量下获得良好的制剂成型性。

2.3 制剂处方筛选研究

制剂处方筛选研究应考虑以下因素：临床用药的要求、制剂成型所用原料和辅料的性质、剂型特点等。通过处方筛选研究，初步确定制剂处方组成，明确所用辅料的种类、型号、规格、用量等。

3. 制剂成型工艺研究

通过制剂成型研究进一步改进和完善处方设计，最终确定制剂处方、工艺和设备，并关注制剂的稳定性。

3.1 制剂成型工艺要求

制剂成型工艺研究一般应考虑成型工艺路线和制备技术的选择，应注意实验室条件与中试和生产的桥接，考虑大生产制剂设备的可行性、适应性。

对单元操作或关键工艺，应进行考察，以保证质量的稳定。应研究各工序技术条件，确定详细的制剂成型工艺流程。在制剂过程中，对于含有毒药物以及用量小而活性强的药物，应特别注意其均匀性。

3.2 制剂技术、制剂设备

在制剂研究过程中，特定的制剂技术和设备往往可能对成型工艺，以及所使用辅料的种类、用量产生很大影响，应正确选用。

在制剂研究过程中，应重点考察设备类型、工艺参数对制剂关键质量属性的影响，可采用多样化的数学建模方法开展制剂成型所用原料性质、工艺参数、关键质量属性评价指标之间的相关性研究，建立关键物料属性、关键工艺参数、制剂成型所用原料关键评价指标的设计空间，并探索相应的过程控制技术，以减少批间质量差异，保证药品质量的稳定，进而保障药品的安全、有效。先进的制剂技术以及相应的制剂设备，是提高制剂水平和产品质量的重要方面，也应予以关注。

（四）包装选择研究

中药复方制剂的包装选择研究主要指制剂成品、中间体/中间产物（如适用）直接接触药品的包装材料（容器）的选择研究，也包括次级包装材料（容器）的选择研究。

应根据产品的影响因素及稳定性研究结果，选择直接接触药品的包装材料（容器）。直接接触药品的包装材料（容器）的选择，应符合直接接触药品的包装材料（容器）、药品包装标签管理等相关要求。

在某些特殊情况或文献资料不充分的情况下，应加强药品与直接接触药品的包装材料（容器）的相容性考察。特别是含有有机溶剂的液体制剂或半固体制剂，一方面可以根据迁移试验结果，考察包装材料中的成份（尤其是包材的添加剂成份）是否会渗出至药品中，引起产品质量的变化；另一方面可以根据吸附试验结果，考察是否会由于包材的吸附/渗出而导致药品浓度的改变、产生沉淀等，从而引起安全性担忧。采用新的直接接触药品的包装材料（容器）或特定剂型直接接触药品的包装材料（容器），在包装材料（容器）的选择研究中除应进行稳定性试验需要进行的项目外，还应增加适宜的考察项目。

（五）中试研究

中试研究是对实验室工艺合理性的验证与完善，是保证工艺达到生产稳定性、可操作性的必经环节。完成中药复方制剂生产工艺系列研究后，应采用与生产基本相符的条件进行工艺放大研究，为实现商业规模的生产工艺验证提供基础。中试研究应考虑与商业规模生产的桥接。中试研究过程要制定详细的工艺规程，并做好记录。

通过中试研究，探索关键步骤、关键工艺参数控制范围和中间体/中间产物（如浸膏等）的得率范围等，发现工艺可行性、劳动保护、环保、生产成本等方面存在的问题，为实现商业规模的生产提供依据。

中试研究设备与生产设备的工作原理一般应一致，主要技术参数应基本相符。中试样品如用于临床试验，应当在符合药品生产质量管理规范条件的车间制备。

由于药品剂型不同，所用生产工艺、设备、生产车间条件、辅料、包装等有很大差异，因此在中试研究中要结合剂型，特别要考虑如何适应生产的特点开展工作。

中试研究的投料量应考虑与商业规模生产研究的桥接，为商业规模生产提供依据。投料量、中间体/中间产物得率、成品率是衡量中试研究可行性、稳定性的重要指标。中试研究的投料量应达到中试研究的目的。中间体/中间产物得率、成品率应相对稳定。

中试研究一般需经过多批次试验，以达到工艺稳定的目的。

（六）商业规模生产研究

商业规模生产重点考察在规模化条件下，产品质量的均一性、稳定性，特别是与临床试验用样品质量的一致性，并进行对比与评估。通过研究，明确适于商业规模生产的所有工艺步骤及其工艺参数控制范围，明确饮片、中间体/中间产物、质量风险点，保障工艺稳健、环保、经济。

商业规模生产应关注与设备的匹配性、生产各环节的流畅与便捷。产品质量的均一稳定及生产效率是衡量规模化生产的重要指标。

商业规模生产的稳定，一般需经过多批次试验。试验中注意工艺参数、质量属性关联性，关注质量的波动性。相关记录应完善、规范、可追溯。

（七）工艺验证

应在开展临床试验前完成关键环节、关键工艺参数的验证，在申请上市许可前完成完整的工艺验证。工艺验证的生产环境要符合药品生产质量管理规范的要求，生产设备要与拟定的生产规模相匹配。

进行工艺验证时，应进行工艺验证方案的设计，按验证方案进行验证。验证结束后应形成工艺验证报告。应针对中试工艺或商业生产规模，选择适宜的指标，设计工艺验证方案，考察在拟定的生产规模以及工艺条件和参数下，人员、设备、材料、生产环境、管控措施等各方面对产品质量带来的影响。若拟定了设计空间或工艺参数范围，工艺验证中应对拟定设计空间或工艺参数范围的极值进行考察，验证工艺的可行性和产品质量的一致性。

Guideline for Pharmacognosy, Chemistry, Manufacturing and Controls (PCMC) Study in Various Phases of Study on New Traditional Chinese Medicines (TCMs) (Trial)

I. Overview

The study of new TCMs encompasses a comprehensive approach that integrates various disciplines such as PCMC, pharmacology, toxicology, and clinical studies. The PCMC study primarily focuses on the analysis of ingredients and their quality, dosage forms, manufacturing processes, quality study, quality standards, and stability, etc. Under the guidance of TCM theories, and in accordance with distinctive characteristics of TCMs, the general laws of new TCMs research and development, and the main objectives of different study phases, it is imperative to conduct targeted studies on new TCMs. Additionally, the implementation of whole life cycle management of TCMs and the promotion of inheritance and innovation of TCMs are essential in order to ensure the safety, efficacy and quality control of the TCMs.

This guideline primarily outlines the fundamental criteria for the essential components of PCMC study that need to be fulfilled during different stages of new TCMs, including clinical trial application, pre-phase III clinical trials, application for marketing authorization and post-market studies. The purpose of this guideline is to serve as a reference for the study of new TCMs. The limitations imposed by the phased requirements outlined in the guidelines may not apply to studies conducted on specific products. Instead, it is recommended that the study contents be organized in a scientific and rational manner, taking into consideration the unique characteristics of the product.

II. General Principles

(I) Adhering to the principles of TCM theories

PCMC studies on new TCMs should be conducted with adherence to TCM theories, while also demonstrating respect for traditional experience and clinical practices. It is highly recommended to employ modern science and technology for the purposes of research and fostering innovation.

(II) Adhering to distinctive characteristics of TCMs and the general rules of R&D

In order to improve the R&D quality and efficiency of new TCMs and facilitate the inheritance and innovative development of TCMs, it is essential to conduct corresponding studies in a phased manner, taking into account distinctive characteristics of TCMs and the general rules of R&D. This approach requires a comprehensive understanding of the complexity of TCMs, the gradual nature of R&D process of new TCMs, and the primary objectives of each phase of the study. Research should be conducted to reflect the concept of quality by design, emphasize the integrity and systematic nature of the study.

(III) Practicing whole life cycle management

The PCMC study of new TCMs should encompass the whole life cycle management. It should focus on enhancing the whole-process quality control study of TCM crude drugs, prepared slices/decoction pieces, intermediates, and preparations. Furthermore, it is crucial to establish and enhance a comprehensive quality control system that aligns with distinctive characteristics of TCMs. In conjunction with advancements in product cognition and continuous progress in science and technology, efforts should be made to continually enhance the manufacturing process, quality control methods, and means of the TCMs. This will facilitate the ongoing improvement of drug quality.

III. Basic Contents

(I) Submission of clinical trial applications

The completion of the following PCMC study is necessary in order to ensure the provision of clinical trial samples of basically consistent quality that meet the necessary requirements for conducting clinical trials. The study encompasses the determination of ingredients and administration route. It involves specifying the origin and medicinal parts of TCM crude drugs, as well as the processing method and preparation process of decoction pieces. Additionally, it aims to establish quality standards and conduct safety-related quality control studies to achieve a basically controllable level of quality. The ultimate goal is to ensure the stability of the samples used in clinical trials.

1. Ingredients and their quality

Ingredients of new TCMs should be standardized, encompassing decoction pieces, extracts, and other relevant components. The origin, medicinal parts, and quality requirements of TCM crude drugs, as well as the processing method and quality standards of decoction pieces, should be specified. Consideration should be given to the places of origin and harvesting periods of TCM crude drugs, including the specific year and time of harvesting, among other factors.

In order to ensure the consistent quality of new TCMs, it is imperative to focus on the quality of TCM crude drugs used in TCMs production and their sustainable utilization. A comprehensive evaluation study of wild TCM crude drugs should be conducted in accordance with the relevant requirements. In studies that involve the utilization of valuable, rare and endangered wild TCM crude drugs, it is imperative to adhere to the stipulations outlined in pertinent laws and regulations. Additionally, careful consideration should be given to the feasibility of cultivating and breeding these materials, with a particular emphasis on sustainability.

2. Dosage form and preparation process

Studies on the preparation process of new TCMs should be conducted under the guidance of TCM theories, and in conjunction with the application experience in humans, the physiochemical properties and pharmacological actions of the chemical components found in various ingredients, among other factors.

Studies pertaining to the selection of dosage form, process route, and main process parameters should be conducted. It is essential to specify the dosage form and preparation process, while also providing a rationale for the selection. The pre-treatment, extraction, purification, concentration, and drying methods as well as the main process parameters need to be specified. Additionally, it is important to basically specify on the yield rate, yield quantity, and other key process indicators of intermediates, such as extracts. It is imperative to conduct studies on the formula design and molding process of preparations. This entails specifying the excipients, molding process, and main process parameters.

The determination of the preparation process should be based on a pilot scale-up study, and it is essential to specify the main process parameters. The consideration of the feasibility and adaptability of manufacturing equipment at a commercial scale is crucial.

Samples used for the non-clinical safety study should be derived from a pilot or larger scale manufacture.

3. Quality study and quality standards

A study should be conducted on the quality control of TCM crude drugs and prepared slices/decoction pieces, intermediates, preparations, and excipients of new TCMs to establish quality standards for these TCMs. A comprehensive study should be conducted to assess the safety and efficacy of the drug. Special attention should be given to studying the quality control aspects, particularly those which have a direct impact on safety, such as toxic components and their control. Additionally, it is crucial to establish a robust quality control method. With the continuous advancement of the study, there is a need for a gradual improvement in the quality study and quality standards.

4. Stability study

Preliminary stability studies should be conducted to ensure the consistent quality of samples for clinical trials. This involves selecting suitable immediate packaging materials/containers for the TCMs, and studying and determining appropriate storage conditions.

(II) Pre-phase III clinical trial

Samples used for clinical trials should be prepared on a manufacturing scale, and the manufacturing process must adhere to the requirements outlined in the *Good Manufacturing Practice.*

1. Ingredients and their quality

Based on preliminary studies conducted on the origins and medicinal parts of TCM crude drugs, as well as the processing methods of decoction pieces, it is necessary to enhance and establish comprehensive information regarding the TCM crude drugs through systematic studies, including literature surveys. These studies should focus on the places of origin, harvesting periods, processing and manufacturing methods employed in the places of origin (such as wild, cultivation, breeding, and other means), storage methods and conditions, and other factors that may impact the quality of the TCM crude drugs in the formula. The objective of these studies is to ensure a consistent and stable quality of the TCM crude drugs. In addition, it is imperative to continuously study and enhance the quality standards for TCM crude drugs and decoction pieces, among other aspects. For new TCMs that necessitate the utilization of valuable, rare and endangered wild TCM crude drugs, it is imperative to conduct study on cultivation and breeding technologies.

2. Manufacturing process

In line with the initial conditions of the clinical trial and findings from the study, large-scale production research should be completed; the production process should be fixed; and detailed process parameters should be clarified to ensure the quality stability of samples. The aim is to ensure the consistent quality of the samples used in Phase III clinical trials. Under the condition that the process route and key process parameters remain unchanged, any modifications to the process parameters, molding process, excipients, and specification, etc. should be thoroughly studied based on the actual changes and in accordance with relevant technical guidelines. The purpose of this study is to provide a rational and necessary explanation for the proposed changes. Additionally, if deemed necessary, a supplementary application should be submitted.

3. Quality study and quality standards

The pursuit of quality study and the enhancement of quality standards should be an ongoing endeavor. This can be achieved by incorporating specific identification of ingredients and implementing multi-marker assays, among other measures. Additionally, it is crucial to conduct studies on safety-related indicators such as heavy metals, harmful elements, pesticide residues, and mycotoxins. These studies should be tailored to the specific conditions of the product, and the findings should inform the development of standards. By doing so, the quality of the product can be effectively controlled and improved.

4. Stability study

The continuation of stability studies is necessary in order to ensure the consistent quality of the samples used in confirmed clinical trials.

(III) Submission of marketing authorization applications

In the field of PCMC study, it is imperative to ensure the completion of all necessary work. This includes specifying the manufacturing process and determining a reasonable range of key process parameters. Additionally, it is essential to establish a comprehensive quality control method to ensure consistent quality between post-market drugs and the samples used in confirmed clinical trials.

1. Ingredients and their quality

In accordance with the requirements for the TCM crude drugs and prepared slices/decoction pieces used in samples for non-clinical safety tests and clinical trials, it is necessary to establish specific information regarding the origin, medicinal parts, places of origin, harvesting period, and processing method of TCM crude drugs, and processing parameters of decoction pieces. Such information should be determined based on relevant study results of TCM crude drugs and prepared slices/decoction pieces. In conjunction with the conditions of clinical trials and the requirements for preparations, there is a need to enhance the quality standards for TCM crude drugs and decoction pieces.

In order to ensure the quality of TCM crude drugs and promote sustainable resource utilization, it is necessary to conduct resource evaluation of the TCM crude drugs in accordance with relevant requirements. Additionally, any valuable, rare and endangered wild TCM crude drugs, if utilized, should meet the post-market production demands.

2. Manufacturing process

In line with the preparation process for samples used in confirmed clinical trials, it is essential to establish control indicators for the production process, conduct a comprehensive verification of the manufacturing process at a commercial scale, determine the manufacturing process and its associated parameters for marketing authorization, and establish the acceptable range of yield rate/yield quantity for intermediates (such as extracts). These measures are crucial for ensuring better control over the consistency of product quality. The stability and feasibility of the manufacturing process are crucial, and the manufacturing conditions must adhere to the requirements outlined in the *Good Manufacturing Practice*. The excipients used must adhere to the pertinent criteria for associated review and approval.

3. Quality study and quality standards

Efforts should be made to enhance study on the quality of TCM crude drugs and prepared slices/decoction pieces, intermediates, preparations, excipients, and immediate packaging materials/containers of the drugs. Special attention should be given to monitoring changes in quality throughout the production process. It is imperative to establish a comprehensive quality standard system in order to achieve complete quality control of the drugs.

Quality standards for preparations should be established based on the test results of samples obtained from confirmed clinical trials, thereby reflecting the quality status of the samples used in clinical trials. In order to ensure consistent quality of the preparations, it is essential to establish a reasonable range for assay and other test indicators. Based on the product characteristics, it is necessary to study and establish various items such as fingerprint or characteristic chromatogram, bioactivity test, and other relevant factors.

4. Stability study

The determination of the expiry date and storage conditions should be based on the stability study results obtained from production-scale samples.

The specification of immediate packaging materials and containers for the samples, as well as their quality control requirements, should be provided. The immediate packaging materials and containers of the samples must adhere to the pertinent criteria for associated review and approval.

(IV) Post-market studies

Continuous efforts should be made to strengthen quality control studies, including conducting large-scale cultivation and breeding studies on wild TCM crude drugs. Additionally, it is essential to establish cultivation and breeding bases for TCM crude drugs in order to ensure stable quality and sustainable utilization of the TCM crude drugs. With advancements in science and technology, upgrading of manufacturing equipment and enhancement in product recognition, the need for conducting relevant studies arises. It is crucial to accumulate relevant data by considering practical production conditions and clinical application requirements. Attention should be given to ensuring the efficacy, safety, and quality control of drugs. Furthermore, it is essential to establish and enhance a comprehensive quality control system throughout the entire production process, aiming to continuously improve the overall product quality.

IV. References

1. *Drug Administration Law of the People's Republic of China*, 2019.

2. State Administration for Market Regulation. *Provisions for Drug Registration*, 2020.

3. *Opinions of the CPC Central Committee and the State Council on Promoting the Preservation, Innovation, and Development of Traditional Chinese Medicine*, 2019.

4. Center for Drug Evaluation, NMPA. *Guideline for Quality Control Study of TCM crude drugs of New Traditional Chinese Medicines (TCMs) (Trial)*, 2020.

5. Center for Drug Evaluation, NMPA. *Guideline for Quality Standard Study of New Traditional Chinese Medicines (TCMs)(Trial)*, 2020.

6. Center for Drug Evaluation, NMPA. *Guideline for Processing Study of Decoction pieces for New Traditional Chinese Medicines (TCMs) (Trial)*, 2020.

7. State Food and Drug Administration. *Guideline for Extraction and Purification Study of Traditional Chinese Medicines and Natural Medicines*, 2005.

8. State Food and Drug Administration. *Guideline for Study on Preparations of Traditional Chinese Medicines and Natural Medicines*, 2005.

中药新药研究各阶段药学研究
技术指导原则（试行）

一、概述

中药新药研究是一项涉及药学、药理毒理、临床等多学科研究的系统工程。药学研究主要包括处方药味及其质量、剂型、生产工艺、质量研究及质量标准、稳定性等研究内容。中药新药研究应在中医药理论指导下，根据中药特点、新药研发的一般规律及不同研究阶段的主要目的，开展针对性研究，落实药品全生命周期管理，促进中药传承与创新，保证药品安全、有效、质量可控。

本指导原则主要针对中药新药申请临床试验、Ⅲ期临床试验前、申请上市许可及上市后研究各阶段需要完成的药学主要研究内容提出基本要求，为中药新药研究提供参考。对于具体产品不必拘泥于本指导原则提出的分阶段要求，应根据产品特点，科学合理安排研究内容。

二、一般原则

（一）遵循中医药理论指导

中药新药药学研究应在中医药理论指导下，尊重传统经验和临床实践，鼓励采用现代科学技术进行研究创新。

（二）符合中药特点及研发规律

应根据中药的特点及新药研发的一般规律，充分认识中药的复杂性、新药研发的渐进性及不同阶段的主要研究目的，分阶段开展相应的研究工作，体现质量源于设计理念，注重研究的整体性和系统性，提高新药的研发质量和效率，促进中药传承和创新发展。

（三）践行全生命周期管理

中药新药药学研究应体现全生命周期管理，加强药材、饮片、中间体、制剂等全过程的质量控制研究，建立和完善符合中药特点的全过程质量控制体系，并随着对产品认知的提高和科学技术的不断进步，持续改进药品生产工艺、质量控制方法和手段，促进药品质量不断提升。

三、基本内容

（一）申请临床试验

应完成下列药学研究工作，为临床试验提供质量基本稳定的样品，满足临床试验的需求。研究内容包括固定处方药味和给药途径；明确药材基原及药用部位、饮片炮制方法、制备工艺；建立质量标准，基本完成安全性相关的质量控制研究，达到质量基本可控；保证临床试验用样品质量稳定。

1. 处方药味及其质量

中药新药的处方药味（包括中药饮片、提取物等）应固定。明确药材的基原、药用部位、质量要求、饮片的炮制方法及质量标准等。关注药材的产地、采收期（包括采收年限和采收时间，下同）等。

为保证中药新药质量稳定，应关注所用药材的质量及其资源可持续利用，对野生药材应按照相关要求开展资源评估研究。对于确需使用珍稀濒危野生药材的，应符合相关法规要求，并重点考虑种植养殖的可行性。

2. 剂型及制备工艺

在中医药理论指导下，结合人用经验、各药味所含化学成份的理化性质和药理作用等，开展中药新药制备工艺研究。

应进行剂型选择、工艺路线及主要工艺参数研究，明确剂型和制备工艺，说明其选择的合理性。明确前处理、提取、纯化、浓缩、干燥等方法及主要工艺参数，基本明确中间体（如浸膏等）的得率/得量等关键工艺指标。进行制剂处方设计及成型工艺研究，明确所用辅料、成型工艺及其主要工艺参数。

制备工艺应经中试放大研究确定，明确主要工艺参数。考虑商业规模生产设备的可行性和适应性。

非临床安全性试验用样品应采用中试及以上生产规模的样品。

3. 质量研究及质量标准

对中药新药用药材/饮片、中间体、制剂及辅料开展质量控制研究，建立质量标准。应围绕药品的安全性、有效性开展质量研究，重点对影响安全性的质控项目进行研究，如毒性成份及其控制，建立质量控制方法。随着研究的不断深入，质量研究及质量标准应逐步完善。

4. 稳定性研究

进行初步稳定性研究，选择适宜的直接接触药品的包装材料/容器，研究确定贮藏条件，保证临床试验用样品的质量稳定。

（二）Ⅲ期临床试验前

临床试验所用样品一般应采用生产规模制备的样品，生产应符合药品生产质量管理规范的要求。

1. 处方药味及其质量

在前期固定药材基原及药用部位、饮片炮制方法等研究基础上，通过对处方中药材的产地、采收期及产地加工、生产方式（野生、种植养殖、其他方式）、贮藏方法和条件等对药材质量影响的系统研究（包括文献研究），完善并确定药材相关信息，保证药材质量稳定。并应对药材、饮片等的质量标准进行不断研究完善。对于确需使用珍稀濒危野生药材的，应开展种植养殖技术研究。

2. 生产工艺

根据前期临床试验情况和研究结果，完成规模化生产研究，固定生产工艺并明确详细的工艺参数，确保Ⅲ期临床试验用样品质量稳定。在工艺路线及关键工艺参数不变的前提下，若需要对工艺参数、成型工艺、辅料、规格等进行变更的，应根据实际发生变更情况，参照相关技术指导原则开展研究工作，说明其合理性、必要性，必要时提出补充申请。

3. 质量研究及质量标准

继续开展质量研究和质量标准完善工作，如增加专属性鉴别药味、多指标的含量测定等。根据产品具体情况开展安全性相关指标（如重金属及有害元素、农药残留、真菌毒素）的研究，视结果列入标准，以更好地控制产品质量。

4. 稳定性研究

继续进行稳定性研究，保证确证性临床试验用样品的质量稳定。

（三）申请上市许可

应完成全部药学研究工作，明确生产工艺及关键工艺参数的合理范围，建立基本完善的质量控制方法，保证上市后药品与确证性临床试验用样品质量一致。

1. 处方药味及其质量

根据非临床安全性试验用样品、临床试验用样品所用药材/饮片情况，结合药材/饮片相关研究结果，固定药材基原、药用部位、产地、采收期、加工方法及饮片炮制工艺参数等。结合临床试验情况及制剂需要，完善药材、饮片等质量标准。

为保证药材质量及资源可持续利用，应按照相关要求完成药材资源评估；

对于使用的珍稀濒危野生药材，应满足上市后生产的需要。

2. 生产工艺

根据确证性临床试验用样品的制备工艺，建立生产过程的控制指标，完成商业规模的生产工艺验证，确定申请上市的生产工艺及工艺参数，确定中间体（如浸膏等）的得率/得量范围等，更好地控制产品质量的一致性。生产工艺应稳定可行，生产条件应符合药品生产质量管理规范的要求。所用辅料应符合关联审评审批相关要求。

3. 质量研究及质量标准

应加强药材/饮片、中间体、制剂及辅料、直接接触药品的包装材料/容器的质量研究，关注生产过程的质量变化，构建完善的质量标准体系，实现药品全过程质量控制。

制剂质量标准的制定应根据确证性临床试验用样品的检测结果，反映临床试验用样品的质量状况，含量测定等检测指标应制定合理的范围，确保制剂质量稳定。根据产品特点，探索建立指纹或特征图谱、生物活性检测等项目。

4. 稳定性研究

根据生产规模样品的稳定性考察结果，确定有效期及贮藏条件。

明确直接接触样品的包装材料/容器及其质量控制要求。所用直接接触样品的包装材料/容器应符合关联审评审批相关要求。

（四）上市后研究

继续加强质量控制研究，对野生药材开展规模化种植养殖研究，建立药材种植养殖基地，保障药材质量稳定和资源可持续利用。随着科学技术的进步、生产设备的更新以及对产品认识的不断深入等，开展相关研究；结合生产实际和临床使用情况，不断积累相关数据，关注药品有效性、安全性及质量可控性，建立完善全过程质量控制体系，推动药品质量不断提升。

四、参考文献

1.《中华人民共和国药品管理法》，2019年.

2. 国家市场监督管理总局.《药品注册管理办法》，2020年.

3.《中共中央 国务院关于促进中医药传承创新发展的意见》，2019年.

4. 国家药品监督管理局药品审评中心.《中药新药用药材质量控制研究技术指导原则（试行）》，2020年.

5. 国家药品监督管理局药品审评中心.《中药新药质量标准研究技术指导原则（试行）》，2020年.

6. 国家药品监督管理局药品审评中心.《中药新药用饮片炮制研究技术指导原则（试行）》，2020 年.

7. 国家食品药品监督管理局.《中药、天然药物提取纯化研究技术指导原则》，2005 年.

8. 国家食品药品监督管理局.《中药、天然药物制剂研究技术指导原则》，2005 年.

Guideline for Quality Study of New Traditional Chinese Medicines (TCMs) (Trial)

I. Overview

Quality study of new TCMs refers to the process of determining critical quality attributes of the TCMs by studying relevant factors related to drug safety and efficacy by using various technologies, methods and means under the guidance of TCM theories. The purpose of quality study is to determine the quality control indicators and their acceptable ranges, and provide basis for manufacturing process control and quality standards establishment of the TCMs, so as to guarantee the safety, efficacy and quality control of the TCMs.

Based on characteristics of the multi-component complex system of TCMs, the quality study of new TCMs should be oriented by clinical value and needs, abide by TCM theories, insist on integrating inheritance and innovation, and utilize new physical, chemical or biological technologies and methods to study and analyze quality characteristics of the TCMs from multiple perspectives. In the meantime, quality study should also reflect the concepts of quality by design, whole-process quality control and risk management. Through studies of quantitative and qualitative transfer of medicinal substances and critical quality attributes across TCM crude drugs, prepared slices/decoction pieces, intermediates (intermediate products) and preparations in different stages, as well as the interaction between medicinal substances and excipients/pharmaceutical packaging materials, the quality control level of TCMs is constantly improved.

This guideline aims to provide reference for the quality study of new TCMs, and relevant contents will continue to be improved in accordance with scientific researches and the development of TCM.

II. Basic Principles

(I) Abiding by the guidance of TCM theories

TCMs have complex medicinal substances, especially compound preparations. Therefore, the quality study should respect traditional theories and practices of TCM, and various study technologies and methods should be selected in accordance with characteristics of different medicines to conduct targeted quality studies and reflect the overall quality of TCMs.

(II) Laying equal emphasis on traditional quality control methods and modern quality study methods

Traditional experience and method are of important significance to TCM quality study and quality control, and in the meantime, application of modern science and technology in TCM quality study is also encouraged. In accordance with characteristics of the medicines, physical, chemical, biological or other modern study methods should be utilized to analyze quality characteristics of the TCMs, study characterization methods of the quality characteristics, critical quality attributes, quality evaluation method, and quantitative and qualitative transfer laws, to effectively reflect the quality of TCMs.

(III) Taking the medicinal substances as important study contents

During the quality study process of new TCMs, study on medicinal substances should be guided by TCM theories and clinical practices, and pay attention to association study of safety and efficacy. Studies on relevant attributes of medicinal substances should be carried out to provide scientific support for manufacturing process control and quality standard development.

(IV) Taking safety, efficacy and quality controllability as the objective

Quality control method and indicators of new TCMs should be able to reflect the safety, efficacy, stability and quality controllability of the TCMs. Medicinal substances and critical quality attributes, and quantitative and qualitative transfer laws of TCM crude drugs, prepared slices/decoction pieces, intermediates and preparations, as well as the interaction between medicinal substances and excipients/pharmaceutical packaging materials are main contents for quality study. Appropriate study methods and quality control indicators should be selected centering on the safety and efficacy, to objectively characterize TCM quality characteristics and provide scientific basis for TCM quality control.

(V) Running throughout the whole life cycle of the TCMs

Quality study of the TCMs should not be only embodied in the entire manufacturing process including the quality of medicinal substances and excipients, manufacturing processes and equipment selection, process control and management, development of quality standards for preparations, risk control and assessment, etc., and should also run throughout the whole life cycle of the TCMs. Post-market quality studies of the TCMs should be strengthened to constantly improve product quality, establish a quality control system aligned with TCM characteristics that spans the entire process and whole life cycle, thus guaranteeing the quality controllability, stability and uniformity of new TCMs.

III. Main Contents

(I) TCM crude drugs and prepared slices/decoction pieces

As the source of preparations, the quality of TCM crude drugs and prepared slices/decoction pieces has a direct influence on drug quality. Therefore, quality research and control of the entire manufacturing process for TCM crude drugs and prepared slices/decoction pieces should be strengthened, and modern information technologies are encouraged to be applied to establish a traceability system of TCM crude drugs and prepared slices/decoction pieces.

The quality control of TCM crude drugs and prepared slices/decoction pieces used in new TCMs should be performed in reference to their systematic study results and in combination with TCM crude drugs and prepared slices/ decoction pieces of specific products, as well as study results of its relevance to the intermediates and preparations, to determine the quality control indicators and their ranges of TCM crude drugs, prepared slices/decoction pieces, so as to meet quality design requirements for new TCMs.

Attention should be paid to impacts on the safety of TCM crude drugs from pesticide residues, heavy metals and harmful elements, and mycotoxin, etc. introduced during planting and cultivation, manufacturing, processing, circulation and storage of TCM crude drugs. If the formula contains animal-derived ingredients, attention should be paid to the possibility of introducing pathogens; in the meantime, attention should be paid to use of hormones and antibiotics in animal-derived ingredients, as well as mycotoxin contamination from some TCM crude drugs due to being infected with toxic fungi, and special safety control methods should be established when necessary; if the formula contains realgar, cinnabar and other mineral ingredients, reasonable purity control indicator of minerals should also be set, and safety influence of the valence state of its heavy metals and harmful elements that may be dissolved and absorbed in human body should also be studied; in addition, if the formula contains toxic ingredients, attention should be paid to its safety and efficacy, and reasonable limits or content ranges should be established as appropriate.

(II) Intermediates

Study on intermediates is one of the important contents of the quality study of new TCMs. The quality of the intermediates (such as powdered prepared slices/decoction pieces, concentrates, and extracts, etc.) should be studied, especially the intermediates directly used for TCM preparations, combined with the preparation process characteristics. In accordance with different characteristics of the TCMs, their physiochemical properties, chemical components, and bioactivity, etc. and influence factors related to safety and efficacy should be studied.

1. Physiochemical properties

Physiochemical properties are of important significance for intermediate quality control and subsequent preparation study, etc. For compound preparations of TCMs with complex chemical components and unclear active components, attention should be paid to studies on overall physiochemical properties of intermediates.

For fluids and semi-solids, critical quality attributes influencing the drug quality should be determined in accordance with the subsequent preparation needs and studies of medicinal substance composition, from quality information of description, relative density, pH value, clarity, flowability, and total solids, etc.

For powdered prepared slices/decoction pieces used directly as medicine, special attention should be paid to its particle size, particle size distribution and mixing uniformity, etc.

For extract powder, flowability, bulk density, solubility and hygroscopicity, etc. should be studied, and its critical quality attributes should be determined in accordance with properties of the medicine itself and subsequent preparation requirements.

2. Chemical components

TCMs have complex and diverse chemical components, and therefore, focused and systematic research on chemical components should be conducted based on the characteristics of new TCMs.

2.1 Compound preparations

For quality studies of compound preparations, a systematic study of chemical components should be conducted under the guidance of TCM theories and in combination with functions and indications, and previous use conditions.

Emphasis should be laid on literature research on chemical components of ingredients, to understand chemical categories, structures, contents, assay and measurement methods, etc. for various components.

Attention should be paid to chemical components related to TCM safety and efficacy, and to chemical components of sovereign drug, precious drugs, toxic drugs or ingredients with large dose in the formula.

Targeted studies should be conducted toward medicinal substances obtained from the confirmed manufacturing process, to identify critical quality attributes.

2.2 Extracts obtained from single plant, animal or mineral materials and their preparations

Since these extracts have been enriched with chemical components related to pharmaceutical effect during the preparation process, emphasis should be placed on systematic research on the composition and chemical component content, etc. of the extracts, and providing full characterization via multiple means of single component content, major chemical classes contents, and fingerprint/ characteristic chromatogram, etc.

Categories of other components contained in the extracts should also be studied, to guarantee the stability and uniformity of the medicinal substances of the extracts.

3. Safety-related factors

3.1 Endogenous toxic components

If the formula contains toxic ingredients, the endogenous toxicity should be analyzed in combination with toxicology study results, and in the meantime, attention should also be paid to ingredients containing structurally similar components with discovered toxic ingredients, as well as the ingredients belonging to the same family and genus with known toxic ingredients.

For ingredients containing known toxic components, limit test methods of toxic components should be established, to define safety limits or non-detection criteria; while if the toxic components are also active, content ranges (upper and lower limits) of such toxic components should be set in accordance with literature report and study results of safety and efficacy.

For ingredients with known toxicity but unclear toxic components, the safety dose range should be studied and determined in accordance with TCM theories and traditional clinical use, or the definitive study on toxic components and in-depth toxicology study on medicinal substances could be conducted, to strengthen quality control.

3.2 Exogenous pollutants

Exogenous pollutants primarily include pesticide residues (including plant growth regulators and their degradants), heavy metals, harmful elements, mycotoxin and sulfur dioxide, etc. introduced from TCM crude drugs and prepared slices/decoction pieces, and also include organic solvent residues and resin residues, etc. introduced during the extraction and processing, as well as the microorganisms grown during the storage process (if applicable). In addition, attention should also be paid to possible pollutants from the equipment and its components.

By the systematic study and analysis of the exogenous pollutants contained in the intermediates, for any pesticide residues, heavy metals, harmful elements and mycotoxin that might be introduced from TCM crude drugs and prepared slices/decoction pieces, their retention in intermediates should be analyzed, and necessary test methods should be studied and established.

If resin and/or organic solvent are used during the extraction and processing, their residue or enrichment in intermediates should be studied and analyzed, safety risks should be evaluated, and reasonable control methods should be established.

4. Bioactivity

It is encouraged to carry out studies on exploring bioactivity assay for new TCMs. It is suggested to combine pharmacological or toxicological research results to establish bioactivity assay method as alternatives or supplements to conventional physical and chemical methods, so as to improve the correlation between quality evaluation and functions and indications (indications for use), and safety of new TCMs.

(III) Preparations

In accordance with characteristics of new TCMs, based on studies on TCM crude drugs and prepared slices/decoction pieces, intermediates, the manufacturing process of preparations and stability, etc., and in combination with studies on medicinal substances, and safety and efficacy study results, the preparation quality study should be conducted with emphasis on the following aspects:

1. Dosage form

Dosage form is one of the important factors influencing the quality of new TCMs. For new TCMs, the administration route is selected and dosage form determined generally based on clinical use needs, and by comprehensively considering formula composition, physiochemical properties of medicinal substances, drug loading quantity of different dosage forms, clinical administration dose, and patient compliance, etc.

For new TCMs, corresponding quality control items should be studied and established according to the characteristics and requirements of different dosage forms, to characterize the characteristics of the dosage form selected. For different types of preparations, it is generally required to set key control indicators in reference to regulations in the General Rules on Preparations in *Chinese Pharmacopoeia*, e.g., disintegration time for oral solid preparations and softening time for suppositories, etc.

2. Formula and molding process of preparations

The formula of preparations should be determined in reference to study results of physiochemical properties, chemical components and bioactivity of intermediates. The properties of intermediates, functions of selected excipients and interaction between medicinal substances and excipients should also be considered comprehensively in combination with characteristics of the dosage form, to study impacts of the molding process on medicinal substances and the quality control method.

It should be noted that medicinal substances are affected by solvents, excipients and various processing conditions during the preparation process. In particular, loss and other changes of active components, volatile components, heat-sensitive components, and other unstable components may be induced by excessive temperature or heating time during drying and sterilization.

The critical control points and control objectives of the manufacturing process of preparations should be determined in reference to the stability of medicinal substances, to guarantee stable quality of the medicine.

3. Microorganism control

Microbial contamination (including primary contamination and secondary contamination) may occur during the manufacturing process of TCM crude drugs and prepared slices/decoction pieces and their preparations. Appropriate microbial control measures or appropriate microorganism removal method (e.g., autoclave, instantaneous high temperature) should be studied and taken into consideration based on ingredients, processing or manufacturing process characteristics, administration route, and drug properties, etc. Methods for removing microorganisms should be validated and ensure that they have no significant impact on the medicinal substances.

Microbiological tests must be carried out toward the preparations, and the microbial limit depends on the dosage form and administration route. The microbial limit test should conform to relevant regulations in the *Chinese Pharmacopoeia*.

4. Others

For new TCMs using extracts from single plants, animals, minerals, or other substances, it is suggested to conduct dissolution studies according to the requirements of dosage form and establish corresponding dissolution test method; moreover, it is encouraged to carry out relevant studies on other types of innovative TCMs in accordance with their own characteristics. For medicinal substances with low content in the preparations or accounting for a small proportion in the formula of preparations, attention should be given to their content uniformity, and relevant study and validation should be performed.

(IV) Relevance of quality study

1. Relevance to safety and efficacy

The quality study of new TCMs should aim to guarantee the safety and efficacy of the TCMs, and specific study methods and quality control indicators are chosen to characterize quality characteristics of new TCMs.

2. Relevance to manufacturing process study

Different preparation processes will get different medicinal substances with different properties, directly affecting the safety and efficacy of the medicine. Quality study should run through the entire process of the manufacturing process study and manufacturing quality control, to ensure consistent quality of the products.

3. Relevance to stability study

Stability study is also an important content of quality study. The stability study indicators should be able to reflect the intrinsic quality changes of the medicine and also reflect the quality study results.

Quality study should pay attention to changes in volatile, heat-sensitive, easily oxidized and other unstable components, and active components, especially changes in toxic components. Attention should be paid to changes in mycotoxin and other pollutants of powdered prepared slices/decoction pieces directly used as medicine, TCM crude drugs and prepared slices/decoction pieces with relatively high contamination risk from fermentation process, etc., and their preparations during storage process, and then corresponding control measures should be taken.

中药新药质量研究技术指导原则（试行）

一、概述

中药新药的质量研究是在中医药理论的指导下，采用各种技术、方法和手段，通过研究影响药品安全性和有效性的相关因素，确定药品关键质量属性的过程。质量研究的目的是确定质量控制指标和可接受范围，为药品生产过程控制和质量标准建立提供依据，保证药品的安全性、有效性和质量可控性。

基于中药多成份复杂体系的特点，中药新药的质量研究应以临床价值和需求为导向，遵循中医药理论，坚持传承和创新相结合，运用物理、化学或生物学等新技术、新方法从多角度研究分析药品的质量特征。同时，质量研究还应体现质量源于设计、全过程质量控制和风险管理的理念，通过对药材/饮片、中间体（中间产物）、制剂的药用物质及关键质量属性在不同环节之间的量质传递研究，以及药用物质与辅料、药包材相互影响的研究，不断提高中药的质量控制水平。

本技术指导原则旨在为中药新药的质量研究提供参考，相关内容将根据科学研究和中医药发展情况继续完善。

二、基本原则

（一）遵循中医药理论指导

中药尤其是复方制剂的物质基础复杂，在进行质量研究时应尊重传统中医药理论与实践，根据不同药物的特点，采用各种研究技术和方法，有针对性地开展质量研究，反映中药整体质量。

（二）传统质量控制方法与现代质量研究方法并重

传统经验方法对中药的质量研究和质量控制具有重要意义，同时鼓励现代科学技术在中药质量研究中的应用。应根据药物自身特点，运用物理、化学或生物学等现代研究方法分析药品的质量特征，研究质量特征的表征方法、关键质量属性、质量评价方法和量质传递规律，有效地反映药品的质量。

（三）以药用物质基础为重要研究内容

在中药新药质量研究过程中，药用物质基础研究应以中医药理论和临床实践为指导，同时关注与安全性、有效性的关联研究。通过药用物质基础相关属性的研究为生产过程控制和质量标准制定提供科学依据。

（四）以保证安全有效、质量可控为目标

中药新药的质量控制方法和指标应能反映药品的安全、有效、稳定、可控。药材/饮片、中间体、制剂的药用物质及关键质量属性、量质传递规律以及药用物质与辅料、药包材相互影响是质量研究的主要内容，应围绕安全性和有效性选择适宜的研究方法和质量控制指标，以客观地表征中药质量特征，为中药质量控制提供科学依据。

（五）贯穿药品全生命周期

中药质量研究不仅应体现在原辅料质量、生产工艺及设备选择、过程控制与管理、制剂质量标准制定、风险控制与评估等药品生产全过程，还应贯穿于药品全生命周期。应加强药品上市后质量研究，不断提升产品质量，构建符合中药特点的全过程和全生命周期的质量控制体系，保证中药新药质量的可控性和稳定均一。

三、主要内容

（一）药材/饮片

药材/饮片作为制剂源头，其质量直接影响药品的质量，应加强药材/饮片生产全过程质量研究与控制，鼓励应用现代信息技术建立药材/饮片的追溯体系。

中药新药用药材/饮片的质量控制应参考其系统研究结果，并结合具体品种的药材/饮片及其与中间体、制剂的相关性研究结果，确定药材/饮片的质量控制指标及范围，以满足中药新药的质量设计要求。

应关注药材种植养殖、生产、加工、流通、贮藏过程中包括农药残留、重金属及有害元素、真菌毒素等对药材安全性的影响。如处方中含有动物药味，应关注引入病原体的可能性；同时，应关注动物药味中激素、抗菌素使用的问题，以及一些药材感染产毒真菌而发生的真菌毒素污染等，必要时建立专门的安全性控制方法；处方若含雄黄、朱砂等矿物药时，还应建立合理的矿物纯度控制指标，并研究其可能在人体溶出被吸收的重金属及有害元素价态对安全性的影响；处方若含毒性药味，应关注其安全性和有效性，必要时制定合理的限量或含量范围。

（二）中间体

中间体研究是中药新药质量研究的重要内容之一，应结合制备工艺特点，研究中间体（如生药粉、浓缩液、浸膏等）的质量，特别是直接用于药物制剂

的中间体。根据药品的不同特点，研究其理化性质、化学成份、生物活性等以及与安全性、有效性相关的影响因素。

1. 理化性质

理化性质研究对于中间体的质量控制、后续的制剂研究等具有重要意义。对于化学成份复杂、有效成份不明确的中药复方制剂，应关注中间体整体理化性质研究。

对于液体和半固体，应根据后续制剂的需要和药用物质组成研究情况，从性状、相对密度、pH 值、澄明度、流动性、总固体等质量信息中确定影响药品质量的关键质量属性。

对于直接入药的生药粉，应重点关注其粒度、粒径分布及混合均匀度等。

对于浸膏粉，应对流动性、堆密度、溶解性、吸湿性等进行研究，根据药物本身的性质和后续制剂的要求，确定其关键质量属性。

2. 化学成份

中药的化学成份复杂多样，应根据中药新药的特点，进行有重点的系统化学成份研究。

2.1 复方制剂

复方制剂的质量研究应在中医药理论指导下，结合功能主治、既往使用情况开展系统的化学成份研究。

应重视处方药味化学成份文献研究，了解各种成份的化学类别、结构、含量以及分析测定方法等。

重点关注与中药安全性、有效性相关的化学成份，关注处方中君药、贵细药、毒剧药或用量较大药味的化学成份。

对确定的工艺所得的药用物质进行有针对性的研究，识别关键质量属性。

2.2 从单一植物、动物、矿物等物质中提取得到的提取物及其制剂

由于此类提取物在制备过程中富集了与药效有关的化学成份，应重点系统研究提取物的组成、化学成份含量等，并通过单体成份含量、大类成份含量及指纹/特征图谱等多种方式予以充分表征。

还应对提取物中其他成份的种类等进行研究，以保证提取物药用物质基础的稳定均一。

3. 与安全性有关的因素

3.1 内源性毒性成份

处方中若含有毒性药味时，应结合毒理学研究结果分析内源性毒性情况，同时还应关注含有与已发现的毒性成份化学结构类似成份的药味，以及与已知

毒性药味相同科属的药味。

对于含毒性成份明确的药味时，应建立毒性成份的限量检查方法，明确安全限量或规定不得检出；若毒性成份又是有效成份时，则应根据文献报道和安全性、有效性研究结果制定毒性成份的含量范围（上下限）。

对于含毒性明确但毒性成份尚不明确的药味时，应根据中医药理论和临床传统使用方法，研究确定其安全剂量范围，或开展毒性成份的确定性研究和药用物质毒理的深入研究，加强质量控制。

3.2 外源性污染物

外源性污染物主要包括由药材/饮片中引入的农药残留（包括植物生长调节剂及其降解物）、重金属及有害元素、真菌毒素、二氧化硫等，还包括提取加工过程中引入的有机溶剂残留、树脂残留等以及贮藏过程中（如适用）滋生的微生物。此外，还应关注可能来自设备及其组件的污染。

通过系统研究和分析中间体中所含外源性污染物的情况，对于可能由药材/饮片中引入农药残留、重金属及有害元素、真菌毒素的，应分析其在中间体中的保留情况，研究建立必要的检查方法。

若提取加工过程中有使用树脂及/或有机溶剂时，应研究分析其在中间体中的残留或富集情况，评估安全性风险，并制定合理的控制方法。

4. 生物活性

鼓励开展探索中药新药的生物活性测定研究。建议结合药理学或毒理学研究结果，建立生物活性测定方法以作为常规物理化学方法的替代或补充，提高中药新药的质量评价与功能主治（适应症）、安全性的关联性。

（三）制剂

应根据中药新药特点，在药材/饮片、中间体、制剂生产过程以及稳定性等研究基础上，结合药用物质基础研究、安全性和有效性研究结果，开展制剂质量研究，重点关注以下方面：

1. 剂型

剂型是影响中药新药质量的重要因素之一。中药新药一般基于临床使用需求，综合考虑药物处方组成、药用物质的理化性质、不同剂型的载药量、临床用药剂量、患者的顺应性等因素选择给药途径并确定剂型。

中药新药应根据不同剂型特点和要求，研究建立相应的质量控制项目以表征所选剂型的特点。不同类型制剂一般要求可参照《中国药典》制剂通则的规定设定关键控制指标，如口服固体制剂的崩解时限、栓剂的融变时限等。

2. 制剂处方、成型工艺

制剂处方的确定应参考中间体的理化性质、化学成份和生物活性的研究结果，还应结合剂型特点综合考虑中间体的性质、所选辅料的作用及原辅料间的相互作用，研究成型工艺过程对药用物质的影响和质量控制方法。

应关注药用物质在制剂过程中受到溶剂、辅料以及各种加工条件的影响，特别是有效成份、易挥发性成份、热敏性成份、其他不稳定成份在干燥、灭菌过程中由于温度过高或受热时间过长造成的成份损失等质量影响。

应参考药用物质稳定性情况，确定制剂工艺关键控制点和控制目标，以保证药品质量稳定。

3. 微生物控制

药材/饮片及其制剂过程中可能会产生微生物污染（包括初级污染、次级污染），应结合处方药味、加工或工艺特点、给药途径、药品特性等情况综合考虑，研究采取适当的微生物控制措施或采用适当的去除微生物的方法（如热压处理、瞬时高温等）。去除微生物的方法应经过验证，并保证其对药用物质基础无明显影响。

对于制剂必须进行微生物检验，其微生物限度取决于剂型和给药途径。微生物限度检查应符合《中国药典》的相关规定。

4. 其他

对从单一植物、动物、矿物等物质中提取得到的提取物新药，建议根据剂型的要求开展溶出度研究，建立相应的溶出度检查方法；鼓励对其他类型创新药物根据自身的特点开展相关研究。对于在制剂中含量较少或在制剂处方中占比较少的药用物质，应关注其含量均匀度，并进行相关研究及验证。

（四）质量研究的关联性

1. 与安全性、有效性的关联性

中药新药的质量研究应以保证药品的安全性和有效性为目的，选择针对性的研究方法和质量控制指标，表征中药新药的质量特征。

2. 与工艺研究的关联性

不同制备工艺获得的药用物质及其性质不同，直接影响药品的安全性和有效性。质量研究应贯穿于工艺研究及生产质量控制的全过程，确保生产出质量一致的产品。

3. 与稳定性研究的关联性

稳定性研究也是质量研究的重要内容。稳定性研究的考察指标应能反映药品内在质量变化、反映质量研究的结果。

质量研究应关注制剂中挥发性、热敏性、易氧化等不稳定成份、有效成份的变化，特别应关注毒性成份的变化。应关注生药粉入药、有发酵过程等污染风险较高的药材/饮片及其制剂贮藏期间真菌毒素等污染的变化并进行控制。

Guideline for Study on Bioassay of Traditional Chinese Medicines (TCMs) (Trial)

I. Overview

Bioassay is a method used to reflect the efficacy and safety of medicines relying on the biological effect of the medicines to test systems in the context of a specific test design, so as to evaluate and control the quality of medicines.

TCMs are characterized by multiple components, multiple targets and overall actions which are used under the guidance of TCM theories. To make up for the shortcomings of current quality control methods, it is necessary to study and explore bioassay methods when it is difficult to reflect the quality of TCMs by current quality control means such as physicochemical assay.

The guideline is developed to encourage the study and exploration of bioassay methods and optimize the TCMs quality control system. With the advance of science and technology and continuous deepening of studies on TCMs, the relevant contents in the guideline will be updated.

II. Basic Principles

(I) Reflecting the characteristics of TCMs and demonstrating the efficacy and safety of TCMs

Studies on bioassay should reflect the characteristics of TCMs, such as multiple components, multiple targets, and overall actions. The tests should demonstrate the efficacy, safety, and quality consistency of TCMs. Studies on bioassay should also fully consider the functions and indications of TCMs and adopt multiple indicators.

(II) Complementing the current quality test methods and improving the quality control of TCMs

TCMs contain complex components with limited research and information about the active components. Although the current quality control methods relying on chemical component tests are simple and easy to implement, they cannot comprehensively reflect the efficacy and safety of TCMs. Bioassay methods are relatively complex, but they can compensate for the shortcomings of the current quality control methods, and are conducive to improving the quality control of TCMs. It is encouraged to conduct studies on bioassay of TCMs and include mature and feasible methods into standards.

(III) The methods should be scientific and feasible

To objectively reflect the clinical efficacy and safety of TCMs, rigorous control measures for test conditions and operating procedures should be developed, and detailed methodological investigations and validations should be performed to ensure the specificity, accuracy, and reproducibility of the methods. The methods should be simple and feasible.

III. Basic Contents

Considering the difficulty in establishing bioassay methods, the complexity of the study object, and the limitations of application, it is preferable to explore and study the use of bioassay on TCMs that are difficult to be fully evaluated with routine physicochemical detection methods, including, but not limited to, the following situations: (1) with clear pharmacological effect, significant activity, and clear dose-effect relationship, but unclear active components; (2) involving toxic ingredients and/or where modern studies show strong toxicity to humans, but the components causing toxic reactions are not clear; and (3) chemical components detected do not have strong correlation with clinical efficacy and safety.

Studies on bioassay of TCMs mainly cover the selection of test methods, the selection and preparation of test articles, the selection and calibration of reference substances, the selection of test systems, the selection of endpoints, evaluation criteria, methodological validation, result statistics, and analysis and evaluation, etc. These Guidelines mainly include the following contents.

(I) Selection of test methods

When evaluating the quality of TCMs, the bioassay should focus on efficacy and safety. It is recommended to select the well-studied (highly recognized in the industry) methods that have a close correlation with clinical efficacy and safety (with a certain dose-effect relationship). It can generally be divided into in vivo testing and in vitro testing; quantitative, semi-quantitative, and qualitative testing; and specific testing and non-specific testing, etc. According to the purpose and requirements of evaluation, multiple bioassay methods can be selected for comprehensive evaluation.

The intensity of biological effects can generally be measured using biological potency assay. Biological potency refers to the intensity unit of biological effect of the test article relative to the reference substance under specific experimental conditions calculated by biostatistics through comparing the specific biological effect of the test article with the reference substance to the test system. Biological potency for the purpose of assessing toxicity is also known as biological toxicity.

In the cases where it is difficult to select appropriate reference substances, a quality control method can also be adopted which involves measuring the dosage of the test article that generates certain biological effects (including toxic reactions) to determine whether the test article complies with prescribed standards based on the dosage.

It is encouraged to study and develop new technologies and methods in conjunction with the characteristics of TCMs and the development in modern biotechnology.

(II) Preparation of test articles

The sample used for preparing the test article should be representative. Test articles should be prepared and studied based on comprehensive considerations of the overall action of TCMs, clinical medication features, manufacturing process, and the selected test system. If an in vitro test system is used, attention should be paid to the interference of substances such as tannins in the test article on the test results. When necessary, artificial gastric fluid, artificial intestinal fluid and other biomimetic extracts can be used for preparing test articles, or medicine-containing serum can be used as a test article.

(III) Selection and calibration of reference substances

The reference substance for the bioassay of TCMs should generally be homogeneous with the test article in terms of chemical composition and/ or biological effects, and samples with quality consistent with those used in confirmed clinical trials should be chosen. For TCMs with complicated components, it is generally difficult to obtain reference substances with good chemical homogeneity. Based on the purpose and needs of bioassay of TCMs, TCM crude drugs, prepared slices/decoction pieces, extracts, Chinese proprietary medicines, or chemical drugs can be selected as the reference substances according to the following conditions: (1) It has the same or similar biological effects to the test article on the selected biological test system; (2) The biological potency/toxicity can be measured, and is stable; and (3) The quality is uniform and stable, and the source can be traced. Calibration method for reference substances of TCMs is generally the same as or similar to the quality control methods for the test article, including bioassay and physicochemical assay.

Studies should be conducted on the preparation methods of reference substances, quality identification, calibration methods, storage conditions, stability, and bioassay results, etc. The reference substances included in registration standards should be calibrated for biological effects.

(IV) Selection of test system

Under the premise of ensuring that the evaluation results are associated with clinical efficacy and safety, priority should be given to relatively simple, cost-effective, and user-friendly test systems.

Available test systems for bioassay include integral animals, isolated tissues, organs, cells, subcellular organelles, receptors, ion channels, enzymes, and microorganisms, etc. Integral animal test results are generally closer to clinical effects, whereas in vitro testing is suitable for cases with obvious effects and good dose-effect relationships. When there is a good correlation between the biological effects of in vitro and in vivo tests, in vitro tests should be prioritized considering animal ethics, economics, and ease of operation.

Standardization studies should be carried out for the test system. The selection of laboratory animals, isolated organs, or cells and other test systems should be closely related to the test principles and endpoints, and have good reproducibility.

(V) Selection of endpoints

Biological effect endpoints should reflect or be associated with the pharmaceutical effect and/or toxicity of TCMs. Evaluation indicators with known or expected pharmacological actions should be selected. In addition, alternative biological effect endpoints may also be considered. In principle, the selected biological effect endpoints should be specific, accurate , reproducible and present certain dose-effect relationships.

A certain function of TCMs is generally related to multiple pharmacological actions, so it is difficult to reflect the primary clinical efficacy or toxicity with a single endpoint. Multiple biological effect endpoints can be observed in the same test system, and the same or different biological effect endpoints can be studied through multiple tests to comprehensively assess its efficacy or toxicity. It is encouraged to explore and use biomarkers and biological effect expression patterns as the biological effect endpoints.

(VI) Others

The selection of test articles, test design, result statistics, evaluation criteria, and methodological validation for studies on biological assay of TCMs should refer to relevant contents in the *Pharmacopoeia of the People's Republic of China*.

中药生物效应检测研究技术指导原则（试行）

一、概述

生物效应检测是利用药物对试验系所产生的生物效应，运用特定的实验设计，反映药物有效性、安全性的一种方法，从而达到评价和控制药品质量的目的。

中药在中医药理论指导下使用，具有多成份、多靶点，发挥整体作用等特点。当以理化检测方法等质量控制手段难以充分反映中药质量时，有必要研究探索生物效应检测方法，以弥补现行质量控制方法的不足。

为鼓励探索研究中药生物效应检测方法，完善中药质量控制体系，制定本技术指导原则。随着科学技术的进步和中医药研究的不断深入，相关内容将不断完善。

二、基本原则

（一）体现中医药特点，反映中药有效性和安全性

生物效应检测研究应尽可能体现中药多成份、多靶点及整体作用等特点，反映中药的有效性、安全性和质量一致性。应结合中医药特点，尽可能选择多个指标进行生物效应检测研究，并与中药的功能主治相关。

（二）与现行质量检测方法相互补充，提高中药质量可控性

中药成份复杂、药效物质基础研究薄弱，现行以化学成份检测为主的质量控制方法虽简单易行，但难以很好地反映中药的有效性、安全性；生物效应检测方法相对复杂，但可以较好地弥补现行质量控制方法的不足，有利于提高中药质量的可控性。鼓励开展中药生物效应检测研究，将成熟可行的方法列入标准。

（三）方法应科学可行

应对试验条件、操作规范等建立严格的控制措施，并进行详细的方法学考察和验证，保证方法专属、准确、可重复，客观真实地反映中药临床有效性和安全性。方法应简便、可行。

三、基本内容

考虑到生物效应检测方法建立的难度、研究对象的复杂性及应用的局限性，可优先考虑将生物效应检测用于常规理化检测方法难以充分评价的中药进

行探索研究，包括但不限于以下情形：（1）药理作用清楚、活性明显、量效关系明确，但有效成份不清楚的；（2）涉及毒性药味和/或现代研究表明对人体具有较强的毒性反应，但产生毒性反应的成份尚不明确的；（3）检测的化学成份与临床疗效和安全性关联性不强的。

中药生物效应检测研究主要包括检测方法的选择、供试品的选择和制备、参照物的选择和标定、试验系的选择、检测指标的选择、判定标准、方法学验证、结果统计与分析评价等。本指导原则主要包括以下内容。

（一）检测方法的选择

在用于中药质量评价时，生物效应检测应围绕有效性、安全性开展研究，尽可能选择与临床的有效性、安全性关联较强（存在一定量效关系）的、研究较成熟（业界认可度较高）的方法。一般可分为体内检测、体外检测；定量、半定量及定性检测；特异性检测、非特异性检测等。根据评价的目的和需求，可选择多种生物效应检测方法进行综合评价。

生物效应的强度，一般可以采用生物效价的方法测定。生物效价是指在特定的试验条件下，通过对比供试品与参照物对试验系的特定生物效应，按生物统计学方法计算出供试品相当于参照物的生物效应强度单位。以评价毒性为目的的生物效价，又称为生物毒价。

在难以选择合适参照物的情况下，也可以采用通过产生一定生物效应（包括毒性反应）的供试品剂量测定，并以此为指标判定供试品是否符合规定的一种质量控制方法。

鼓励针对中药的特点，结合现代生物技术的发展，研究建立新技术和新方法。

（二）供试品的制备

用于制备供试品的样品应具有代表性。综合考虑中药整体作用、临床用药特点、生产工艺及选择的试验系等研究制备供试品。如采用体外试验系时，应充分关注供试品中的鞣质等物质对测定结果的干扰。必要时，可采用人工胃液、人工肠液等仿生提取制备供试品，或采用含药血清等作为供试品。

（三）参照物的选择和标定

中药生物效应检测的参照物，一般应与供试品在化学组成和/或生物效应方面具有同质性，选择与验证性临床试验用样品质量一致的样品。对成份复杂的中药，化学同质性好的参照物一般难以获得，基于中药生物效应检测的目的和需要，也可根据以下条件选择药材/饮片、提取物、中成药或化学药品作为参照物：（1）在选定的生物试验系上，与供试品具有相同或相近的生物效应；

（2）生物效价/毒价可标定，稳定性好；（3）质量均一稳定，可溯源。

中药参照物的标定方法一般选择与该供试品质量控制相同或相近的方法，包括生物效应测定和理化测定。应对参照物制备方法、质量鉴定、标定方法、贮存条件、稳定性和生物效应测定结果等进行研究。列入注册标准的参照物应经过生物效应的标定。

（四）试验系的选择

在能够保证评价结果与临床疗效和安全性相关联的前提下，优先选择相对简便、经济、可操作性强的试验系。

生物效应检测可选择的试验系包括整体动物、离体组织、器官、细胞、亚细胞器、受体、离子通道、酶和微生物等。整体动物试验结果一般与临床效应更接近，体外试验适用于效应明显且有良好量效关系的情况。当体外试验和体内试验的生物效应相关性较好时，从动物伦理、经济学及操作简便性方面考虑，可优先选择体外试验。

应对试验系进行标准化研究。实验动物、离体器官或细胞等试验系的选择应与实验原理及测定指标密切相关，并有良好的可重复性。

（五）检测指标的选择

生物效应检测指标应反映或关联中药的药效和/或毒性，选取已知或预期药理作用的评价指标，也可考虑采用替代的生物效应检测指标。生物效应指标的选择原则上应具有专属性、准确性、可重复性和一定的量效关系。

中药的某一功效一般与多种药理作用相关，采用单一指标通常难以反映其临床主要疗效或毒性情况，可在同一试验系中观察多个生物效应指标，也可通过多项试验考察相同或不同的生物效应指标，综合考察其疗效或毒性。鼓励探索采用生物标志物、生物效应表达谱等作为生物效应检测指标。

（六）其他

中药生物效应检测研究涉及的供试品的选择、实验设计、结果统计、判定标准、方法学验证等内容可参考中国药典相关内容。

Guideline for Quality Standard Study of New Traditional Chinese Medicines (TCMs) (Trial)

I. Overview

The quality standards of TCMs are an important study subject for new TCMs. The study should follow the discipline of TCM development, adhere to a way of inheritance in combination with innovation, and reflect the concept of life-cycle management on TCM quality. Scientific, reasonable, and feasible quality standards should be established through an in-depth study by applying modern science and technology to ensure quality control of the TCMs.

Researchers should select and determine the markers of the quality standards in a targeted manner according to the formula composition, preparation process, physical and chemical properties of medicinal substances, and stability of the preparation. The quality standards should also be continuously improved in combination with the development of relevant science and technology, so as to improve the quality control level of new TCMs and ensure their safety and efficacy.

This guideline aims to provide technical guidance for quality standard study on new TCMs and focus on the basic requirements for study and establishment of quality standards. It also can be applicable to those of natural medicines.

II. Basic Principles

(I) Quality standards should reveal the quality of TCMs

The quality standards should embody the quality of TCM preparations as per their characteristics and be linked to their safety and efficacy. It is encouraged to carry out exploratory study through various approaches on the active component in TCMs, and the identification method corresponding to all ingredients in a formula should be established. Generally, active components, toxic components, and other chemical components that possess obvious indicative characteristics should be selected as the quality marker. In the development of quality standards, the settings of test items and requirements should be assessed on their scientificity and rationality, and test methods should be assessed on their applicability and feasibility. In the process of quality standard study, it is encouraged to explore the correlation between the results from clinical trials or non-clinical studies and each marker selected from the components existing in the test samples, and quality studies on the safety and efficacy of TCMs should be undertaken so that adequate evidence can be provided for the rationale behind the adoption of markers in the quality standard.

(II) Quality standards' relevance should be considered

The quality standards for prepared slices/decoction pieces, extracts, intermediates, and preparations constitute the quality standard system of TCM preparations. An integral quality standard system is the basis of traceability for TCM quality, which reflects the medicinal substance's quantity and quality transfer from decoction pieces, extracts, and intermediates to preparations during the producing process of TCM preparations. The system also reveals the relationship between quality standards,process design, and stability studies, etc.

(III) The quality standard study should reveal the characteristics of TCM preparations

Targeted study on quality standard should be carried out as per the characteristics of formula composition, active marker or analytical marker, excipients, and dosage forms of preparations. Due to the differences in medicinal substances of TCM preparations, quality standards should reflect different characteristics conveyed by quality markers, methods, and relevant requirements set in each item of standards. Quality control methods for TCMs should be tailored to the specific drug requirements,and integration of multiple methods are encouraged. The ingredients existing in a compound preparation of TCMs are closely related to the formula and the manufacturing process; multiple markers, if necessary, should be properly set up in the quality standard. The limit or limit range for each marker in a quality standard should be determined based on the study data obtained from the samples used in clinical trials.

(IV) Quality standards should be scientific, standardized, and feasible

The quality standards for new TCMs should be developed in compliance with the relevant requirements under the General Notices, the General Rules on Preparations, and chapters for the development of various test methods in the *Chinese Pharmacopoeia*. Study on quality standards should be undertaken by following the *National Drug Standard Work Manual*. Systematic study and validation should be performed by consulting the *Guideline for Validation of Analytical Method* in the *Chinese Pharmacopoeia* for the requirements, so that the rationality and feasibility behind the establishment of analytical methods are proven. Representative samples should be applied in quality standard study, and each test method should be simple and feasible. Reference substances should be reasonably selected to meet the needs of the tests, and reference extracts are encouraged to be used in multi-marker assay. The newly applied reference substances should be subject to assignment-related studies such as structure validation and purity analysis in accordance with the requirements of the *Guideline for the Study on Pharmaceutical Reference Substances*, and the candidate reference substances should be submitted to the National Institutes for Food and Drug Control following the *Measures for the Application and Filing of Medicinal Substances of Pharmaceutical Reference Substances*.

(V) Phases of study on quality standards of TCMs

Study on the quality standards of new TCMs is a process of gradual improvement. In the study phase before clinical trials, emphasis should be placed on study and establishment of test methods in terms of major markers, including toxic components, and the markers related to safety should be considered as all-around as possible for inclusion in a quality standard. During clinical trials, it is necessary to study and establish the markers and methods that comprehensively embody the quality of TCM preparations to improve the quality control of TCMs. In the study phase before a new TCM is marketed, attention should be paid to the consistency between markers adopted in the quality standard for preparations and the corresponding ones adopted in the quality standard for samples used in confirmed clinical trials.

Based on the consideration regarding risk assessment, the test items should be reasonably selected for inclusion in the quality standard, and reasonable limits and content ranges should be formulated based on the test data from samples that are used in clinical trials. After a TCM preparation is marketed, the quality standard should be continuously revised and improved based on the accumulation of production data.

(VI) Quality standards should be processing

The methods adopted in quality standards should be scientific, advanced, and practical, and also fulfill the requirements for simplicity, sensitivity, accuracy, and reliability. The development of modern science and technology has provided new technologies and methods for the study on quality standards of new TCMs. If the actual conditions allow and need modern scientific and technological achievements to be applied in quality standard study and testing, the relevant new technologies and methods are encouraged to be applied in quality standards to better embody the TCMs' inherent quality. If it comes to the case that a new method is applied to replace an old one, the requirements on relevant markers for quality control should be reasonably defined through studies comparing the two methods.

III. Main Contents

The contents of quality standards for new TCMs generally encompass items such as the name of medicine, formula, preparation method, description, identification, test, extract, fingerprint or characteristic chromatogram, assay, functions and indications, usage and dosage, precautions, specifications, and storage, among others. The following is a brief description of the main study contents and general requirements for some items in the quality standards of new TCMs.

(I) Name of medicine

The name includes the formal name of the medicine and its name in Chinese Pinyin. Naming should comply with the relevant provisions required by the National Medical Products Administration.

(II) Formula

The formula includes the names and amounts of the ingredients, such as decoction pieces and extracts. The ingredients of a compound preparation should generally be arranged in the order of sovereign, minister, adjuvant and courier. The amount unit is gram (g) for solid ingredients and gram (g) or milliliter (ml) for liquid ingredients. The amount of each ingredient in a formula is generally converted by the amount that is used for manufacturing 1000 units of preparation (tablets, granules, g, ml, etc.); except for special circumstances, integer digits are generally adopted for the numerical value of each ingredient amount.

The names of ingredients should be adopted in accordance with those in the national drug standards or drug registration standards; aliases or synonyms should be avoided. For detailed requirements in this regard, refer to the *Chinese Pharmacopoeia* for the relevant provisions. If there is no national drug standard or drug registration standard for certain decoction pieces or extracts contained in the formula of a compound preparation, it is necessary to additionally establish their quality standards as attachments to the quality standard of the preparation. Furthermore, the preparation process must be included in the quality standard of extract.

(III) Procedure

The preparation method is a brief description of the manufacturing process and generally includes process procedures and major process parameters such as pre-treatment, extraction, purification, concentration, drying, and molding, among others. The preparation method should be normatively described by consulting the *Chinese Pharmacopoeia* and the *National Drug Standard Work Manual* for requirements on formats and terms. The description requires accurate wording, concise language, and rigorous logic, and should avoid using sentences that are prone to misunderstanding or ambiguity.

(IV) Description

The description embodies the characteristics of TCM quality to a certain extent, and the appearance, shape, smell, taste, solubility, and physical constants, etc. should be described based on the preparation itself and its contents.

Generally, the range of color differences should not be too wide when describing the color of an appearance. Composite colors should be described by hyphenated compound words with subsidiary color as a preceding word and dominant color as a following word. For example, yellow-brown means brown is the dominant color. The other descriptions should refer to relevant requirements under the General Notices of the *Chinese Pharmacopoeia*.

(V) Identification

Commonly used identification methods include microscopic identification, chemical reactions, chromatographic, spectroscopic, and biological methods. The identification test should generally adopt a method with high specificity, high sensitivity, good reproducibility, rapidity, and operational convenience. A method that can simultaneously identify multiple ingredients in one test is encouraged to be developed.

If raw drug powders, as an ingredient, are directly fed into a preparation, a microscopic identification method should generally be developed. If raw drug powders, as multi-ingredients, are directly fed into a preparation, the specific characteristics of each ingredient should be described in the microscopic identification method. The identification method of chemical reaction is usually applicable to the mineral ingredients and the ingredients containing major chemical classes in the preparation. Chromatographic methods mainly include the thin-layer chromatographic (TLC/HPTLC), the gas chromatographic (GC), and the high-performance liquid chromatographic (HPLC/UPLC) methods, etc. The TLC method can perform identification as per the retention factor (Rf) value and features of the separated spots/streaks by visualizing a developed plate. The consistency of characteristic spots/streaks between the sample and reference substances in terms of numbers, Rf values, colors, and manifestation under ultraviolet (UV) absorption/fluorescence should be detailed. The HPLC and GC methods should perform identification as per chromatographic features such as retention time. If a formula contains an ingredient from animal origin whose biological macromolecular components, such as protein and polypeptide, etc., are the only feature of that ingredient in the preparation, the identification method specific to the ingredient should be established accordingly in the study.

(VI) Test

1. Test items regarding dosage form

It is required to formulate the test method that is capable of reflecting the preparation characteristics as per the natures of dosage forms and the needs of clinical medication by consulting the *Chinese Pharmacopoeia* for the relevant provisions under the General Rules on Preparations. If there are two or more methods for option in the test items regarding dosage form under the General Rules of the *Chinese Pharmacopoeia*, the method should be logically selected according to the preparation characteristics, followed by an explanation.

2. Test items regarding safety

If an ingredient contained in a formula is likely to be contaminated by heavy metals and harmful elements, or if harmful elements are likely to be introduced by the equipment, excipients, and materials used for separation in the production process, limit test methods should be established accordingly for heavy metals and harmful elements. Limits should be reasonably determined on the basis of sufficient study and risk assessment, which should also fulfill the requirements under the relevant provisions in the *Chinese Pharmacopoeia* and other standards.

If an organic solvent (except ethanol) is used for extraction or processing in the preparation process, a test method for organic solvent residue should be established in the quality standard; if macroporous adsorption resin is used for separation and purification, a limit test method for organic resin residues that likely exist in extracts should be studied and established according to the type of resin, possible degradation products of the resin, and the solvent used. For example, the possible degradation products of styrene-type macroporous adsorption resins mainly include, but are not limited to, benzene, *n*-hexane, toluene, xylene, styrene, and diethyl benzene, among others. Limits for the above-mentioned solvent residues or organic resin residues should comply with the relevant provisions of the *Chinese Pharmacopoeia*, or be determined as per the relevant requirements of the International Council for Harmonization of Technical Requirements for Pharmaceuticals for Human Use (ICH).

If an ingredient in a formula contains one or a group of toxic components which are unrelated to the indication of the TCM, a limit test method for the relevant toxic components should be established for that ingredient, and limits need to be reasonably determined based on the data obtained from toxicology or literature studies.

3. Test items regarding characteristics of medicinal substance

Test items should be established in a targeted manner as per characteristics of TCMs. For example, test methods for related substances and dissolution should be established for oral solid preparations made from a single extracted compound; for oral solid preparations containing insoluble extracts, dissolution studies should be carried out. For preparations whose major marker is polysaccharides, study should be undertaken to establish a test method that specifically reflects the structural features of macromolecular substances, such as the molecular weight distribution of polysaccharides.

4. Determination of test limit

Test methods and limits for each test item in a quality standard should be elaborated. In general, for test items included in a quality standard, the rationality of test methods and their limits should be fully demonstrated from the perspective of safety and actual manufacturing conditions. Test limits, especially those for hazardous substances, should be determined within the allowed range that is backed by safety data.

(VII) Extracts

The total amount of the extract obtained from the extract test can be used as an marker to control the quality consistency among different batches of the same TCM preparation. The method for extract test can be established by the selection of an appropriate solvent (not limited to one solvent) as per the physical and chemical properties of the major compounds contained in the preparation. According to different categories of solvents, an extract can be divided into water-soluble extract, alcohol-soluble extract, ethyl acetate extract, and ether extract. The impact of various influencing factors on the result of extract test should be investigated through a systematic study, e.g., the influence of excipients. The method for extract test should indicate the category and amount of solvent, test method, and temperature parameter, etc., and a limit range for the extract amount should be reasonably specified.

(Ⅷ) Fingerprint/characteristic chromatogram

For a new TCM preparation (except that containing a single extracted compound), generally, the fingerprint/characteristic chromatogram should be subject to study and the establishment of a standard. The study generally encompasses the establishment of analytical methods, the identification of chromatographic peaks, the establishment of a reference chromatogram, and data analysis and evaluation, etc.

There are a variety of chromatographic methods available for fingerprint/characteristic chromatogram study, e.g., the HPLC/UPLC method, the HPTLC method, and the GC method, among others. The method for preparing a test sample should be appropriately established according to the properties of the major compounds contained in the preparation. If a TCM preparation contains numerous categories of components with disparities in physical and chemical properties, it can be considered to separately prepare the test sample in a targeted manner as per the component category, and multiple fingerprints/characteristic chromatograms can be established to provide information on different categories of components. If single method cannot fully reveal the characteristics of the test sample, two or more methods can be employed to obtain different fingerprints/characteristic chromatograms for analysis.

The selection of test methods and parameters for the fingerprint/characteristic chromatogram should be performed based on the principle of maximizing the information on the components contained in the preparation. Generally, if one or more major active or analytical markers are available, they should be selected as reference substances. When an appropriate reference substance is unavailable, the steady chromatographic peak available on the chromatogram is an alternative to the reference, which should be identified as much as possible.

The chromatographic peaks presenting on the fingerprints/characteristic chromatograms of all batches of samples are selected as common peaks through the analysis of representative chromatograms. Chromatographic peaks with high content and strong specificity (with priority for known effective/ active components, markers, and other known components) can be selected as characteristic peaks. In the process of conducting study on the fingerprint/ characteristic chromatogram, the major chromatographic peaks should be identified as much as possible.

The fingerprint/characteristic chromatogram generally uses similarity, relative retention time and peak area ratio of characteristic peaks, etc. as quality markers. Based on the results tested from multiple batches of samples, the computer software of the fingerprint similarity evaluation system is used to acquire the pattern of common peaks, followed by the establishment of a reference fingerprint chromatogram. The software is further used to analyze and compare the similarity between the fingerprint of test samples and the reference chromatogram, and the features of non-common peaks also need attention. The relative retention time and its range for each characteristic peak need to be defined for a characteristic chromatogram. The similarity, relative retention time, peak area ratio, and its range for the fingerprint/characteristic chromatogram in a quality standard must be formulated based on the evaluation of the data tested from multiple batches of samples.

(IX) Assay

1. Selection of assay markers

Where the formula composition of preparations is different, the selection of assay markers will also be different. For a preparation containing a single extracted compound, this component is selected for assay. The assay methods of one or more major markers should be established for the preparation containing an extract with a basically clear composition, and the assay methods of major chemical classes should also be studied and established.

Assay methods for multiple ingredients should be studied and established as much as possible for compound preparations. The chemical components related to the safety and efficacy of a preparation should be given priority in selection according to the functions and indications of the preparation. Generally, effective/ active components, toxic components, and markers contained in sovereign medicines, etc. are prior choices as markers for assays. In addition, it is necessary to take into consideration the correlation between the assay markers and both the manufacturing process and product stability, and the assay method for multi-components or multi-ingredients should be established as much as possible. If a manufacturing process includes multiple process routes, the assay method should be established for the effective/active or markers relevant to each process route; while if a manufacturing process involves the extraction of volatile oil, the assay method for the total amount of volatile oil or corresponding markers should be developed, and the method should be included in the quality standard as appropriate. If an ingredient contains a specific heat-sensitive component, study on assay method that can reflect the degree how the component endures heating and the stability of the component during the production process should be conducted, and the assay method should be included in the quality standard as appropriate.

2. Assay method

The assay methods encompass the volumetric (titration) method, the chromatographic method, and the spectroscopic method, among others. The chromatographic methods include the GC method, the HPLC/UPLC method, and others. The GC or GC-MS method is preferred for volatile components, and the HPLC/UPLC method is preferred for non-volatile components. For the inorganic components contained in mineral ingredients, the volumetric method, the atomic absorption spectrometric method (AAS), the inductively coupled plasma atomic emission spectrometric method (ICP-AES), and the inductively coupled plasma mass spectrometric method (ICP-MS), etc. can be adopted for assay.

The adopted assay method should be validated.

3. Content range

In general, the content range of a major compound should be specified for the single extracted compound and its preparation; the percentage range of content equivalent to the labeled amount per unit of preparation for the component should be specified based on its actual content and the preparation requirements.

For extracts, the content ranges for major markers and for major chemical classes contained in extracts should be specified in the quality standards; one or more components can be assigned as markers to a major compounds as well as to a major chemical classes. For preparations made from extracts, the content ranges for major markers and for major chemical classes should be specified in the quality standards of preparations based on the actual content in the extracts and the preparation requirements.

For compound preparations, multiple markers are encouraged to be adopted for an assay, and the content range for each marker should be specified in the assay method. Where a formula contains ingredients with components that are likely effective as well as toxic, assays must be performed, and the content ranges of these components should be specified.

(X) Bioactivity assay

Bioactivity assay methods generally encompass biological potency assays and bioactivity limit assays. Due to the limitations of the existing conventional physical and chemical methods applied in quality control on TCM preparations, it is encouraged to explore study on bioactivity assay and establish bioactivity assay methods as a substitute or supplement for conventional physical and chemical methods.

The application of bioactivity assay methods should comply with the basic principles of randomization, control, and reproducibility in pharmacology studies, and the established methods should be simple, precise, feasible, and controllable, and also have explicit criteria for judgment. The selection of the test system is closely related to the experimental principle and the establishment of markers. A test system with clear background information, few influencing factors, sensitive quality markers, and high cost performance ratio should be selected. The assay/potency determination method that characterizes the bioactivity intensity of TCM preparations should be validated according to the requirements of the bioactivity assay method. For detailed requirements of the bioactivity assay methods for different medicines, please refer to the relevant guidelines.

(XI) Specifications

Specifications for TCM preparations should refer to the *Guideline for on*

Writing of Specification Expression of for Chinese Proprietary Medicines for the relevant requirements.

(XII) Storage

The descriptions under the storage item listed in a quality standard are the basic requirements for the storage and preservation of TCM preparations. The stability of TCM preparations is not only related to their own properties, but also affected by many external factors. The storage conditions should be defined through systematic study of the immediate packaging materials for TCM crude drugs (decoction pieces), extracts, and preparations based on the factors that influence stability of TCM preparations and the stability study results of TCM preparations.

IV. Main References

1. National Medical Products Administration. *Technical Requirements for Study on New-registered Traditional Chinese Medicines*, 1999.

2. State Food and Drug Administration. *Technical Requirements for Study on New-registered Natural Medicines*, 2013.

3. Chinese Pharmacopoeia Commission. *National Drug Standard Work Manual*, 2012.

中药新药质量标准研究技术指导原则（试行）

一、概述

中药质量标准是中药新药研究的重要内容。中药质量标准研究应遵循中医药发展规律，坚持继承和创新相结合，体现药品质量全生命周期管理的理念；在深入研究的基础上，运用现代科学技术，建立科学、合理、可行的质量标准，保障药品质量可控。

研究者应根据中药新药的处方组成、制备工艺、药用物质的理化性质、制剂的特性和稳定性的特点，有针对性地选择并确定质量标准控制指标，还应结合相关科学技术的发展，不断完善质量标准的内容，提高中药新药的质量控制水平，保证药品的安全性和有效性。

本指导原则旨在为我国中药新药质量标准研究提供技术指导，重点阐述中药新药质量标准研究及质量标准制定的基本要求，天然药物的质量标准研究也可参照本指导原则。

二、基本原则

（一）质量标准应能反映中药质量

质量标准应根据中药的特点反映中药制剂的质量，并与药物的安全性、有效性相关联。鼓励采用多种形式开展中药活性成份的探索性研究，对处方中所有药味均应建立相应的鉴别方法；通常应选择所含有效（活性）成份、毒性成份和其他指标特征明显的化学成份等作为检测指标。建立质量标准应对检验项目及其标准设置的科学性及合理性、检验方法的适用性和可行性进行评估。在质量标准研究过程中，鼓励探索临床试验及非临床研究结果与试验样品中各指标成份的相关性，开展与中药安全性、有效性相关的质量研究，为质量标准中各项指标确定的合理性提供充分的依据。

（二）质量标准研究的关联性

中药饮片或提取物、中间产物、制剂等质量标准构成了中药制剂的质量标准体系，完善的质量标准体系是药品质量可追溯的基础；反映了中药制剂生产过程中，定量或质量可控的药用物质从饮片或提取物、中间体到制剂的传递过程，这种量质传递过程符合中药制剂的质量控制特点，也体现了中药制剂质量标准与工艺设计、质量研究、稳定性研究等的关系。

（三）质量标准研究应反映制剂特点

质量标准应结合制剂的处方组成、有效成份或指标成份、辅料以及剂型的特点开展针对性研究。不同药物制剂的药用物质基础各不相同，其质量标准的各项检测指标、方法及相关要求等也应分别体现各自不同的特点。中药质量控制方法选择应因药制宜，鼓励多种方法融合。中药复方制剂所含成份与其处方、工艺密切相关，应在其质量标准中建立多种指标的检验检测项目。质量标准各项指标限度及其范围应根据临床试验用样品等的研究数据来确定。

（四）质量标准应科学、规范、可行

中药新药质量标准应符合《中国药典》凡例、制剂通则和各检验检测方法等的要求。质量标准研究应参照《国家药品标准工作手册》的规范，按照《中国药典》中的《药品质量标准分析方法验证指导原则》的要求进行系统研究和验证，以证明分析方法的合理性、可行性。质量标准研究用样品应具有代表性，各检验检测方法应简便、可行。应根据检验检测的需要，合理地选择标准物质，鼓励选择对照提取物用于多指标成份的含量测定方法的研究。新增的标准物质应按照《药品标准物质研究技术指导原则》的要求，进行结构确证、纯度分析等标定相关研究，并按《药品标准物质原料申报备案办法》的要求送中国食品药品检定研究院对标准物质进行备案。

（五）质量标准研究的阶段性

中药新药质量标准研究是随着新药研究的不断推进而逐步完善的过程。在临床试验前的研究阶段，应着重研究建立包括毒性成份在内的主要指标的检验检测方法，质量标准涉及安全性的指标应尽可能全面。在临床试验期间，应研究建立全面反映制剂质量的指标、方法，提高药品质量的可控性。新药上市前的研究阶段，应重点考虑制剂质量标准的各项指标与确证性临床试验样品质量标准相应指标的一致性。基于风险评估的考虑，合理选择纳入质量标准的检验检测项目，并根据临床试验用样品的检验检测数据制定合理的限度、含量范围等。药品上市后，还应积累生产数据，继续修订完善质量标准。

（六）质量标准应具有先进性

质量标准采用的方法应具有科学性、先进性和实用性，并符合简便、灵敏、准确和可靠的要求。现代科学技术的发展为中药新药的质量标准研究提供了更多的新技术、新方法。若现代科学技术发展的成果符合中药质量标准研究及检验检测实际需要，鼓励在质量标准中合理利用有关的新技术、新方法，以利于更好地反映中药的内在质量。对于提高和完善质量标准的研究，若有采用

新方法替换标准中的原方法的情况，则应开展二者的对比研究，合理确定相关指标的质量控制要求。

三、主要内容

中药新药质量标准的内容一般包括：药品名称、处方、制法、性状、鉴别、检查、浸出物、指纹/特征图谱、含量测定、功能与主治、用法与用量、注意、规格、贮藏等。以下就中药新药质量标准中部分项目的主要研究内容及一般要求进行简要说明：

（一）药品名称

包括药品正名与汉语拼音名，名称应符合国家药品监督管理部门的有关规定。

（二）处方

处方包括组方饮片和提取物等药味的名称与用量，复方制剂的处方药味排序一般应按君、臣、佐、使的顺序排列。固体药味的用量单位为克（g），液体药味的用量单位为克（g）或毫升（ml）。处方中各药味量一般以1000个制剂单位（片、粒、g、ml等）的制成量折算；除特殊情况外，各药味量的数值一般采用整数位。

处方药味的名称应使用国家药品标准或药品注册标准中的名称，避免使用别名或异名，详细要求参照《中国药典》的有关规范。如含有无国家药品标准且不具有药品注册标准的中药饮片、提取物，应单独建立该药味的质量标准，并附于制剂标准中，提取物的质量标准应包括其制备工艺。

（三）制法

制法为生产工艺的简要描述，一般包含前处理、提取、纯化、浓缩、干燥和成型等工艺过程及主要工艺参数。制法描述的格式和用语可参照《中国药典》和《国家药品标准工作手册》的格式和用语进行规范，要求用词准确、语言简练、逻辑严谨，避免使用易产生误解或歧义的语句。

（四）性状

性状在一定程度上反映药品的质量特性，应按制剂本身或内容物的实际状态描述其外观、形态、嗅、味、溶解度及物理常数等。通常描述外观颜色的色差范围不宜过宽。复合色的描述应为辅色在前，主色在后，如黄棕色，以棕色为主。性状项的其他内容要求应参照《中国药典》凡例。

（五）鉴别

鉴别的常用方法有显微鉴别法、化学反应法、色谱法、光谱法和生物学方法等。鉴别检验一般应采用专属性强、灵敏度高、重现性好、快速和操作便捷的方法，鼓励研究建立一次试验同时鉴别多个药味的方法。

制剂中若有直接入药的生药粉，一般应建立显微鉴别方法；若制剂中含有多种直接入药的生药粉，在显微鉴别方法中应分别描述各药味的专属性特征。化学反应鉴别法一般适用于制剂中含有矿物类药味以及有类似结构特征的大类化学成份的鉴别。色谱法主要包括薄层色谱法（TLC/HPTLC）、气相色谱法（GC）和高效液相色谱法（HPLC/UPLC）等。TLC法可采用比移值和显色特征等进行鉴别，对特征斑点的个数、比移值、斑点颜色、紫外吸收/荧光特征等与标准物质的一致性予以详细描述；HPLC法、GC法可采用保留时间等色谱特征进行鉴别。若处方中含有动物来源的药味并且在制剂中仅其蛋白质、多肽等生物大分子成份具备识别特征，应研究建立相应的特异性检验检测方法。

（六）检查

1. 与剂型相关的检查项目

应根据剂型特点及临床用药需要，参照《中国药典》制剂通则的相应规定，建立反映制剂特性的检查方法。若《中国药典》通则中与剂型相关的检查项目有两种或两种以上的方法作为可选项，应根据制剂特点进行合理选择，并说明原因。

2. 与安全性相关的检查项目

处方含易被重金属及有害元素污染的药味，或其生产过程中使用的设备、辅料、分离材料等有可能引入有害元素，应建立相应的重金属及有害元素的限量检查方法，应在充分研究和风险评估的基础上制定合理的限度，并符合《中国药典》等标准的相关规定。

制剂工艺中若使用有机溶剂（乙醇除外）进行提取加工，在质量标准中应建立有机溶剂残留检查法；若使用大孔吸附树脂进行分离纯化，应根据树脂的类型、树脂的可能降解产物和使用溶剂等情况，研究建立提取物中可能的树脂有机物残留的限量检查方法，如苯乙烯型大孔吸附树脂可能的降解产物主要包括但不限于苯、正己烷、甲苯、二甲苯、苯乙烯、二乙基苯等。上述溶剂残留限度或树脂有机物残留限度应符合《中国药典》的规定，或参照国际人用药品注册技术协调会（ICH）的相关要求制订。

若处方中的药味含有某一种或一类毒性成份而非药效成份，应针对该药味建立有关毒性成份的限量检查方法，其限度可根据相应的毒理学或文献研究资料合理制定。

3. 与药品特性相关的检查项目

应根据药品的特点建立有针对性的检查项目，如提取的天然单一成份口服固体制剂应建立有关物质、溶出度等的检查方法；含难溶性提取物的口服固体制剂，应进行溶出度的检查研究。主要指标成份为多糖类物质的制剂，应研究建立多糖分子量分布等反映大分子物质结构特征的专属性检查方法。

4. 检查限度的确定

质量标准中应详细说明各项检查的检验方法及其限度。一般列入质量标准的检查项目，应从安全性方面及生产实际充分论证该检验方法及其限度的合理性。设定的检查限度尤其是有害物质检查限度应在安全性数据所能支持的水平范围以内。

（七）浸出物

浸出物检查可用作控制提取物总量一致性的指标。浸出物的检测方法可根据制剂所含主要成份的理化性质选择适宜的溶剂（不限于一种），基于不同的溶剂可将浸出物分为水溶性浸出物、醇溶性浸出物、乙酸乙酯浸出物及醚浸出物等。应系统研究考察各种影响因素对浸出物检测的影响，如辅料的影响等。浸出物的检测方法中应注明溶剂的种类及用量、测定方法及温度参数等，并规定合理的浸出物限度范围。

（八）指纹/特征图谱

中药新药制剂（提取的天然单一成份制剂除外）一般应进行指纹/特征图谱研究并建立相应的标准。内容一般包括建立分析方法、色谱峰的指认、建立对照图谱、数据分析与评价等过程。

指纹/特征图谱一般采用各种色谱方法，如 HPLC/UPLC 法、HPTLC 法、GC 法等。应根据所含主要成份的性质研究建立合适的供试品制备方法。若药品中含多种理化性质差异较大的不同类型成份，可考虑针对不同类型成份分别制备供试品，并建立多个指纹/特征图谱以分别反映不同类型成份的信息。若一种方法不能完整体现供试品所含成份特征，可采用两种或两种以上的方法获取不同的指纹/特征图谱进行分析。

指纹/特征图谱的检测方法、参数等的选择，应以反映制剂所含成份信息最大化为原则。一般选取容易获取的一个或多个主要活性成份或指标成份作为参照物；若无合适的参照物，也可选择图谱中稳定的色谱峰作为参照峰，并应尽可能对其进行指认。

通过对代表性样品指纹/特征图谱的分析，选择各批样品中均出现的色谱峰作为共有峰。可选择其中含量高、专属性强的色谱峰（优先选择已知有效/活性成份、含量测定指标成份及其他已知成份）作为特征峰。指纹/特征图谱研究过程中，应尽可能对图谱中主要色谱峰进行指认。

指纹/特征图谱一般以相似度或特征峰相对保留时间、峰面积比值等为检测指标。可根据多批样品的检测结果，采用指纹图谱相似度评价系统计算机软件获取共有峰的模式，建立对照指纹图谱，采用上述软件对供试品指纹图谱与对照指纹图谱进行相似度分析比较，并关注非共有峰的特征。特征图谱需确定各特征峰的相对保留时间及其范围。应在样品检测数据的基础上进行评价，制定指纹/特征图谱相似度或相对保留时间、峰面积比值及其范围。

（九）含量测定

1. 含量测定指标的选择

制剂的处方组成不同，其含量测定指标选择也不相同。提取的天然单一成份制剂选择该成份进行含量测定。组成基本明确的提取物制剂应建立一个或多个主要指标成份的含量测定方法，应研究建立大类成份的含量测定方法。

复方制剂应尽可能研究建立处方中多个药味的含量测定方法，根据其功能主治，应首选与药品安全性、有效性相关联的化学成份，一般优先选择有效/活性成份、毒性成份、君药所含指标成份等为含量测定指标。此外，需考虑含量测定指标与工艺、稳定性的相关性，并尽可能建立多成份或多组分的含量测定方法。若制法中包含多种工艺路线，应针对各种工艺路线研究建立相关有效/活性成份或指标成份的含量测定方法；若有提取挥发油的工艺，应进行挥发油总量或相应指标成份的含量测定方法研究，视情况列入标准；若含有明确的热敏感成份，应进行可反映生产过程中物料的受热程度及稳定性的含量测定方法研究，视情况列入标准。

2. 含量测定方法

含量测定方法包括容量（滴定）法、色谱法、光谱法等，其中色谱方法包括 GC 法和 HPLC/UPLC 法等，挥发性成份可优先考虑 GC 法或 GC–MS 法，非挥发性成份可优先考虑 HPLC/UPLC 法。矿物类药味的无机成份可采用容量法、原子吸收光谱法（AAS）、电感耦合等离子体原子发射光谱法（ICP–AES）、电感耦合等离子体质谱法（ICP–MS）等方法进行含量测定。

含量测定所采用的方法应通过方法学验证。

3. 含量范围

提取的天然单一成份及其制剂一般应规定主成份的含量范围；应根据其含量情况和制剂的要求，规定单位制剂中该成份相当于标示量的百分比范围。

提取物质量标准中应规定所含大类成份及主要指标成份的含量范围，大类成份及主要指标成份可以是一种或数种成份；制剂应根据提取物的含量情况和制剂的要求，规定大类成份和主要指标成份的含量范围。

复方制剂鼓励建立多个含量测定指标，并对各含量测定指标规定含量范围。处方若含有可能既为有效成份又为有毒成份的药味，应对其进行含量测定并规定含量范围。

（十）生物活性测定

生物活性测定方法一般包括生物效价测定法和生物活性限值测定法。由于现有的常规物理化学方法在控制药品质量方面具有一定的局限性，鼓励探索开展生物活性测定研究，建立生物活性测定方法以作为常规物理化学方法的替代或补充。

采用生物活性测定方法应符合药理学研究的随机、对照、重复的基本原则，建立的方法应具备简单、精确、可行、可控的特点，并有明确的判断标准。试验系统的选择与实验原理和制定指标密切相关，应选择背景资料清楚、影响因素少、检测指标灵敏和性价比高的试验系统。表征药物的生物活性强度的含量（效价）测定方法，应按生物活性测定方法的要求进行验证。不同药物的生物活性测定方法的详细要求，可参照相关指导原则。

（十一）规格

制剂规格表述应参照《中成药规格表述技术指导原则》的相关要求。

（十二）贮藏

贮藏项目表述的内容系对药品贮藏与保管的基本要求。药品的稳定性不仅与其自身的性质有关，还受到许多外界因素的干扰。应通过对直接接触药材（饮片）、提取物、制剂的包装材料和贮藏条件进行系统考察，根据稳定性影响因素和药品稳定性考察的试验结果，确定贮藏条件。

四、主要参考文献

1. 国家药品监督管理局.《中药新药研究的技术要求》，1999 年.

2. 国家食品药品监督管理局.《天然药物新药研究技术要求》，2013 年.

3. 国家药典委员会.《国家药品标准工作手册》，2012 年.

Common Format and Guidelines on Writing of Manufacturing Process and Quality Standard for Traditional Chinese Medicines (TCMs)

I. Common Format and Writing Guideline of Manufacturing Process for TCMs

Common format and Writing Guideline of Manufacturing Process for TCMs is only to be provided as a reference for the format and writing of manufacturing process for TCMs. The manufacturing process of specific TCMs should be written in accordance with the actual situation and needs.

Manufacturing Process of TCMs

Acceptance No.:_____ Name of medicine: _____

Marketing Authorization Holder: _____

Manufacturer:_____

Manufacturing address (detailed to the plant/workshop, manufacturing line): _____

(If product manufacturing involves multiple manufacturers, the name, address, and duty of each manufacturer should be listed; for the products manufactured overseas, information should be added as appropriate, such as the name and address of the sub-packaging plant and the name of the domestic contact agency)

I. Formula

The categories and amounts of all TCM materials in a formula should be listed, and their feeding forms should be indicated.

Table 1 Formula of TCMs

Name[1]	Amount of 1000 preparation units	Amount of the proposed commercial scale	Note[2]
TCM material 1			
TCM material 2			
…			
Total amount of finished TCM preparation			

Notes: 1. TCM materials include prepared slices/decoction pieces and extracts, etc.

2. The form of TCM materials in a formula should be indicated, relying on descriptions in the pre–treatment part of the manufacturing process, e.g., prepared TCM slices and powders, etc. The writing of a formula can generally refer to the relevant provisions in the *Chinese Pharmacopoeia*.

II. TCM Materials and Excipients, Other Materials Used in Preparation, and Primary Pharmaceutical Packaging Materials

Table 2 Information for TCM materials, excipients, and primary pharmaceutical packaging materials

TCM material	Name	Place of origin of TCM crude drugs	Manufacturer of decoction pieces, and the other TCM materials	Current standard	Note[1]	
Excipient	Name	Specification	Manufacturer	Current standard	Registration No. and status	Note

continued

Material used during manufacturing [2]	Name	Specification	Manufacturer	Current standard	Note	
Primary pharmaceutical packaging material and container	Name	Specification	Manufacturer	Current standard	Registration No. and status	Note

Notes: 1. Information on TCM material can be listed as an attachment, including origin, harvesting period, and quality requirements, etc.

2. Materials used during manufacturing, e.g., macro−porous resin and diatomaceous earth, etc.

III. Manufacturing Process

As the process may vary among TCM products, this part only gives examples of the methods, parameters, conditions and requirements involved in common process steps.

1. Flowchart of manufacturing process

The flowchart of manufacturing process should be complete, intuitive, and concise. It is recommended that the flowchart be provided in the form of rectangular text boxes and arrows.

2. Treatment of TCM materials and excipients

(1) Pre-treatment of TCM materials: The methods and conditions for pre-treatment of TCM crude drugs and/or decoction pieces and the storage period and conditions for the treated materials should be indicated. For those to be cut after being processed with infiltration, softening, or other treatment methods, the specific method and conditions as well as the size of cutting, etc., should be indicated; for those that need to be crushed before feeding, the crushing method,

grain size or granularity, etc., should be indicated; for those that need to be smashed, the smashing method and size of the smashed pieces, etc. should be indicated; and for those that need to be processed with supplementary materials, the method and conditions for processing with supplementary materials should be indicated (the basis for processing with supplementary materials should be indicated), e.g., the heating temperature and time, and the amount of the supplementary material used.

(2) Treatment of excipients and other materials used in preparation: If the excipients and other materials used in preparation need to be processed, the processing method and conditions, the processing procedure and process parameters, and the resulted material's storage period and conditions etc., should indicated. The quality standards should be provided as well.

3. Extraction

Specify the method and conditions of extraction, the category and amount of the solvent used for extraction, the extraction times, the temperature and time of extraction, the filtration method and conditions of the extract, and the storage conditions and period of the extract, etc. For the TCM material that is treated by blending different batches to pursue quality uniformity, the method, conditions, quality indicators, and requirements for the treatment should be specified accordingly.

4. Concentration

The method and conditions of concentration should be specified, for instance, the applied temperature, pressure, time, storage conditions and period of the concentrate, etc. In addition, the relative density, the ratio of the weight (volume) of the concentrate to that of the decoction pieces used accordingly, and the yielded range of the concentrate or extract, should be specified.

5. Purification

The method and conditions of purification should be specified, and the parameters should be described in detail. For example, for ethanol precipitation, the ethanol concentration, the relative density of the extract used with measuring temperature, the weight/volume ratio of the concentrate, and the temperature need to be specified. It is required to specify the stirring method and conditions applied during ethanol precipitation. It is also required to specify the holding time and temperature of the ethanol precipitation, as well as the ethanol content to be achieved. It is also necessary to specify the final purified extract's storage conditions and duration.

6. Drying

The drying method and conditions, drying equipment, etc., as well as the yielded range of dry extract, should be defined.

7. Other treatments

List relevant methods, conditions, and requirements for operational procedures for each unit of the manufacturing process in accordance with the specific situation. Solutions to the problems that are likely to occur in each part of the procedures can be supplemented in an attachment, e.g., the relevant provisions and quality control methods for replacing or repairing filter materials. In the case of online testing and control during manufacturing, relevant indicators, methods, and requirements should be defined.

8. Pharmaceutic formulation

The category and amount of the excipient in the preparation should be specified. See Table 3 for details.

Table 3 Pharmaceutic formulation

Name[1]	Amount of 1000 preparation units	Amount of proposed commercial scale
Intermediate 1		
Intermediate 2		
Excipient 1		
Excipient...		

Note: 1. The intermediate refers to the extract, dry extract, and volatile oil, etc., used for the pharmaceutic formulation. Extracts and powders, etc. that are used directly for the preparation should also be listed. The amount range for the excipient could be reasonably determined, as the case may be.

9. Manufacturing process of preparation

The pharmaceutic formulation should be defined, and the method and parameters of the molding process should be detailed, including the adding method and conditions and order for TCM materials and excipients, as well as the method and conditions of molding.

For granules, the method and conditions of granulation, the category and adding method of the excipient, the drying method and conditions, and the grain size, etc. should be specified.

Ⅳ. Main Equipment

For major equipment used for operation in each step of the manufacturing process (e.g., powdering, extraction, concentration, purification, fluid mixing, filtration, filling and sealing, sterilization, drying, granulation, and tableting, etc.), a list of information should be provided with regard to name, model, manufacturer, working principle, key technical parameters, and yielded range, etc.

V. Other Manufacturing Information

If special equipment is used in the manufacturing process, the operational method or control requirements for the equipment in relevant processes should be clearly described. If nitrogen charging is required, the nitrogen-making method or quality requirements for nitrogen and nitrogen charging method, etc. should be described. The production scale should be specified, and the process parameters should fall into the specified ranges. Additional pages can be added as needed.

Ⅵ. Attachment

The data relevant to the quality of TCM preparations can be indicated under "Manufacturing Process" as an attachment, e.g., internal control standards for TCM materials, quality standards for intermediates, treatment methods and quality standards for excipients and materials used in the preparation process, etc.

II. Common Format and Writing Guideline of Quality Standard for TCMs

(I) Format of quality standard for TCMs

National Medical Products Administration
(size 2 in boldface)

Drug Registration Standard
(size 1 in boldface)

Name of Medicine

Name in Chinese Pinyin

[Formula]

[Procedure]

[Description]

[Identification]

[Test]

[Extractives] (if applicable)

[Characteristic Chromatogram or Fingerprint] (if applicable)

[Assay]

[Functions and Indications]/[Indications for Use]

[Usage and Dosage]

[Precautions] (if applicable)

[Specifications]

[Storage]

[Institution for Verification] (if applicable)

[Marketing Authorization Holder]

Notes: 1. Paper size: A4; additional A4 paper can be used as needed.

2. Typeface: size 4 in boldface for the title; size 5 in Song for the text.

(II) Guidelines on writing of quality standard for TCMs

I. Name

The name refers to the generic name of TCMs, including the formal name and the Chinese Pinyin. It should comply with the *Naming Principle for Generic Names of Drugs*.

II. [Formula]

The names and amounts of ingredients in a formula should be described by consulting the *Chinese Pharmacopoeia* for the norms and requirements with regard to formats and terms. The names of ingredients should be written in accordance with those in the national drug standards or drug registration standards; aliases or synonyms should be avoided. The amount unit should be gram (g) for a solid ingredient and gram (g) or milliliter (ml) for a liquid ingredient. The amount of each ingredient should be generally converted by the amount that is used for manufacturing 1000 units of preparation (tablet, granule, g, ml, etc.).

III. [Procedure]

The essential steps and necessary technical parameters in the manufacturing process should be described by consulting the *Chinese Pharmacopoeia* for norms and requirements with regard to formats and terms. Generally, it includes the manufacturing processes and key process parameters, such as pre-treatment, extraction, purification, concentration, drying, and molding, etc.

IV. [Description]

Based on the preparation itself and its contents, appearance, shape, smell, taste, solubility (if applicable), and physical constants (if applicable), etc. should be described in accordance with the actual condition by consulting the *Chinese Pharmacopoeia* for the norms and requirements with regard to formats and terms. Generally, the range of color differences should not be too wide when describing the color of an appearance. Composite colors should be described by hyphenated compound words with subsidiary color as a preceding word and dominant color as a following word.

V. [Identification]

The methods of microscopic and physiochemical identification should be set forth in turn as per the order of identification items by consulting the *Chinese Pharmacopoeia* for the norms and requirements with regard to formats and terms. Powder identification under the item of microscopic identification refers to the characteristics observed under a microscope upon preparation by a certain method. Physiochemical identification encompasses physical, chemical, spectral, and chromatographic methods, etc.

VI. [Test]

The test method and limit for each item in a quality standard should be detailed by consulting the *Chinese Pharmacopoeia* for the norms and requirements with regard to formats and terms.

All kinds of preparations, should comply with the relevant provisions under the general rules in the *Chinese Pharmacopoeia* unless otherwise specified.

VII. [Extractives]

The category and amount of the solvent used for the extractives test, test method, and test parameters should be detailed by consulting the *Chinese Pharmacopoeia* for the norms and requirements with regard to formats and terms. The range for the extractives should be reasonably determined.

VIII. [Characteristic Chromatogram or Fingerprint]

The analytical method of a characteristic chromatogram or fingerprint, identified chromatographic peaks, reference chromatogram, data analysis and evaluation method (relevant parameters or other special provisions should be listed when necessary), etc. should be detailed by consulting the *Chinese Pharmacopoeia* for the norms and requirements with regard to formats and terms. Similarity and/or relative retention time and its range for the target peaks on the fingerprint/characteristic chromatogram should be defined by testing qualified samples.

IX. [Assay]

All the assay methods for each item in a quality standard should be elaborated by consulting the *Chinese Pharmacopoeia* for the norms and requirements with regard to formats and terms. The range of content for the assay item should be determined accordingly.

X. [Functions and Indications]/[Indications for Use]

It should be consistent with the package insert.

XI. [Usage and Dosage]

It should be consistent with the package insert.

XII. [Precautions]

Major contraindications and adverse reactions should be listed. Those that are commonly contraindicated from the perspective of TCM theories could be omitted.

XIII. [Specifications]

The text creation and normative wordings for specifications should refer to the relevant requirements in the *Guideline on Writing of Specification for Chinese Proprietary Medicines* issued by the National Medical Products Administration.

XIV. [Storage]

Storage conditions should be described in a normative manner by consulting the *Chinese Pharmacopoeia* for the norms and requirements. Special requirements for storage conditions of TCM preparations need to be explained.

XV. Others

For the "Institution for Verification" of the quality standard, the full name of the institution should be provided, such as "National Institutes for Food and Drug Control" or "** Provincial (Municipal, Autonomous Regional) Institute (Research Institute) for Drug Control".

中药生产工艺、质量标准通用格式和撰写指南

一、中药生产工艺通用格式和撰写指南

中药生产工艺通用格式和撰写指南仅为撰写中药生产工艺提供参考，具体品种应根据品种的实际情况和需要确定。

中药生产工艺

受 理 号：_____   药品名称：_____

药品上市许可持有人：_____

生产企业：_____

生产地址（具体到厂房/车间、生产线）：_____

（如产品的生产涉及到多个生产企业，请列表分别说明每个生产企业的名称、地址以及职责；境外生产的药品，视情况增加药品分包装厂名称和地址、境内联系机构名称等内容）

一、处方

列出所用全部原料的种类及用量，标明投料形式。

表 1　中药处方

名称[1]	1000 个制剂单位处方剂量	拟定商业规模处方剂量	备注[2]
原料 1			
原料 2			
……			
制成总量			

注：1. 原料包含饮片、提取物等。

2. 结合工艺中药材（饮片）前处理部分，注明处方原料的投料形式，如饮片、药粉等。处方的撰写一般可参照《中国药典》的相关规定。

二、原辅料、制备过程中所用材料、直接接触药品的包装材料

表 2　原辅料及包材信息表

原料	名称	药材产地	饮片等的生产企业	执行标准	备注[1]	
辅料	名称	规格（或型号）	生产企业	执行标准	登记号及登记状态	备注
生产过程所用材料[2]	名称	规格（或型号）	生产企业	执行标准	备注	
直接接触药品的包装材料和容器	名称	规格（或型号）	生产企业	执行标准	登记号及登记状态	备注

注：1. 药材基原、采收期、质量要求等内容可以附件的形式分别列出。

2. 如生产过程中使用到的大孔吸附树脂、硅藻土等。

三、制备工艺

由于具体品种的实际工艺情况不同，以下仅举例说明部分常见工艺步骤的方法、参数、条件及要求等。

1. 工艺流程图

工艺流程图应完整、直观、简洁。建议以矩形文本框和箭头的形式提供产品的工艺流程图。

2. 原辅料处理

（1）原料的前处理：明确药材（饮片）前处理的方法和条件，明确处理

后原料的保存时间和条件等。如需经过浸润或软化等处理后切制的，应明确浸润或软化等处理的方法和条件，及切制规格等；需粉碎后投料的，应明确粉碎方法、粒径或粒度等；需破碎的应明确破碎方法、破碎后药材大小等；需炮炙的，应明确炮炙方法和条件（注明炮炙的依据），如加热温度、时间、辅料用量等。

（2）辅料及所用材料的处理：辅料及所用材料需处理的，应明确处理方法和条件，说明处理的操作流程和工艺参数，明确处理后辅料及所用材料的保存时间和条件等，并提供处理后辅料及所用材料的质量标准。

3. 提取

明确提取方法及条件，提取用溶媒的种类、用量，提取次数，提取温度、时间，提取液过滤的方法及条件，以及提取液的贮存条件和期限等。如采用质量均一化方法处理后投料的，应明确相应的方法、条件、质量指标及要求。

4. 浓缩

明确浓缩的方法、条件，如温度、压力、时间，浓缩液的贮存条件和期限等。明确浓缩液的相对密度或浓缩液重量（体积）与饮片的比例，明确浓缩液或浸膏的得率范围。

5. 纯化

明确纯化的方法及条件，详述相关工艺参数。如醇沉，需明确醇沉用乙醇的浓度，醇沉前浸膏的相对密度（明确测定温度）或浓缩液重量（体积）与饮片的比例，醇沉前浸膏的温度，搅拌方法和条件，醇沉需达到的含醇量，醇沉静置时间和温度等，并明确醇沉液的贮存条件和期限等。

6. 干燥

明确干燥的方法、条件及设备等，明确干浸膏得率范围。

7. 其他处理

需根据具体品种的实际工艺情况，列出各单元操作步骤的相关方法、条件及要求。对各环节易出现的问题及处理方法，可以附件的形式进行补充。如滤材阻塞、损坏时更换滤材或维修处理的相关规定和质控方法等。生产中如有在线检测与控制的，应明确相关指标、方法及要求。

8. 制剂处方

应明确辅料种类及用量。具体见表3。

9. 制剂工艺

明确制剂处方，详述成型工艺的方法及参数，包括原辅料的加入方法、条件和投料顺序，以及成型方法及条件。

表 3　制剂处方

名称[1]	1000 个制剂单位的剂量	拟定商业规模的剂量
中间体 1		
中间体 2		
辅料 1		
辅料……		

注：1. 制剂处方中的中间体指制剂成型前的浸膏、干浸膏、挥发油等。如有直接用于制剂的提取物、药粉等也列入制剂处方，可根据实际情况确定合理的辅料用量范围。

如颗粒剂应明确制粒的方法和条件、辅料的种类及加入方法、干燥方法及条件、颗粒粒度等。

四、主要设备

应提供生产工艺中各单元操作（如粉碎、提取、浓缩、纯化、配液、过滤、灌封、灭菌、干燥、制粒、压片等）中使用到的主要设备名称、设备型号、生产厂、工作原理、关键技术参数、产量范围等，应列表说明。

五、其他生产信息

对于生产工艺中的特殊设备、操作方法或相关过程的控制要求，应明确说明。如需充氮的，应说明制氮方法或氮气质控要求、氮气充入方式等。应明确生产规模，工艺参数应不超出规定的范围。如有其他需要说明的内容可另外增加附页。

六、附件

在"生产工艺"后可附上与药品质量有关的资料作为附件，如原料的内控标准、中间体质量标准、辅料及制备过程中所用材料的处理方法及质量标准等。

二、中药质量标准通用格式和撰写指南

（一）中药质量标准格式

国家药品监督管理局（黑体二号）

药品注册标准（黑体一号）

药品名称

汉语拼音

【处方】

【制法】

【性状】

【鉴别】

【检查】

【浸出物】（如适用）

【特征图谱或指纹图谱】（如适用）

【含量测定】

【功能与主治】/【适应症】

【用法与用量】

【注意】（如适用）

【规格】

【贮藏】

【复核单位】（如适用）

【药品上市许可持有人】

注：1. 纸型：A4，此页不够时，另用 A4 型空白纸。

2. 标题：四号黑体；正文：五号宋体。

（二）中药质量标准撰写指南

一、药品名称

列入中药质量标准中的药品名称为其通用名称，包括药品正名与汉语拼音名，名称应符合药品通用名称命名原则。

二、【处方】

参照中国药典格式要求和用语规范等，描述组方药味的名称与用量。药味的名称应使用国家标准或注册标准中的饮片名称，避免使用别名和异名。固体药味的用量单位为克（g），液体药味的用量单位为克（g）或毫升（ml），各药味量一般以 1000 个制剂单位（片、粒、g、ml 等）的制成量折算。

三、【制法】

参照中国药典格式要求和用语规范等，描述生产工艺中的主要步骤和必要的技术参数，一般包含前处理、提取、纯化、浓缩、干燥和成型等工艺过程及主要工艺参数。

四、【性状】

参照中国药典格式要求和用语规范等，按照制剂本身或内容物的实际状态描述其外观、形态、嗅、味、溶解度（如适用）及物理常数（如适用）等。通常描述外观颜色的色差范围不宜过宽。复合色的描述应为辅色在前，主色在后。

五、【鉴别】

参照中国药典格式要求和用语规范等，根据鉴别项目依次描述显微鉴别、理化鉴别方法。显微鉴别中的粉末鉴别指经过一定方法制备后在显微镜下观察的特征。理化鉴别包括物理、化学、光谱、色谱等鉴别方法。

六、【检查】

参照中国药典格式要求和用语规范等，详细描述各项检查的检验方法及其限度。

各类制剂，除另有规定以外，均应符合中国药典各制剂通则项下有关的各项规定。

七、【浸出物】

参照中国药典格式要求和用语规范等，详细描述浸出物检查的溶剂种类及用量、测定方法及参数等，并规定合理的浸出物限度范围。

八、【特征图谱或指纹图谱】

参照中国药典格式要求和用语规范等，详细描述特征图谱或指纹图谱的分析方法、指认的色谱峰、对照图谱、数据分析与评价方法（必要时，列出相关

参数或其他特殊规定）等，并制定合格样品的指纹/特征图谱相似度及或相对
保留时间等及其范围。

九、【含量测定】

参照中国药典格式要求和用语规范等，依次详细描述各含量测定项的测定
方法，并制定相应的含量范围。

十、【功能与主治】/【适应症】

与说明书一致。

十一、【用法与用量】

与说明书一致。

十二、【注意】

列出主要的禁忌和不良反应。属中医一般常规禁忌者从略。

十三、【规格】

制剂规格内容设定和规范表述，应参照国家局颁布的《中成药规格表述技
术指导原则》等的相关要求。

十四、【贮藏】

贮藏条件的表示方法应参照中国药典要求规范书写，对贮藏条件有特殊要
求的制剂需要予以说明。

十五、其他

质量标准的"复核单位"根据实际情况填写"中国食品药品检定研究院"、
"** 省（市、自治区）药品检验所（研究院）"等单位全称。

Guideline on Writing of Specification for Chinese Proprietary Medicines

I. Overview

Specifications are usually defined as the amounts of medicinal components per unit preparation (e.g., per capsule, tablet, gram, milliliter, or pill). However, most Chinese proprietary medicines (CPMs) are of complex components, which is difficult to directly indicate. Currently, the specifications of CPMs are defined in the weight or volume per unit, which might result in inaccurate use of the medicine in clinical practice. The Guideline intends to standardize the specification of CPMs.

Specifications, as an important part of the package insert, should provide as accurate amounts of medicinal components as possible to facilitate the sales, storage, distribution, and use of medicines. Although the amounts of medicinal components are hard to be directly defined in the specifications of CPMs, the dosage of ingredients in a unit preparation could be indicated. Therefore, the specifications for CPMs should generally include the theoretical amounts (or labeled amounts) of the ingredients equivalent in the unit preparation, including prepared slices/decoction pieces, extracts, and active component, etc.

Generally, it is suggested to define the specifications of CPMs according to the guideline. Where it is impractical, other reasonable ways are permitted due to the complexity of CPMs.

II. General Principles for Specification of CPMs

(I) The principle of correspondence with ingredients

For preparations of which the ingredients are decoction pieces, the specification should generally include their amounts equivalent in the unit preparation. e.g., for tablets the specifications should be defined as "** g per tablet" (equivalent to ** g of decoction pieces); for liquid preparations, the specifications should be defined as "Each ml is equivalent to ** g of decoction pieces".

For preparations which are of active component, the specifications should be directly defined with their labeled amounts in the unit preparation. e.g., the specification of Breviscapine Dripping Pills should be defined as "Each pill contains 4 mg of breviscapine".

For preparations which are of extracts such as solid extracts, fluid extracts, and plant oils, the specifications should be defined as the theoretical amounts of relevant ingredients in the unit preparation. e.g., for granules of which the ingredients are ** solid extracts and decoction pieces, the specifications should be defined as "Each g is equivalent to ** g of decoction pieces, contains ** mg of ** solid extracts".

For preparations containing various types of ingredients, they should generally be defined one by one. When it is impractical, they should be merged according to the ingredient type. If the ingredients of a preparation contain multiple decoction pieces and different extracts, the equivalent total amounts of decoction pieces and extracts contained in unit preparation should be calculated separately, and the specification should be defined as "Each tablet is equivalent to ** g of decoction pieces and contains ** mg of extracts".

If the formula contains chemical drugs and active component, the labeled amounts should be clearly indicated, respectively.

Table 1 Examples of specification for different types of ingredients

Product name	Type of ingredient	Specification
Banlangen Granules	decoction pieces	Each bag is equivalent to 7 g of decoction pieces.
Breviscapine Injection	active component	Each vial contains 4 mg of breviscapine.
Gypenosides Dripping Pills	extracts	Every ** pill weighs ** g (each g contains 6 mg of gypenosides).
Component Berberine Hydrochloride Tablets	decoction pieces and chemical drugs	Each tablet weighs ** g (equivalent to 0.318 g of decoction pieces, contains 30 mg of berberine hydrochloride).
Keteling Tablets	dry extracts and chemical drugs	Each tablet weighs ** g (contains 180 mg of dry extract of *Ficus macrocarpa* and 0.7 mg of chlorpheniramine maleate).

If the amount of decoction pieces per unit preparation of one drug variety is the same, it could be regarded as the same specification. If the unit volume or weight of preparations of the same variety contains the same amounts of ingredients (except for injections, metered dose aerosols, and sprays, etc.), they are generally considered to share the same specification. If preparations of the same drug variety contain different amounts of ingredients, they are generally considered to have different specifications.

Specifications of medicines generally do not include information regarding excipients. If the unit preparations (sugar-free granules and lactose-containing granules, sugar-coated tablets and film-coated tablets) of the same variety have equivalent amounts of decoction pieces, they are considered to share the same specification regardless of the different excipients used. Due to the particularity of TCM pills, honeyed pills and water-honeyed pills are still considered to belong to different specifications.

(II) The principle of coordination with usage and dosage and package specification

The package specifications are mainly used to indicate the amounts of medicinal preparations contained in the smallest packaging container, such as 12 tablets per sheet, 100 ml per bottle, and 10 g per bag. The specifications should be coordinated with the [Usage and Dosage] item and the package specifications under the [Package] item.

Specifications should be expressed in a way that facilitates accurate administration. Except for pediatric medicines, taking only one third (1/3) or one fourth (1/4) of a bag (bottle) at a time should be generally avoided in the specification.

Specifications should be consistent with the usage and dosage. For example, when the [Usage and Dosage] of a pill is expressed as "Take ** g orally each time...", the [Specification] should be expressed as "Every ** pill weighs ** g (equivalent to ** g of decoction pieces)", and at the same time, the package specification under the [Package] item should be expressed as "Each bottle contains ** g". When the [Usage and Dosage] is expressed as "Take 1 bag orally each time...", the [Specification] should be expressed as "Each bag is equivalent to ** g of decoction pieces", and the package specification under the [Package] item should be expressed as "Each bag contains ** g". When the [Usage and Dosage] is expressed as "Take ** pills orally each time...", the [Specification] should be expressed as "Every ** pill weighs ** g (equivalent to ** g of decoction pieces)", and at the same time, the package specification under the [Package] item should be expressed as "Each bottle (bag) contains ** pills".

(III) The principle of language standardization

The dosage units such as gram and milliliter etc. of specifications are respectively expressed in English g, ml, e.g. each pill is equivalent to **g of decoction pieces , and each ml is equivalent to **g of decoction pieces. Other dose units such as pills, bags and pellets etc. are expressed in Chinese. The grams and milliliters of specifications of OTC are also expressed in Chinese.

For preparations of which the ingredients are decoction pieces, the term "equivalent to" should be used. For preparations of which the ingredients are active components or extracts, the term "contain(s)" should be used. For preparations of which the ingredients are fed in various forms (decoction pieces, active components, and extracts, etc.), the term "equivalent to ** g of decoction pieces, and contain(s)..." should be used in specification .

If the specification of a medicine is not an integer, it is usually retained for no more than two decimal places.

III. Examples of Specification Expression of CPMs in Different Dosage Forms

In principle, it is recommended that the specifications of TCM component preparations should be classified and defined based on the characteristics of solid, semi-solid, and liquid, etc. For solid preparations such as granules, tablets, and capsules, the specifications should be expressed as "Each g, tablet, or capsule is equivalent to ** g of decoction pieces". For tablets and capsules, it is also suggested to clarify the tablet weight or the capsule content weight, e.g., "Each tablet weighs ** g (equivalent to ** g of decoction pieces)". For liquid preparations (other than injections, metered dose aerosols and sprays) such as mixtures (oral solutions) and lotions, the concentrations should be stated as "Each ml is equivalent to ** g of decoction pieces". For semi-solid preparations such as ointments, their specifications should be expressed as "Each g is equivalent to ** g of decoction pieces".

The specifications of injections are defined by the loading quantity and the theoretical amounts of corresponding ingredients in the packaging container. If an injection has two specifications, i.e., 2 ml and 10 ml per vial (each ml is equivalent to 1 g of decoction pieces), its specification should be expressed as follows: (1) 2 ml per vial: equivalent to 2 g of decoction pieces; or (2) 10 ml per vial: equivalent to 10 g of decoction pieces. Although the concentrations of the two are the same, they are still considered to belong to different specifications.

The specifications of TCM pills should be expressed separately according to different types of pills. For large honeyed pills, the specifications should be expressed as "Each pill is equivalent to ** g of decoction pieces", and the pill weight should also be indicated. For dripping pills, the specifications should be expressed as "Each g of the dripping pill is equivalent to ** g of decoction pieces", and the pill weight should also be indicated. For small honeyed pills, water pills, and condensed pills, etc., the specifications should be expressed according to the usage and dosage. when such medicine is taken by the pill weight, the specification should be expressed as "Each ** g of pills is equivalent to ** g of decoction pieces", and the pill weight should also be indicated; when taken by the number of pills, the specification should be expressed as "Each ** pills are equivalent to ** g of decoction pieces", and the pill weight should also be indicated. The pill weight in brackets is a supplementary requirement for the pill size. The size of the pills can, to a certain extent, reflect the amount of decoction pieces contained in the pills, which can be used as a basis for testing and clinical dosage division. If the specifications of pills of the same variety are expressed as "Each 10 pills weigh 0.25 g (each g is equivalent to 0.5 g of decoction pieces" and "Every 20 pills weigh 0.25 g (each g is equivalent to 0.5 g of decoction pieces)", respectively, the two should be considered to share the same specification.

For metered dose aerosols and sprays, the theoretical amounts of corresponding ingredients for each delivery should be specified as well as the loading quantity and the theoretical amounts of corresponding ingredients in the packaging container. For example: The specification of a metered dose aerosol is "10 ml: equivalent to 6 g of decoction pieces (0.1 g of decoction pieces × 60 deliveries)", where: "10 ml" is the quantity of the aerosol, "equivalent to 6 g of decoction pieces" is the equivalent amount of decoction pieces for 10 ml of the aerosol; "0.1 g of decoction pieces" is the equivalent amount of decoction pieces for each delivery of the aerosol, and "60 deliveries" is the number of deliveries available for 10 ml of the aerosol.

Refer to Table 2 for the specification of CPMs in different dosage forms.

Table 2 Examples of specification for CPMs in different dosage forms [#]

No.	Dosage form	Specification	Package specification	Single dose
1	Pills (large honeyed pills)	Each pill weighs ** g (equivalent to ** g of decoction pieces)	Each box contains ** pills	** pill(s) each time
	Pills (small honeyed pills, water–honeyed pills, water pills, and condensed pills)	Every ** pills weigh ** g (Each g is equivalent to ** g of decoction pieces); Every ** pills weigh ** g (equivalent to ** g of decoction pieces)	Each bottle contains ** g; Each box contains ** pills	** g each time; ** pill(s) each time
	Pills (dripping pills)	Every ** pills weigh ** g (Each g is equivalent to ** g of decoction pieces)	Each bottle contains ** g; Each bottle contains ** pills	** g each time; ** pill(s) each time
2	Granules	Each g is equivalent to ** g of decoction pieces	Each bag contains ** g	** bag(s) each time
3	Tablets	Each tablet weighs ** g (equivalent to ** g of decoction pieces). Sugar–coated tablets: Each tablet weighs ** g (equivalent to ** g of decoction pieces)	Each bottle contains ** tablets	** tablet(s) each time

continued

No.	Dosage form	Specification	Package speci-fication	Single dose
4	Capsules	Each capsule contains ** g (equivalent to ** g of decoction pieces)	Each bottle contains ** capsules	** capsule(s) each time
5	Mixtures (oral solutions)	Each ml is equivalent to ** g of decoction pieces; Each vial is equivalent to ** g of decoction pieces	Each bottle contains ** ml; Each vial contains ** ml	** ml each time ** vial(s) each time
6	Syrups	Each ml is equivalent to ** g of decoction pieces	Each bottle contains ** ml (graduated)	** ml each time
7	Powder	Each g is equivalent to ** g of decoction pieces	Each bag contains ** g	** g each time
8	Injections	** ml per vial: equivalent to ** g of decoction pieces	Each vial contains ** ml	** ml each time
9	Sterile powder for injection	** g per bottle: equivalent to ** g of decoction pieces	Each bottle contains ** g	** bottle(s) each time
10	Condensed decoctions	Each g is equivalent to ** g of decoction pieces	Each bottle contains ** g	** g each time
11	Liquors, tinctures	Each ml is equivalent to ** g of decoction pieces	Each bottle contains ** ml	** ml each time
12	Emplastrum, plaster, and applicator	Each patch is equivalent to ** g of decoction pieces (with size indicated)	Each box contains ** patch(es)	1 patch each time
13	Ointment, cream	Each g is equivalent to ** g of decoction pieces	Each vial contains ** g	** g each time
14	Gels	Each g is equivalent to ** g of decoction pieces	Each vial contains ** g	** g each time
15	Suppository	Each capsule is equivalent to ** g of decoction pieces	Each box contains ** capsule(s)	** capsule(s) each time
16	Fluid extracts and extracts	Each g is equivalent to ** g of decoction pieces	Each bottle contains ** g	** g each time

continued

No.	Dosage form	Specification	Package specification	Single dose
17	Aerosols and sprays	Quantitative: ** ml: equivalent to ** g of decoction pieces (** mg of decoction pieces × ** deliveries or sprays); Non–quantitative: Each ml is equivalent to ** g of decoction pieces	Each bottle contains ** ml	Quantitative: ** ml each time; Non–quantitative: ** delivery(ies) or spray(s) each time
18	Eye drops	Each ml is equivalent to ** g of decoction pieces	Each bottle contains ** ml	** ml each time
19	Pastille	Each pastille is equivalent to ** g of decoction pieces	Each box contains ** pastille(s)	** pastille(s) each time
20	Moxa and pression	Each g is equivalent to ** g of decoction pieces	Each box contains ** bag(s)	** bag(s) each time
21	Paints	Each ml is equivalent to ** g of decoction pieces	Each bottle contains ** ml	** ml each time
22	Films	Each piece is equivalent to ** g of decoction pieces (with size indicated)	Each box contains ** piece(s)	**piece(s) each time
23	Medicated tea	Each g is equivalent to ** g of decoction pieces	Each bag contains ** g	** bag(s) each time
24	Other solid and semi–solid preparations (pastes and colloids, etc.)	Each g is equivalent to ** g of decoction pieces	Each vial (bag/box) contains ** g	** g each time
25	Other liquid preparations (distillates, liniments, enemas, lotions, and perfusate, etc.)	Each ml is equivalent to ** g of decoction pieces	Each bottle contains ** ml	** ml each time

#: For the specification in the table, decoction pieces are used as examples of ingredients.

中成药规格表述技术指导原则

一、概述

药品规格通常以单位制剂（每粒、片、克、毫升、丸）中所含药物成份的量表示。但是，中成药大多为复方制剂，所含成份复杂，难以直接在规格项下直接标示所含成份的量。目前，中成药的规格大多仅以单位制剂的重量或体积等表述，给临床准确用药带来不便。为规范中成药规格的表述内容及表述方式，制定本技术指导原则。

规格是药品说明书内容的重要组成部分，其表述应尽可能提供准确的药物成份量的信息，以便于药品的销售、贮运、分发、使用。中成药的药品规格虽无法直接标明所含药物成份的量，但可以标示出制成单位制剂所需处方药味的剂量。鉴于以上认识，中成药的药品规格标示内容中一般应包含单位制剂中所相当的处方药味（包括饮片、提取物、有效成份等）的理论量（或标示量）。

中成药的药品规格建议参照本指导原则进行规范表述。由于中成药的情况比较复杂，实际工作中难以按本指导原则规范的，可以具体问题具体分析，采用其他合理的方式标示单位制剂中所含药物量的信息。

二、中成药规格表述的一般原则

（一）与处方药味相对应的原则

处方药味为饮片的制剂，其药品规格标示内容一般应包含单位制剂相当于饮片的重量。如处方药味为饮片的片剂，其药品规格可标示为"每片重 **g（ 相当于饮片 **g ）"；液体制剂，其药品规格可标示为"每 1ml 相当于饮片 **g"。

处方药味为有效成份等的制剂，其药品规格可直接以单位制剂中所含有效成份等的标示量标示。如处方为有效成份的灯盏花素滴丸，其规格可标示为"每丸含灯盏花素 4mg"。

处方药味为浸膏、流浸膏、植物油脂等提取物的，其药品规格可以单位制剂中所含相应药味的理论量标示。如某颗粒剂处方含 ** 浸膏及饮片，其规格可标示为：每 1g 相当于饮片 **g，含 ** 浸膏 **mg。

处方药味包含多种类型的制剂，在规格中一般需一一表述。难以在规格项下一一表述的，可按处方药味的类型合并后表述。如某药的处方药味有多个饮片及多种提取物，可分别计算单位制剂中相当的饮片总量及所含提取物的总量，规格标示为："每片相当于饮片 **g，含提取物 **mg"。

处方含化学药、有效成份的应——注明标示量。

表 1 不同投料药味类型的规格表述举例

品名	处方药味类型	规格表述
板蓝根颗粒	饮片	每袋相当于饮片 7g
灯盏花素注射液	有效成份	每支含灯盏花素 4mg
绞股蓝总苷滴丸	提取物	每 ** 丸重 **g（每 1g 含绞股蓝总苷 6mg）
复方黄连素片	饮片、化学药	每片重 **g（相当于饮片 0.318g，含盐酸小檗碱 30mg）
咳特灵片	干浸膏、化学药	每片重 **g（含小叶榕干浸膏 180mg、马来酸氯苯那敏 0.7mg）

如同品种单位制剂相当的饮片量等相同，一般视为相同药品规格。同品种单位体积或重量制剂中的药物量相同（注射剂、定量型气雾剂及喷雾剂等除外）的，一般视为相同的药品规格；同品种浓度不同的，一般视为不同的药品规格。

药品规格一般不表述与辅料相关的内容。如同品种单位制剂相当的饮片量等相同，因辅料不同而形成的无糖颗粒与乳糖型颗粒，糖衣片与薄膜衣片等均视为相同的药品规格。由于中药丸剂的特殊性，蜜丸、水蜜丸仍视为不同的药品规格。

（二）与用法用量、装量规格相协调的原则

药品的装量规格主要用于标示最小包装容器内所装药物制剂的量，如每板装 12 片、每瓶装 100ml、每袋装 10g，等等。药品规格应与说明书的【用法用量】、【包装】的装量规格等协调。

规格表述应便于准确用药。除儿童用药外，一般不应出现一次服用 1/3 袋（瓶）或 1/4 袋（瓶）等情形。

规格等的表述应与用法用量相符。例如，当丸剂的【用法用量】为"口服。一次 **g……"时，【规格】可表述为"每 ** 丸重 **g（相当于饮片 **g）"，同时【包装】的装量规格表述为"每瓶装 **g"；当其【用法用量】为"口服。一次 1 袋……"时，【规格】可表述为"每袋相当于饮片 **g"，同时【包装】的装量规格表述为"每袋装 **g"；当【用法用量】为"口服。一次 ** 丸……"时，【规格】可表述为"每 ** 丸重 **g（相当于饮片 **g）"，同时【包装】的装量规格表述为"每瓶（袋）装 ** 丸"。

（三）用语规范的原则

中药规格中的克、毫升等剂量单位分别用英文 g、ml 等表示，如每粒相当于饮片 **g，每 1ml 相当于饮片 **g 等。其他丸、袋、粒等剂量单位均用中文表示。OTC 中药规格中的克、毫升等也均用中文表示。

处方药味为饮片的制剂，用"相当于"表述；处方药味为有效成份、提取物的制剂，用"含"表述；处方药味为饮片、有效成份、提取物等多种形式投料的药物，在规格表述中采用"相当于饮片 **g，含……"表述。

如药品规格不是整数，一般保留不多于两位的小数。

三、不同剂型中成药规格的表述举例

中药复方制剂的药品规格原则上建议按照固体、半固体、液体等的特点分类表述。颗粒剂、片剂、胶囊等固体制剂，其规格可表述为每 1g、每片或每粒相当于饮片 **g。片剂、胶囊剂建议同时明确片重或胶囊内容物量，如每片重 **g（相当于饮片 **g）。合剂（口服液）、洗液等液体制剂（注射剂、定量气雾剂及喷雾剂等除外），其规格可按浓度标示为每 1ml 相当于饮片 **g。软膏等半固体制剂，其规格标示为每 1g 相当于饮片 **g。

注射剂等的药品规格以包装容器内的装量及其所相当的药味理论量标示。如某注射剂有每支 2ml 及 10ml 两种规格（每 ml 相当于饮片量 1g），其药品规格可标示为：（1）每支 2ml：相当于饮片 2g；（2）每支 10ml：相当于饮片 10g。虽然二者药物浓度相同，但仍视为不同药品规格。

中药丸剂的规格可根据丸剂的不同情形分别表述。大蜜丸以每丸相当 **g 饮片表述，同时标明丸重。滴丸以每 g 滴丸相当 **g 饮片表述，同时标明丸重。小蜜丸、水丸、浓缩丸等根据用法用量的情况确定，按丸剂重量服用的，规格以每 **g 丸剂相当于 **g 饮片表述，同时标明丸重；按丸数服用的，以每 ** 丸相当于 **g 饮片表述，同时标明丸重。括号内的丸重为对丸剂大小的补充规定。丸剂大小的信息一定程度上可以反映出丸剂所含饮片的量，可作为检验的依据，并为临床用药分剂量提供依据。如同品种丸剂的规格表述为"每 10 丸重 0.25g（每 1g 相当于饮片 0.5g）""每 20 丸重 0.25g（每 1g 相当于饮片 0.5g）"，二者应视为相同的药品规格。

定量气雾剂及喷雾剂等，在规定包装容器内的装量及其所相当的药味理论量的同时，还应规定每揿所相当的药味理论量。如某定量气雾剂的规格为：

10ml：相当于饮片 6g（0.1g 饮片 ×60 揿）。其中，"10ml"为气雾剂的装量，"相当于饮片 6g"为 10ml 气雾剂所相当的饮片量；"0.1g 饮片"为每揿气雾剂所相当的饮片量，"60 揿"为 10ml 气雾剂的可揿次数。

不同剂型药品规格的表述参见表 2。

表 2　不同剂型中成药的药品规格表述举例 #

序号	剂型	药品规格	装量规格	一次用量
1	丸剂（大蜜丸）	每丸重 **g（相当于饮片 **g）	每盒装 ** 丸	一次 ** 丸
	丸剂（小蜜丸、水蜜丸、水丸、浓缩丸）	每 ** 丸重 **g（每 1g 相当于饮片 **g）；每 ** 丸重 **g（相当于饮片 **g）	每瓶装 **g；每盒装 ** 丸	一次 **g；一次 ** 丸
	丸剂（滴丸）	每 ** 丸重 **g（每 1g 相当于饮片 **g）	每瓶装 **g；每瓶装 ** 丸	一次 **g；一次 ** 丸
2	颗粒剂	每 1g 相当于饮片 **g	每袋装 **g	一次 ** 袋
3	片剂	每片重 **g（相当于饮片 **g）；糖衣片：每片心重 **g（相当于饮片 **g）	每瓶装 ** 片	一次 ** 片
4	胶囊剂	每粒装 **g（相当于饮片 **g）	每瓶装 ** 粒	一次 ** 粒
5	合剂（口服液）	每 1ml 相当于饮片 **g；每支相当于饮片 **g	每瓶装 **ml；每支装 **ml	一次 **ml；一次 ** 支
6	糖浆剂	每 1ml 相当于饮片 **g	每瓶装 **ml（有刻度）	一次 **ml
7	散剂	每 1g 相当于饮片 **g	每袋装 **g	一次 **g
8	注射液	每支 **ml：相当于饮片 **g	每支装 **ml	一次 **ml
9	注射用无菌粉末	每瓶 **g：相当于饮片 **g	每瓶装 **g	一次 ** 瓶
10	煎膏剂	每 1g 相当于饮片 **g	每瓶装 **g	一次 **g
11	酒剂、酊剂	每 1ml 相当于饮片 **g	每瓶装 **ml	一次 **ml

序号	剂型	药品规格	装量规格	一次用量
12	贴膏剂、膏药、贴敷剂	每贴相当于饮片 **g（标明尺寸）	每盒装 ** 贴	一次 1 贴
13	软膏剂、乳膏剂	每 1g 相当于饮片 **g	每支装 **g	一次 **g
14	凝胶剂	每 1g 相当于饮片 **g	每支装 **g	一次 **g
15	栓剂	每粒相当于饮片 **g	每盒装 ** 粒	一次 ** 粒
16	流浸膏与浸膏剂	每 1g 相当于饮片 **g	每瓶装 **g	一次 **g
17	气雾剂、喷雾剂	定量：**ml：相当于饮片 **g（**mg 饮片 ×*** 揿或喷）；非定量：每 1ml 相当于饮片 **g	每瓶装 **ml	定量：一次 **ml；非定量：一次 ** 揿或喷
18	滴眼剂	每 1ml 相当于饮片 **g	每瓶装 **ml	一次 **ml
19	锭剂	每锭相当于饮片 **g	每盒装 ** 锭	一次 ** 锭
20	灸熨剂	每 1g 相当于饮片 **g	每盒装 ** 袋	一次 ** 袋
21	涂膜剂	每 1ml 相当于饮片 **g	每瓶装 **ml	一次 **ml
22	膜剂	每片相当于饮片 **g（标明尺寸）	每盒装 ** 片	一次 ** 片
23	茶剂	每 1g 相当于饮片 **g	每袋装 **g	一次 ** 袋
24	其他半固体及固体制剂（糊剂、胶剂等）	每 1g 相当于饮片 **g	每支（袋、盒）装 **g	一次 **g
25	其他液体制剂（露剂、搽剂、灌肠剂、洗剂、灌注液等）	每 1ml 相当于饮片 **g	每瓶装 **ml	一次 **ml

#：表中药品规格的表述以处方药味均为饮片为例。

Guideline for Studies on Pharmacognosy, Chemistry, Manufacturing and Controls (PCMC) Changes to Marketed Traditional Chinese Medicines (TCMs) (Trial)

I. Overview

This Guideline is intended to provide instructions to marketing authorization holders (hereinafter referred to as "MAHs") and/or manufacturers of medicines on studies and evaluations of proposed changes in production, quality control, and use based on their knowledge about marketed TCMs according to the requirements for risk control and the safety, efficacy and quality control of medicines.

The Guideline specifies the following matters: changes in manufacturing process, changes in excipients in preparation formulas, changes in specification or package specification, changes in registration standards, changes in packaging materials and containers, changes in shelf life or storage conditions, and changes in manufacturing sites of preparations. The work on other changes should be carried out on a case-by-case basis and in accordance with the basic principles of the Guideline.

In the Guideline, the relevant changes are divided into three categories based on risks of the changes on safety, efficacy and quality control of medicines and the degree of influences, which are major changes, moderate changes and minor changes. Major changes refer to changes that may have a significant influence on the safety, efficacy and quality control of medicines. Moderate changes refer to changes that may have a moderate influence on the safety, efficacy and quality control of medicines. Minor changes refer to changes that basically have no influence on the safety, efficacy and quality control of medicines. Where the category of changes may not be clear, the MAHs should determine the category of changes based on characteristics of the medicine and study evaluation results, and then conduct relevant studies.

The Guideline lists common changes items and categories of TCMs from the perspective of technical evaluation, and address relevant studies and validations that should be generally conducted on the proposed changes to marketed TCMs on the basis of relevant regulations and guidelines issued by China, the requirements for risk control and the safety, efficacy and quality control of medicines, the experiences an aehivements acquired by summarizing and learning from the change studies during the production process of TCMs in recent decades and inaccording with the characteristics of TCMs. For the detailed requirements for specific study work, the corresponding guidelines may be referenced.

As the responsible entity for self-assessment of change studies and study results, the MAHs should decide whether to implement changes on the basis of fully investigating and studying the possible risks and influences of the changes on safety, efficacy and quality control of medicines and evaluating the study results scientifically in accordance with the principles and requirements specified in the Guideline.

The classification of changes set forth in the Guideline relies on general considerations of the situations listed and only reflects a current basic understanding on the technical issues involved in the changes. For specific changes, the MAHs should determine the category of changes based on the study results in combination with the characteristics of medicines. In addition, due to the complexity and diversity of changes to marketed TCMs, the Guideline cannot cover all changes, and need to be updated with in-depth understanding as there may be new changes with the continuous development of process technology. If sufficient evidence obtained by other scientific studies can prove that changes do not have adverse effect on the safety, efficacy and quality control of medicines, change studies may not need to be carried out in strict accordance with the Guideline. MAHs are encouraged to learn from the concepts and methods of "Quality by Design (QbD)", "Design Space" and "Established Conditions" in the relevant guidelines of the International Council for Harmonisation of Technical Requirements for Pharmaceuticals for Human Use (ICH), and perform change management in the context of strengthening the studies of pharmaceutical processes and quality.

The MAHs can communicate with corresponding regulatory authorities in a timely manner in the process of pharmaceutical research and development and studies of postapproval changes, especially special changes and new changes due to the use of new technologies, methods, equipment, and dosage forms, etc.

II. Basic Principles

(I) MAHs should fulfill the primary responsibilities

The MAHs should fulfill the primary responsibilities of change studies, evaluation and change management, have a comprehensive and accurate understanding of the R&D, production process, and the properties of medicines, and establish a quality risk management system throughout medicines lifecyle. When considering changes to medicines, the MAHs should be aware of the reasons, extent and influence of the changes on medicines, and carry out corresponding studies in accordance with the basic principles and requirements of the Guideline and in combination with the properties of medicines. In addition, special attention should be paid to strengthening the comprehensive analysis of study results, assessing their influences on the safety, efficacy and quality control of medicines, and submitting supplementary applications, filing applications or reports in compliance with the *Provisions for Drug Registration* and relevant requirements.

(II) Changes should be necessary, scientific and reasonable

Changes to marketed TCMs should be necessary, scientific and reasonable. The proposal of changes should be based on the continuous accumulation and updating of pharmaceutical knowledge (e.g., production experience, retrospective analysis of quality, changes in control methods and application of new technologies). Scientific thinking methods should be used, and scientific decision-making procedures be followed for the purpose of realizing production, improving the quality of medicines, and providing convenience for patients to use. Relevant regulations and common sense should not be violated. Change studies should be based on previous studies and data accumulation in the study stage and the actual production process. Relevant study data from the early quality design stage can be used as the basis for the later change study. More systematical and thorough study work and more abundant data accumulated in production activities will be helpful for the studies on post-market changes. The MAHs should comprehensively analyze the influence of changes on the safety, efficacy and quality control of medicines on the basis of the study results, and explain the necessity, scientific nature and basis of the changes.

(III) MAHs should comprehensively evaluate and validate the influence of changes on the safety, efficacy and quality control of medicines

The quality of TCMs depends on the quality control of the whole process of production. All parts of production are closely related. Changes in certain aspects such as preparation formula, manufacturing process, site and quality standard may have a comprehensive influence on the safety, efficacy and quality control of medicines.

In case of any changes to medicines, it is necessary to study and evaluate the risks and degree of influence of such changes on the safety, efficacy and quality control of medicines through comprehensive studies. Targeted indicators should be selected and studied according to details about changes, properties of medicines and preparation requirements, and the degree of influence of the changes on medicines should be studied and evaluated. The changes listed in the Guidelines and their classification are only based on general considerations. The MAHs should carry out relevant studies and evaluations based on science, risks, the actual situation of changes and the prediction of the degree of influence of such changes on medicines. Specific change category and related studies should be determined based on the study data and comprehensive evaluation results. Medicines after change should have controllable, homogeneous and consistent quality. The changes should not cause significant changes in medicinal substances or absorption and utilization of preparations, or adverse impact on or significant changes in the safety and efficacy of medicines. Otherwise, a comprehensive evaluation should be performed on the efficacy and safety of medicines after change. If changes in manufacturing process or excipients lead to significant changes in medicinal substances or absorption and utilization of preparations, studies should be carried out according to improved new TCMs.

(IV) Follow the characteristics and laws of TCMs

TCMs have a long history and unique theories and technical methods, and have been proved by abundant clinical practice. Changes to TCMs should comply with the characteristics and laws of TCMs. For prepared slices/decoction pieces based on TCM theories and traditional processes, under circumstances of not changing process technologies, the process parameters before and after changes can generally be compared through Pharmacognosy, Chemistry, Manufacturing and Controls (PCMC) studies to evaluate the consistency before and after the change. In general, study contents include, but are not limited to, the comparison of extract yield (dry extract yield), extractives, fingerprints chromatograms (characteristic chromatograms), and the content of multiple markers.

III. Basic Requirements

(I) Requirements for investigational samples

The studies on changes to marketed TCMs are generally conducted using samples that can represent the actual production. The validation of manufacturing process should be performed using production-scale samples. Comparative studies of drug quality before and after change are generally conducted using three (3) consecutive batches of samples before change and three (3) consecutive batches of samples after change.

(II) Associated change requirements

A change application may just involve one or more changes. For example, the change in drug specification may be accompanied by changes in excipients or changes in pharmaceutical packaging materials. For the convenience of expression, the Guideline refer to other changes involved or induced by a change as associated changes.

For associated changes, the study should be comprehensively considered according to the basic thinking of each change study in the Guideline, and relevant studies should be carried out. These changes may have different degrees of influence on the quality, safety and efficacy of medicines and should be studied according to the change category with higher technical requirements on the whole.

(III) Requirements for preparations containing toxic ingredients

For the changes to preparations containing toxic ingredients in formulas, studies should be performed on the influence of the changes on safety of the medicine, especially the safety of changes in the following categories of preparations: (1) preparations containing extremely toxic (highly toxic) ingredients; (2) preparations containing seriously toxic ingredients upon modern studies; (3) preparations containing toxic ingredients for pediatric use and use in pregnant and lactating women; and (4) preparations that contain ingredients contraindicated or used with caution in pregnant women and are indicated for use in pregnant and lactating women. Extremely toxic ingredients refer to 28 toxic TCM products published by the State Council in the *Provisions for Medicinal Toxic Drugs* (1988) and the raw TCM materials/ingredients marked as extremely toxic (or highly toxic) in various editions of *Pharmacopoeia of the People's Republic of China*, ministerial standards, standards for imported raw TCM materials, and standards for raw TCM materials of provinces (autonomous regions and municipalities directly under the Central Government). Toxic ingredients are raw TCM materials/ingredients marked as toxic in various editions of *Pharmacopoeia of the People's Republic of China*, ministerial standards, standards for imported raw TCM materials, and standards for raw TCM materials of provinces (autonomous regions and municipalities directly under the Central Government). Where the classification of toxicity varies across the standards of provinces (autonomous regions and municipalities directly under the Central Government), the classification standard for higher toxicity should prevail.

(IV) Requirements for quality comparative study

Quality comparative study is an important consideration for change studies and critical basis for classification. Quality and drug standard studies should be conducted where a drug standard cannot well reflect the quality of medicines, quality control of medicines is low, and it is difficult to evaluate the influence of changes through quality comparative studies of medicines before and after changes only based on the drug standard. In addition, quality comparative studies should be performed using appropriate evaluation indicators and test methods based on the characteristics of medicines, e.g., extractives, fingerprint chromatograms (characteristic chromatograms), dissolution test, and bioassay. The influence of changes on quality of medicines can be objectively evaluated according to the study of quality before and after change.

(V) Others

Change studies of compound preparations of TCMs and chemical medicines, TCM injections, and sustained/controlled release preparations should take a full consideration of the characteristics of medicines and requirements for preparations, and focus on the influence of changes on the safety, efficacy, and quality control of medicines. In addition, relevant studies should be conducted according to relevant guideline and technical requirements.

IV. Changes in Manufacturing Processes

Process changes to marketed TCMs include: manufacturing process route, methods, and parameters, etc. Changes in the manufacturing process of TCMs may involve pre-treatment, extraction, separation and purification, concentration, drying, and preparation molding, etc. Changes in manufacturing process may involve only one or more of the steps above, and studies should be implemented according to the change category for a higher technical requirement. For the preparations containing extremely toxic (highly toxic) ingredients or ingredients with severe toxicity upon modern studies, if their changes in manufacturing process involve these toxic ingredients, studies should be performed according to major changes. If necessary, studies such as non-clinical safety evaluation should be performed.

Manufacturing equipment is closely associated with manufacturing process. The selected manufacturing equipment should meet manufacturing process requirements. The concept that manufacturing equipment is to serve the quality of medicines should be established. In addition, the influence of changes in manufacturing equipment on quality of medicines should be evaluated based on full consideration of the working principle and suitability of the manufacturing equipment as well as their potential changes.

Generally, the changes in manufacturing process should not cause significant changes in medicinal substances. Safety and efficacy should be comprehensively evaluated where the changes in manufacturing process result in significant changes in medicinal substances, e.g., change in the method of processing of decoction pieces (e.g., changing from stir-baking with honey to no processing or simple processing), change in the type of extraction solvent, and change in the extraction and purification methods.

(I) Minor changes

1. Information on changes

These changes include, but are not limited to, the following circumstances:

(1) Changes in process parameters of pre-treatment caused by changes in manufacturing equipment model and scale under circumstances of not changing the working principle of equipment.

(2) Changes in pulverization method or process parameters in pre-treatment, with little influence on powder yield, particle size distribution of powder, content of active or analytical markers.

(3) Changes in the size and shape of decoction pieces for extraction, with little influence on the extraction yield and the content of active or analytical markers.

(4) Changes only in the standing temperature and time of liquid materials caused by changes in manufacturing equipment and scale, or changes only in parameters such as concentration time and drying time, ect., which have little influence on the content of active or analytical markers and microbial limit.

(5) Change only from allowing decoctions to stand and filtering it to centrifuging (or change only from centrifuging to allowing decoctions to stand and filtering it), which has little influence on the total solid and the content of active or analytical markers in the decoctions.

(6) Change only in the standing time of alcohol precipitation or water precipitation only, which has little influence on the total solid and the content of active or analytical markers in the substance obtained.

(7) Change only from combining and concentrating the extracts obtained from multiple extractions to direct concentrating each extract, or change only from direct concentrating each extract to combining and concentrating the extracts obtained by multiple extractions.

(8) In order to meet the need of subsequent preparation molding process, appropriate decrease or increase in relative density of thin extract, which has little influence on the total solid and the content of active or analytical markers in the thin extract (except for the circumstance where thin extract needs further purification).

(9) Change in concentration and drying process parameters of decoction, which has little influence on the content of active or analytical markers.

(10) Change in the equipment type and parameters in process steps such as mixing, filling, tableting and granulation, etc., which has little influence on preparation quality.

(11) Change in the pill-making method of pills (except for waxed pills and paste pills), which has little influence on disintegration, dissolving or dissolution of medicines, e.g., the mutual change between different methods like water spray rotating method, extrusion-spheronization method, and compressing method, or change from manual pill making to mechanical pill making.

(12) Change in compounding temperature, dripping temperature, and condensate temperature during the dripping process of dripping pills, which has little influence on the content of active or analytical markers.

(13) Change in drying process parameters during the molding process of oral solid preparations, which has little influence on the content of active or analytical markers.

(14) Addition of the polishing process for pills, capsules and tablets.

(15) Addition of the step of charging inert gases in the filling and sealing process.

2. Study and validation

(1) Causes and details of changes, the necessity and basis of changes.

(2) Study data on the change in manufacturing process.

(3) Comparative study data on quality before and after change.

(4) Self-test reports for 3 consecutive batches of samples produced after change.

(5) Study data on stability.

(II) Moderate changes

1. Information on changes

These changes include, but are not limited to, the following circumstances:

(1) Change from separate pulverization of multiple decoction pieces to mixed pulverization, or change from mixed pulverization to separate pulverization ,which doesn't have significant impact on the powder yield, powder particle size distribution, and the content of active or analytical markers.

(2) Change in the particle size of pulverized decoction pieces used for medicinal powder (excluding ultra-micro pulverization) , which doesn't have significant impact on the subsequent molding process.

(3) Addition of high-temperature instant sterilization and differential pressure sterilization for powdered prepared slices/decoction pieces, which doesn't have significant impact on the content of active or analytical markers.

(4) Change of the sterilization method for powdered decoction pieces, which doesn't have significant impact on the content of active or analytical markers.

(5) Change of extraction time, amount of solvent and number of times of water extraction, which doesn't have significant impact on the extraction yield of extract and the content of active or analytical markers.

(6) In the subsequent decoction process after the volatile oil or aromatic aqueous liquid is obtained by the extraction of decoction pieces, change from decocting the drug residue and other decoction pieces to decocting the drug residue separately, or change from the drug residue separately to decocting the drug residue and other decoction pieces, which doesn't have significant impact on the total solid and the content of active or analytical markers in the extract.

(7) Change in the concentration and drying method of decoctions, which doesn't have significant impact on the content of active or analytical markers.

(8) Addition of the processes of common filtration or standing and centrifugation of decoctions, or change in filter materials, pore size and times of filtration for common filtration of decoctions, which doesn't have significant impact on relevant test items (e.g., total solid, content of active or analytical markers).

(9) Change in the order of adding medicinal substances and excipients during the molding process of common oral solid preparations, which has no influence on quality requirements such as preparation uniformity.

(10) Change in the filling process of common oral TCM compound prescription or single-ingredient prescription capsules, e.g., change from powder filling to filling after granulation, or change from filling after granulation to powder filling, which has no influence on the quality of preparations.

(11) Change of the processing method of volatile oil, e.g., change from spraying into to adding after inclusion of β-cyclodextrin.

(12) Change in the granulation method of common oral TCM compound prescription or single-ingredient prescription solid preparations, which has no influence on the quality of preparations.

(13) Change in drying method in the molding process of oral solid preparations, which has no influence on the quality of preparations.

(14) Change of moist heat sterilization for non-sterile preparations to terminal aseptic filling process, or addition of moist heat sterilization process, or adjustment of sterilization process parameters, which meets process design requirements and has little influence on the content of active or analytical markers.

2. Study and validation

(1) Causes and details of changes, the necessity and basis of changes.

(2) Data on change in manufacturing process, including comparative study data before and after change and study data of the process after change, validation

data and batch production records, etc.

(3) Comparative study data on quality before and after change. For oral solid preparations, special attention should be paid to the influence on medicine solubility, dissolution and disintegration time. For preparations made from single extracted compound or the extract, the influence of changes on dissolution should be studied.

(4) Self-test reports for 3 consecutive batches of samples produced after change.

(5) Study data on stability, including comparison with the stability of the medicine before change.

(III) Major changes

1. Information on changes

These changes include, but are not limited to, the following circumstances:

(1) Changes in other process parameters (e.g., extraction time, solvent amount, and frequency) without changing the extraction solvent (excluding water, different concentrations of ethanol are considered different solvents) and extraction methods.

(2) Changes in relative density of the decoctions before alcohol/water precipitation, amount of alcohol after alcohol precipitation/adding amount of water used for water precipitation, and temperature of alcohol/water precipitation (including the temperature of the decoctions during alcohol/water precipitation and the standing temperature after alcohol/water precipitation).

(3) Change from combined extraction to separate extraction, or vice versa, of multiple decoction pieces.

(4) Changes in the granulation method for common oral solid preparations made from single extracted compound or the extract.

(5) Changes in the molding process for preparations for external use, waxed pills, and pasted pills, etc.

(6) Changes in sterilization steps for sterile preparations.

2. Study and validation

Comprehensive study and validation are generally required to demonstrate that a process change will not have a significant influence on the quality of medicines. In addition to studies under moderate changes, dissolution study data should be provided, and when necessary, bioequivalence study be conducted for common oral solid preparations made from single extracted compound or the extract, which are subject to changes in granulation method and other molding processes. For preparations for external use, non-clinical irritation and anaphylaxis data should be provided when necessary. The MAHs should carefully consider the necessity of process changes depending on the circumstances. Given the complexity of changes in manufacturing process of TCMs, the MAHs may communicate with drug regulatory authorities regarding changes and related studies through post-market change communications.

V. Changes of Excipients in Preparation Formulas

Changes of excipients in preparation formulas usually include the change of supplier, type, amount or grade of the excipients. The grade of excipients mainly depends on their model and/or function and impurities. Such changes should be studied based on circumstances, the degree of influence of the changes on medicines and the characteristics of preparations, etc. The following aspects should be focused on: First, the properties of excipients. Whether the excipients involved in changes can affect medicine dissolution or release behaviors of preparations, or are critical excipients that affect *in vivo* medicine absorption of preparations. Second, the characteristics of preparations. For preparations with different characteristics, the changes of excipients may have different effects on the quality, efficacy and safety of medicines.

If changes of excipients involve other changes (e.g., changes in specification and process), an overall study should be conducted according to the change category for higher technical requirements. For common oral solid preparations made from single extracted compound or the extract, dissolution study data should generally be provided. If a new excipient is used, study data should be provided in accordance with the relevant requirements for such new excipient.

For changes of excipients that significantly affect the absorption and utilization of medicinal substances and cause significant changes in efficacy and safety, a comprehensive evaluation of safety and efficacy should be conducted, e.g., changes in special excipients that have TCM crude drugs standards (i.e., honey and rock sugar) and have functions and indications related to the functions or safety of the medicines; addition or removal of excipients in preparations for external use that have a significant effect on absorption and utilization of the preparations. Where the excipients involved in minor and moderate changes are commonly used excipients with national standards or registration standards, and need to be registered according to excipient management requirements, the registration status should be "A".

(I) Minor changes

1. Information on changes

These changes include, but are not limited to, the following circumstances:

(1) Change in materials for appearance polishing of preparations.

(2) Change in the supplier of excipients without lowering the grades and quality standards of the excipients, which does not affect the quality and stability of the medicines.

(3) Removal of essences, coloring agents, and flavor agents or reduction of their amounts; addition or alteration of the types or amounts of essences, coloring agents, and flavor agents (except for pediatric medicines).

(4) Change in the type or amount of fillers, diluents, wetting agents, lubricants, or glidants in common oral TCM compound prescription or single-ingredient prescription preparations.

2. Study and validation

(1) Causes and details of changes, the necessity and basis of changes.

(2) Description of excipients before and after change and their quality standards.

(3) Study data of preparation formulas (if applicable).

(4) Study data of manufacturing processes involved in changes.

(5) Self-test reports for 3 consecutive batches of samples produced after change.

(6) Study data on stability.

(7) Revised and complete package inserts and labels.

(II) Moderate changes

1. Information on changes

These changes include, but are not limited to, the following circumstances:

(1) Change in the type or amount of other excipients (excluding adding or reducing excipients that may affect medicine dissolution or release) except for fillers, diluents, wetting agents, lubricants, and glidants in common oral TCM compound prescription or single-ingredient prescription preparations; for common oral TCM compound prescription or single-ingredient prescription solid preparations, change in the gastric soluble film coating material and change of sugar coated tablets to gastric soluble film coated tablets, etc.

(2) Change in the grade of excipients in common oral solid preparations, which does not affect the quality of medicines.

(3) Addition or alteration of the type or amount of essences, coloring agents, and flavor agents for pediatric medicines without affecting quality of medicines.

(4) Addition of inclusion materials of volatile components, such as β-cyclodextrin.

(5) Change in the type or amount of excipients (excluding penetration enhancers) of preparations for external use that have topical effects (excluding those used for serious ulcers and burns, etc.), e.g., replacing paraffin with beeswax.

Such changes generally should meet the following requirements: not for sustained/controlled release and other special dosage forms; the extent of changes in excipients should be within their permitted application scopes, and the amount of excipients should be minimized as much as possible, and the optimal amount of excipients be selected. Such changes are relatively complex. Regardless of the circumstances, they should be managed according to the requirements for major changes if they may have significant effects on the safety, efficacy, and quality control of medicines.

2. Study and validation

(1) Causes and details of changes, the necessity and basis of changes.

(2) Description of excipients before and after change and their quality standards.

(3) Study data of preparation formulas.

(4) Study and validation data of manufacturing process involved in changes and batch production records, etc.

(5) Comparative study data on quality before and after change, quality study data and literatures, and quality standards.

(6) Self-test reports for 3 consecutive batches of samples produced after change.

(7) Study data on stability, including comparison with the stability of the medicine before change.

(8) When necessary, safety study data should be provided for pharmaceutical excipients such as flavor agents, essences, and coloring agents used for pediatric medicines.

(9) When necessary, non-clinical irritation and anaphylaxis studies should be conducted on preparations for external use based on their characteristics.

(10) Revised and complete package inserts and labels.

(III) Major changes

1. Information on changes

These changes include, but are not limited to, the following circumstances:

(1) Changes in the types and amounts of excipients in preparations made from single extracted compound or an extract, as well as in common oral

preparations with extremely toxic (highly toxic) ingredients or ingredients with severe toxicity upon modern studies.

(2) Change in the type or amount of penetration enhancers in preparations for external use that have topical effects (excluding those used for severe ulcers and burns, etc.); change in the type or amount of excipients (excluding penetration enhancers) in preparations for external use that have topical effects for severe ulcers and burns, etc., or those preparations that have systemic effects.

(3) The excipients used have not been used in the marketed products with the same administration route.

(4) Changes in excipients that are included for registration management, and the excipients after change have not been registered or the registration status is "I".

2. Study and validation

The following study data should also be provided, when necessary, in addition to studies under moderate changes:

(1) For oral solid preparations made from single extracted component or an extract, dissolution study data should generally be provided, and bioequivalence studies be conducted when necessary.

(2) When necessary, study data related to absorption and utilization should be provided for preparations made from single extracted compound or an extract, ophthalmic preparations, inhalation preparations, preparations for external use (e.g., aerosols), sustained/controlled release preparations and those of other special dosage forms.

(3) Non-clinical irritation and anaphylaxis study data should be provided based on the characteristics of preparations.

VI. Changes in Specification or Package Specification

Changes in specification should follow the principles of being scientific, reasonable, necessary, and convenient for clinical use, and should be determined appropriately based on the usage and dosage of medicines. The study should focus on the consistency in formula, process, daily administration/dosage between medicines with the original specification and those after the change in specification. Changing the specification of a medicine should not cause changes in medicinal substances or the originally approved usage and dosage, or target population of the medicine. A comprehensive evaluation of safety and efficacy should be conducted when changes may cause significant changes on medicinal substances or have a significant effect on their absorption and utilization. Any changes in excipients should conform to the relevant requirements for excipient changes.

(I) Minor changes

1. Information on changes

These changes include, but are not limited to, the following circumstances:

Change in the quantity of a medicine per minimum package unit, e.g., changing from A bags per box to B bags per box for granules, and changing from A tablets per blister to B tablets per blister for tablets.

2. Study and validation

(1) Causes and details of changes, the necessity and basis of changes.

(2) Revised and improved package inserts and labels.

(II) Moderate changes

1. Information on changes

These changes include, but are not limited to, the following circumstances:

Changes in the loading quantity of a medicine per minimum package unit for granules, concentrated decoctions, and syrups, etc.

2. Study and validation

(1) Causes and details of changes, the necessity and basis of changes.

(2) Study and validation data of manufacturing process involved in changes and batch production records, etc. (if applicable).

(3) Comparative study data on quality before and after change, quality study data and literatures, and quality standards (if applicable).

(4) Self-test reports for 3 consecutive batches of samples produced after change.

(5) Study data on stability, including comparative study data on the stability of the medicine before and after change. If there is no change in packaging materials, study data on stability is generally not required; however, if factors that affect medicine stability, such as the size of packaging container, are involved, study data on stability should be provided.

(6) Revised and complete package inserts and labels.

(III) Major changes

1. Information on changes

These changes include, but are not limited to, the following circumstances:

(1) The expression of medicine specification should be standardized according to the *Guideline for Specification Expression of Chinese Proprietary Medicines*, and quality standards, package inserts and labels should be revised accordingly.

(2) Actual changes in medicine specification, e.g., changes in the weight and size of tablets, changes in the loading quantity of capsules, and changes in the medicine concentration of liquid preparations (equivalent amount of decoction pieces contained per unit volume), etc.

2. Study and validation (excluding the standardization of specification expression)

(1) Causes and details of changes, the necessity and basis of changes.

(2) Study and validation data of manufacturing process involved in changes and batch production records, etc.

(3) Comparative study data on quality before and after change, quality study data and literatures, and quality standards.

(4) Self-test reports for 3 consecutive batches of samples produced after change.

(5) Study data on stability, including comparative study data on the stability of the medicine before and after change.

(6) Revised and complete package inserts and labels.

VII. Changes in Registration Standard

The changes in registration standard outlined in the Guideline mainly refer to the revision of test items, such as the test, identification, and assay, ect., and their methods or limits/ranges within the registration standard. The modified drug registration standard should at least meet the requirements of national drug standards.

After TCMs are marketed, the MAHs should keep improving the quality standards based on the growing knowledge about medicines in conjunction with the latest progress in the test technology, methods, and means, so as to increase its control. The changes in registration standard should not cause the reduction of quality control level of medicines, and should not have adverse impact on quality assurance of medicines. Usually, based on the current registration standard, addition of test items, tightening limit ranges or improving specificity of test methods can better control and ensure quality of medicines. Studies on changes in test items are mainly the methodological study and validation of test methods, as well as the determination of limits/ranges.

To make a change in registration standard, it is necessary to consider whether the change will affect the shelf life of the medicine. If the registration standard has been improved (e.g., narrowing of limits and addition of test items, etc.), it is required to study whether the medicine complies with the requirements in the new quality standard within the originally established shelf life.

(I) Moderate changes

1. Information on changes

These changes include, but are not limited to, the following circumstances:

(1) Narrowing of limits on the basis of the range specified in the original standard.

These changes refer to narrowing the control limits on the basis of the range specified in the original standard. Narrowing of limit range caused by major changes in manufacturing process of medicines is not within the scope of these changes.

(2) Change in text description in the registration standard should not involve changes in test methods and limits.

(3) Relevant contents in the registration standard should be revised after the application for modifications of the registration standard according to approved items, e.g., change in storage conditions or strength, is approved.

(4) Addition of test items.

The new test items should be able to control product quality more effectively. Methodological validation of the new test items and proposed control limit should comply with the requirements of relevant guidelines. These changes do not include addition of test items due to safety or quality. The addition of test items in the standard, due to changes in PCMC characteristics caused by manufacturing process changes, does not fall into the scope of such changes.

2. Study and validation

(1) Reasons for changes in the registration standard and details about the changes.

(2) Study data related to changes in the registration standard, as well as comparative study data before and after change. If an analytical method is added or changed, methodological study data and comparative study data before and after change should be provided. If there is a change in the specified limit of relevant substances in test items or in the content limit or range, the basis for the change should be provided, e.g., test data of samples for clinical studies or test data of medicines since they were marketed. When necessary, relevant safety study data or literatures should also be provided.

(3) Quality standards before and after change.

(4) Self-test and re-test reports for 3 consecutive batches of samples (if

applicable).

(5) Study data on stability.

(II) Major changes

1. Information on changes

These changes include, but are not limited to, the following circumstances:

(1) Changes in test methods, excluding changes in the registration standard caused by changes in national drug standards.

(2) Widening of control limit.

(3) Deletion of any item in the registration standard.

2. Study and validation

Relevant study data for these changes can be provided with reference to those for moderate changes.

VIII. Changes in Packaging Materials and Containers

Packaging materials and containers are part of the medicines. Packaging materials and containers in the Guideline mainly refer to packages in direct contact with medicines. Changes in packaging materials and containers may have influence on factors related to the safety, efficacy and quality control of medicines. The risks are dependent upon the route of administration of preparations, performance of packaging materials and containers, and compatibility between packages and preparations, etc.

In general, changes in packaging materials and containers of medicines should be beneficial to ensure the quality and stability of medicines, or should at least not reduce the protective effect of pharmaceutical packaging materials and containers, and adverse interactions between medicines and packaging materials should not occur.

Studies should be conducted comprehensively based on the application scope of pharmaceutical packaging materials, characteristics of container closure systems, characteristics of dosage forms, and the administration route of medicines. Studies should focus on whether there is any interaction between medicines and packaging materials or containers, and whether the stability of medicines is affected before and after change.

Changes in packaging materials and containers that directly contact intermediates in the production process of medicines should be evaluated in accordance with relevant requirements of products for the category of changes, and relevant studies be conducted.

(I) Minor changes

1. Information on changes

These changes include, but are not limited to, the following circumstances:

(1) Changes in materials and/or types of packaging materials and containers of non-sterile solid preparations not specified in the Guideline. Packaging materials and containers after change have been used in marketed medicines with the same route of administration and have the same or better applicability.

(2) Changes in suppliers, sizes and/or shapes of packaging materials and containers not specified in the Guideline.

2. Study and validation

(1) Describe the reasons for changes in packaging materials and containers and the information on packaging materials and containers after change in detail. List the quality standards for packaging materials and containers after change.

(2) Provide the comparative study of relevant characteristics of packaging materials and containers before and after change.

(3) Self-test reports for 3 consecutive batches of samples produced after change.

(4) Study data on stability (if applicable).

(II) Moderate changes

1. Information on changes

These changes include, but are not limited to, the following circumstances:

(1) Changes in materials and/or types of packaging materials and containers of liquid/semi-solid preparations (excluding injections, ophthalmic preparations, and inhalation preparations), such as changing PP bottles for oral liquid preparations to PET bottles for oral liquid preparations.

(2) Changes in materials and/or types of packaging materials and containers of non-sterile solid preparations, such as change among blister package, bottle and bag, and changing from double-aluminium blister to aluminium-plastic blister package.

(3) Changes in suppliers, sizes and/or shapes of packaging materials and containers of injections.

2. Study and validation

(1) Describe the reasons for changes in packaging materials and containers and the information on packaging materials and containers after change in detail. List the quality standards for packaging materials and containers after change.

(2) Carry out comparative studies of relevant characteristics of packaging materials and containers before and after change and equivalence/commutability studies on packaging materials.

(3) Carry out compatibility studies on packaging materials according to the products. If changes in sealing parts are involved, tightness studies of package should be carried out.

(4) Perform validation for the packaging process.

(5) Self-test reports for 3 consecutive batches of samples produced after change.

(6) Study data on stability, including comparison with the stability of the medicine before change (if applicable).

(7) Revised and complete package inserts and labels.

(III) Major changes

1. Information on changes

These changes include, but are not limited to, the following circumstances:

(1) Changes in materials and/or types of packaging materials and containers of inhalation preparations, injections, and ophthalmic preparations.

(2) Changes in suppliers, sizes and/or shapes of metered dose delivery devices of inhalation preparations.

(3) Removal of secondary package providing additional protection for medicines (such as high-barrier external bag).

(4) Changes to packaging materials and containers with a completely new material, structure, and intended use with higher risks.

(5) Changes in packaging materials and containers that are included for registration management. Packaging materials and containers after change have not been registered or the registration status is "I".

2. Study and validation

(1) Describe the reasons for changes in packaging materials and containers and the information on packaging materials and containers after change in detail. List the quality standards for packaging materials and containers after change.

(2) Carry out comparative studies on relevant characteristics of packaging materials and containers before and after change and equivalence/commutability studies on packaging materials.

(3) Carry out compatibility studies on packaging materials according to the products. If changes in sealing parts are involved, tightness studies on package should be carried out. A change in the metered dose delivery device necessitates corresponding study depending on characteristics of the delivery device to demonstrate dosing accuracy after change is not lower than that before change.

(4) Perform validation for the packaging process. Aseptic/sterilization process of sterile preparations should be verified, if necessary.

(5) Self-test reports for 3 consecutive batches of samples produced after change.

(6) Study data on stability, including comparison with the stability of the medicine before change.

(7) Revised and complete package inserts and labels.

IX. Changes in Shelf Life or Storage Conditions

Changes in shelf life and/or storage conditions of medicines may include the following circumstances: ① prolongation of shelf life; ② shortening of shelf life; ③ tightening of storage conditions; and ④ loosening of storage conditions. Changes may only involve the change of one of the above situations, and may also involve changes of many of the above situations. In such cases, it is necessary to conduct studies separately. Where the stability study protocol is not consistent with that at the time of marketing authorization of the medicine, the quality control items and test methods are changed, or the manufacturing process or preparation formula is changed, corresponding studies should be conducted on the shelf life or storage conditions according to the changes. The shelf life of the medicine to be changed should not exceed the duration of the long-term stability study. Attention should be paid to the storage duration and storage conditions of intermediates during the production process.

(I) Moderate changes

1. Information on changes

These changes include, but are not limited to, the following circumstances:

(1) Prolongation of the shelf life of medicines

This change only refers to the prolongation of the shelf life of a medicine in the absence of any change in the manufacturing process and production quality control methods, formulas, quality standards, packaging materials and containers in direct contact with the medicine, and storage conditions, etc.

(2) Shortening of the shelf life or tightening of storage conditions of medicines

Generally, quality of medicines can be better guaranteed by shortening the shelf life and tightening the storage conditions. This includes situations where the expiry date needs to be shortened based on changes in the usage region of the medicine and corresponding stability study results.

2. Study and validation

(1) Causes and details of changes, the necessity and basis of changes.

(2) The stability study should be conducted on 3 batches of medicines according to the established stability study protocol.

(3) Revised and complete package inserts and labels.

(II) Major changes

1. Information on changes

These changes include the loosening of storage conditions, etc.

2. Study and validation

(1) Causes and details of changes, the necessity and basis of changes.

(2) The stability study should be conducted on 3 batches of medicines in accordance with the established stability study protocol, including the comparative studies with the stability before change.

(3) Revised and complete package inserts and labels.

X. Changes in the Manufacturing Site of Preparations

Changes in the manufacturing site of TCM preparations (including pre-treatment, extraction and purification, concentration and drying, preparation molding and packaging addresses), including changes or additions to the actual manufacturing address of preparations, or alterations, reconstruction and new construction of the manufacturing site at the same manufacturing address. The same manufacturing address refers to that the new and old plants that are responsible for actual production have the same physical address, which should be indicated in approval documents of medicines. The manufacturing sites of preparations include manufacturing sites owned by the MAHs or those of entrusted manufacturers.

Changes in manufacturing sites of preparations generally require comprehensive studies and validation, which should focus on the consistency of quality control throughout the production process before and after the site change.

Whether there are significant differences in quality of medicines before and after change should be evaluated by comparing and analyzing critical process control parameters of medicines before and after change as well as comparative study and analysis of medicinal substances. The MAHs should ensure that the medicines that meet the intended uses and registration requirements can be continuously and stably manufactured with the production technology after transferring to a new manufacturing site. Changes in the manufacturing sites of preparations should not affect the formula, process, packaging materials and containers that come into direct contact with the medicines, or lower the level of quality control or standards. The technical requirements for changes in the manufacturing site of extracts are the same as those for changes in the manufacturing site of preparations.

The relevant provisions of the *Measures for the Supervision and Administration of Drug Production* and the *Provisions for Post-market Changes of Drugs (Trial)* should be implemented for changing the manufacturing site of preparations. The study and validation may refer to the following contents:

(1) Details of and reasons for changes.

(2) Compare manufacturing process between old and new manufacturing sites. Compare the performance, working principle, production capacity, manufacturer and model of the manufacturing equipment before and after change, carry out quality risk assessment and describe the changes.

(3) Study and validation data of manufacturing process involved in changes and batch production records (if applicable).

(4) Comparative study data on quality before and after change (if applicable).

(5) Self-test reports for 3 consecutive batches of samples produced after change (if applicable).

(6) Study data on stability, including comparison with the stability of the medicine before change (if applicable).

已上市中药药学变更研究技术指导原则（试行）

一、概述

本技术指导原则适用于指导药品上市许可持有人（以下简称为持有人）和/或生产企业根据对已上市中药的认知，基于风险控制和药品安全、有效、质量可控的要求，针对在生产、质量控制、使用等方面拟进行的变更开展研究和评估工作。

本技术指导原则涉及事项包括：变更生产工艺、变更制剂处方中的辅料、变更规格或包装规格、变更注册标准、变更包装材料和容器、变更有效期或贮藏条件、变更制剂生产场地。对于其他变更，应根据其具体情况，按照本技术指导原则的基本原则进行相应工作。

按照变更对药品安全性、有效性和质量可控性的风险和产生影响的程度，本技术指导原则对所述及的变更划分为三类：重大变更、中等变更、微小变更。重大变更是指对药品的安全性、有效性和质量可控性可能产生重大影响的变更。中等变更是指对药品的安全性、有效性和质量可控性可能有中等程度影响的变更。微小变更是指对药品的安全性、有效性和质量可控性基本不产生影响的变更。对于变更类别可能不清晰的，持有人应根据药品特点和研究评估结果确定变更类别，进行相关研究。

本技术指导原则以国家颁布的相关法规及技术指导原则为基础，基于风险控制和药品安全、有效、质量可控的要求，通过研究、总结、吸收近几十年来中药生产过程中变更研究的经验和成果，根据中药特点，从技术评价角度列举了目前中药常见变更事项及其分类，阐述了对已上市中药拟进行的变更在一般情况下应开展的相关研究验证工作。各项研究工作的具体要求可参见相应的技术指导原则。

持有人作为变更研究和研究结果自我评估的责任主体，应按照本技术指导原则的原则和要求，充分考察研究变更对药品安全性、有效性和质量可控性可能产生的风险和影响，在对研究结果进行科学评估的基础上决定是否进行变更的实施。

本技术指导原则所列变更分类是基于对所列情形的一般考虑，仅反映了当前对变更涉及的技术问题的基本认知。对于具体的变更，持有人应结合药品特点，根据研究结果确定变更类别。此外，由于已上市中药变更的复杂性和多样性，本技术指导原则内容无法涵盖所有变更情况，而且随着工艺技术的不断发展可能出现新的变更情况，需要随着认识的不断深入而不断更新。如果通过其他科学研究获得充分的证据，证明变更对药品的安全性、有效性及质量可控性不会产生不利影响，可以不必完全按本技术指导原则的要求进行变更研究。鼓励持有人借鉴国际人用药品注册技术要求协调会（International Council for Harmonisation of Technical Requirements for Pharmaceuticals for Human Use，ICH）相关技术指导原则中的"质量源于设计""设计空间""既定条件"等理念和方法，在加强对药品工艺、质量研究的基础上，开展变更管理相关工作。

在药品研发及上市后变更研究过程中，特别是对于特殊变更问题以及由于新技术、新方法、新设备、新剂型等的使用出现的新的变更情况，持有人可及时与相应监管机构开展沟通交流。

二、基本原则

（一）持有人应履行主体责任

持有人应履行变更研究及其评估、变更管理的主体责任，应对药品的研发和生产过程、药品的性质等有全面和准确的了解，建立药品全生命周期的质量风险管理体系；当考虑对药品进行变更时，持有人应当清楚变更的原因、变更的程度及其对药品的影响，按照本技术指导原则的基本原则和要求，结合药品特点，开展相应研究；并应特别注意加强对研究结果进行全面分析，评估其对药品安全性、有效性和质量可控性的影响，按照《药品注册管理办法》规定及相关要求，提出补充申请、备案或报告。

（二）变更应必要、科学、合理

已上市中药变更应符合变更的必要性、科学性、合理性要求。变更的提出应基于对药品知识的不断积累和更新（例如：生产经验、质量回顾分析、控制方法的改变和新技术的应用等），应运用科学思维方法，遵循科学决策的程序，以有助于药品的生产实现、质量提升、利于患者使用等为目的，不得有违相关法规和常识。变更研究应以既往研究阶段以及实际生产过程中的研究和数据积累为基础，前期质量设计阶段的相关研究数据可以作为后期变更研究的依据。研究工作越系统、深入，生产过程中积累的数据越充分，对上市后的变更研究越有帮助。持有人应根据研究结果全面分析变更对药品安全性、有效性和质量可控性的影响，说明变更的必要性、科学性和合理性。

（三）持有人应全面评估、验证变更事项对药品安全性、有效性和质量可控性的影响

中药质量取决于生产全过程的质量控制，生产各环节是紧密关联的，制剂处方、生产工艺、场地、质量标准等某一方面的变更可能对药品安全性、有效性和质量可控性带来全面的影响。

药品发生变更时，需通过全面的研究工作考察和评估变更对药品安全性、有效性和质量可控性的风险和产生影响的程度。应根据变更的具体情况、药物性质及制剂要求等选择有针对性的指标进行考察，研究评估变更对药品影响程度。本技术指导原则中所列变更情形及其分类，只是基于一般考虑，持有人应基于科学、基于风险，根据变更实际情况、变更对药品影响程度的预判，开展相关研究和评估工作，具体变更类别及相关研究工作应根据其研究数据、综合评估结果确定。变更后的药品应质量可控、均一稳定。变更不应引起药用物质基础或制剂吸收、利用的明显改变，对药品安全性、有效性产生不利影响或带来明显变化，否则应进行变更后药品的安全性和有效性的全面评价。生产工艺或辅料等的改变引起药用物质基础或制剂吸收、利用明显改变的，应按照改良型新药进行研究。

（四）遵循中医药自身特点和规律

中药具有悠久的历史传统和独特的理论及技术方法，并经丰富的临床实践所证明。中药的变更应遵循中医药自身特点和规律。基于中医药理论和传统工艺制备的中药，在工艺方法不变的情况下，其工艺参数的变更一般可通过药学研究进行变更前后的比较，评估变更前后的一致性。研究内容一般包括但不限于出膏率（干膏率）、浸出物、指纹图谱（特征图谱）以及多种成份含量的比较。

三、基本要求

（一）研究用样品要求

已上市中药变更的研究一般应采用能代表生产实际情况的样品。生产工艺验证工作需采用生产规模的样品。变更前后药品质量比较研究，一般采用变更前连续3批样品和变更后连续3批样品进行。

（二）关联变更要求

变更申请可能只涉及某一种情况的变更，也可能涉及多种情况的变更，如：药品规格的变更可能伴随辅料的变更，或同时伴随药品包装材料的变更等。为了叙述的方便，本技术指导原则将一项变更伴随或引发的其他变更称之为关联变更。

对于关联变更，研究工作应按照本技术指导原则中各项变更研究工作的基本思路综合考虑，并进行相关研究。这些变更对药品质量、安全性、有效性影响程度可能不同，总体上需按照技术要求较高的变更类别进行研究。

（三）含毒性药味制剂要求

对于处方中含有毒性药味制剂的变更，应关注变更对药品安全性的影响，尤其应关注以下几类制剂变更的安全性，开展相关研究：（1）含大毒（剧毒）药味的制剂；（2）含有现代研究发现有严重毒性药味的制剂；（3）含有分类为有毒药味，且为儿科用药、妊娠期和哺乳期妇女用药的制剂；（4）含有孕妇禁用或慎用的药味，且功能主治为妊娠期和哺乳期妇女用药的制剂。大毒药味是指国务院《医疗用毒性药品管理办法》（1988 年）公布的 28 种毒性中药品种和历版《中国药典》、部颁标准、进口药材标准、各省（自治区、直辖市）药材标准中标注为大毒（或剧毒）的药材/药味。有毒药味是指历版《中国药典》、部颁标准、进口药材标准、各省（自治区、直辖市）药材标准中标注为有毒的药材/药味。各省（自治区、直辖市）标准中毒性大小分类不一致的，以毒性高的分类标准为依据。

（四）质量对比研究要求

质量对比研究是变更研究工作的重要考量以及分类的重要依据。如果药品标准不能较好地反映药品质量，对于药品质量的可控性低，仅依据药品标准进行变更前后药品质量对比研究难以评估变更影响的，应开展质量及药品标准研究工作，根据药品特点采用合适的评价指标及检测方法，如：浸出物、指纹图谱（特征图谱）、溶出度检查、生物活性测定等，进行质量对比研究，根据变更前后质量研究情况客观评估变更对药品质量的影响情况。

（五）其他

中西复方制剂及中药注射剂、缓释/控释制剂等制剂的变更研究应充分考虑药品特点、制剂要求，全面关注变更对药品安全性、有效性和质量可控性的影响，并参照相关技术指导原则、技术要求开展相关研究工作。

四、变更生产工艺

已上市中药的工艺变更包括：生产工艺路线、方法、参数等变更。中药生产工艺变更可能涉及前处理、提取、分离纯化、浓缩、干燥、制剂成型等工艺的变更。生产工艺变更可能只涉及上述某一环节，也可能涉及多个环节，研究工作应按照技术要求较高的变更类别实施。含大毒（剧毒）药味或现代研究发现有严重毒性药味的制剂，生产工艺变更内容涉及上述毒性药味的，应按照重大变更进行研究，必要时开展非临床安全性评价等研究工作。

生产设备与生产工艺密切相关。生产设备的选择应符合生产工艺的要求，应树立生产设备是为药品质量服务的理念，充分考虑生产设备工作原理、设备的适用性，以及可能引起的变化，评估生产设备的改变对药品质量的影响。

生产工艺变更一般不应引起药用物质基础的明显改变。生产工艺变化引起药用物质基础发生明显改变的，应进行安全性、有效性全面评价，如：改变饮片炮炙方法（如：蜜炙改成生用），改变提取溶剂种类，改变提取纯化方法等。

（一）微小变更

1. 变更情况

此类变更包括但不限于以下情形：

（1）前处理中，在设备工作原理不变的情况下，因生产设备型号、规模的改变而引起的工艺参数变更。

（2）前处理中，变更粉碎方法或粉碎工艺参数，对出粉率、粉末粒度分布、活性成份或指标成份含量等基本不产生影响的。

（3）变更提取用饮片的大小、形状等，对提取得率及活性成份或指标成份含量等基本不产生影响的。

（4）仅因生产设备、规模的改变而引起液体物料静置存放的温度、时间发生变更，或浓缩、干燥所需时间等参数发生变更，对活性成份或指标成份含量、微生物限度等基本不产生影响的。

（5）仅由药液静置、过滤改为离心（或离心改为药液静置、过滤），对药液中的总固体量、活性成份或指标成份含量等基本不产生影响的。

（6）仅变更醇沉或水沉的放置时间，对所得物中总固体量、活性成份或指标成份含量等基本不产生影响的。

（7）仅由多次提取的提取液合并浓缩变更为每次提取液直接浓缩，或仅由每次提取液直接浓缩，变更为多次提取的提取液合并浓缩。

（8）为了适应后续制剂成型工艺需要，清膏相对密度适当降低或提高，对清膏中总固体量、活性成份或指标成份含量等基本不产生影响的（清膏需进一步纯化处理的不在此范畴）。

（9）变更药液浓缩、干燥工艺参数，对活性成份或指标成份含量等基本不产生影响的。

（10）变更混合、充填、压片、制粒等工艺步骤中设备类型及参数，对制剂质量基本不产生影响的。

（11）变更丸剂（蜡丸、糊丸等除外）制丸方法，对药物的崩解、溶散或溶出基本不产生影响的，如：泛制法、挤出滚圆法、压制法等之间的相互转变，或由手工制丸变更为机器制丸。

（12）变更滴丸滴制过程中配料温度、滴制温度、冷凝液温度，对活性成份或指标成份含量等质量基本不产生影响的。

（13）变更口服固体制剂成型工艺中干燥工艺参数，对活性成份或指标成份含量等基本不产生影响的。

（14）增加丸剂、胶囊剂、片剂抛光工序。

（15）增加灌封工序中填充惰性气体步骤。

2. 研究验证工作

（1）变更的原因、具体情况，说明变更的必要性和合理性。

（2）变更工艺研究资料。

（3）变更前后质量对比研究资料。

（4）变更后连续生产的 3 批样品的自检报告书。

（5）稳定性研究资料。

（二）中等变更

1. 变更情况

此类变更包括但不限于以下情形：

（1）多种饮片单独粉碎变更为混合后粉碎，或混合粉碎变更为单独粉碎，对出粉率、粉末粒度分布、活性成份或指标成份含量等不产生明显影响的。

（2）采用药粉入药的，饮片粉碎粒度的改变（不包括超微粉碎），对后续成型工艺不产生明显影响的。

（3）饮片粉末增加高温瞬时灭菌、压差灭菌等方法，对其活性成份或指标成份含量等不产生明显影响的。

（4）变更饮片粉末灭菌方法，对其活性成份或指标成份含量等不产生明显影响的。

（5）变更水提取的提取时间、溶剂用量、次数，对浸膏提取得率、活性成份或指标成份含量等不产生明显影响的。

（6）饮片提取挥发油或芳香水后的后续水提工艺中，由药渣与其他饮片合并提取变更为药渣单独提取，或药渣单独提取变更为与其他饮片合并提取，对提取液的总固体量、活性成份或指标成份含量等不产生明显影响的。

（7）变更药液浓缩、干燥方法，对活性成份或指标成份含量等不产生明显影响的。

（8）增加药液普通过滤或静置、离心工序，或者变更药液普通过滤的滤材材质、孔径及过滤次数等，对相关检测指标（如：总固体量、活性成份或指标成份含量等）不产生明显影响的。

（9）变更普通口服固体制剂成型过程中原辅料的加入顺序，对制剂均匀性等质量要求不产生影响的。

（10）变更普通口服中药复方或单方胶囊剂填充工艺，如：由粉末填充变更为制粒后填充，或由制粒后填充变更为粉末填充，对制剂质量不产生影响的。

（11）变更挥发油的处理方式，如：由喷入变更为β-环糊精包合后加入。

（12）变更普通口服中药复方或单方固体制剂的制粒方式，对制剂质量不产生影响的。

（13）变更口服固体制剂成型工艺中干燥方法，对制剂质量不产生影响的。

（14）非无菌制剂由湿热灭菌变更为终端无菌灌装工艺，或增加湿热灭菌工序，或灭菌工艺参数的调整，符合工艺设计要求且对活性成份或指标成份含量等基本不产生影响的。

2. 研究验证工作

（1）变更的原因、具体情况，说明变更的必要性和合理性。

（2）变更工艺资料，包括变更前后对比研究资料和变更后工艺研究资料、验证资料、批生产记录等。

（3）变更前后质量对比研究资料。口服固体制剂尤其应关注对药物的溶化性、溶散时限或崩解时限的影响。提取的单一成份或提取物制成的制剂，应研究变更对溶出度的影响。

（4）变更后连续生产的3批样品的自检报告书。

（5）稳定性研究资料，包括与变更前药品稳定性情况的比较。

（三）重大变更

1. 变更情况

此类变更包括但不限于以下情形：

（1）提取溶剂（不包括水，不同浓度的乙醇视为不同溶剂）和提取方式不变，其他工艺参数（如：提取时间、溶剂用量、次数）的变更。

（2）醇沉/水沉前药液的相对密度、醇沉含醇量/水沉加水量、醇沉/水沉温度（包括醇沉/水沉时药液的温度、醇沉/水沉后静置的温度）等的变更。

（3）多种饮片合并提取与分开提取的改变。

（4）提取的单一成份或提取物制成的普通口服固体制剂制粒方式的改变。

（5）外用制剂、蜡丸、糊丸等成型工艺方法的改变。

（6）变更无菌制剂灭菌步骤。

2. 研究验证工作

一般需进行全面的研究和验证工作，证明工艺变更不会对药品质量产生重大影响。除中等变更项下研究工作外，提取的单一成份或提取物制成的普通口服固体制剂涉及制粒方式变更等成型工艺改变的应提供溶出度研究资料，必要时应开展生物等效性研究；外用制剂等必要时应有非临床刺激性、过敏性等研究资料。持有人应根据实际情况慎重考虑工艺变更的必要性。鉴于中药生产工艺变更的复杂性，持有人可通过上市后变更沟通交流途径，就变更事项及相关研究工作与药品审评机构进行交流。

五、变更制剂处方中的辅料

变更制剂处方中的辅料一般包括变更辅料供应商、种类、用量或级别等。辅料的级别主要与辅料的型号和/或功能、杂质状况等相关。此类变更应结合变更的具体情况，变更对药品的影响程度、制剂的特性等进行相应的研究工作，重点考察以下方面：第一，辅料的性质。变更涉及的辅料是否会影响制剂药物溶出或释放行为，或是否为影响制剂体内药物吸收的关键性辅料。第二，制剂的特性。对于不同特性制剂，辅料变更可能对药品质量、疗效和安全性产生不同的影响。

辅料变更涉及其他变更的（例如：规格和工艺变更等），总体上需按照技术要求较高的变更类别进行研究。对于提取的单一成份或提取物制成的普通口服固体制剂一般应提供溶出度研究资料。对于使用新辅料的，应按新辅料相关要求提供研究资料。对药用物质吸收、利用有明显影响，引起有效性、安全性发生明显变化的辅料变更，应进行安全性、有效性全面评价，如：具有药材标准的特殊辅料（如：蜂蜜、冰糖等）的改变，且该辅料功能主治与药品功能主治或安全性相关；外用制剂中增加或删除对制剂吸收、利用有明显影响的辅料等。微小和中等变更涉及的辅料应为常用辅料，具有国家标准或注册标准，根据辅料管理要求需要登记的，登记状态应为"A"。

（一）微小变更

1. 变更情况

此类变更包括但不限于以下情形：

（1）变更制剂外观抛光材料。

（2）在辅料的级别及质量标准不降低的情况下，变更辅料供应商，不影响药物质量和稳定性的。

（3）删除香精、色素、矫味剂，或减少其用量；增加或改变香精、色素、矫味剂的种类或用量（儿童用药除外）。

（4）变更普通口服中药复方或单方制剂中填充剂、稀释剂、润湿剂、润滑剂、助流剂的种类或用量。

2. 研究验证工作

（1）变更的原因、具体情况，说明变更的必要性和合理性。

（2）变更前后辅料相关情况的说明及其质量标准。

（3）制剂处方研究资料（如适用）。

（4）变更所涉及的生产工艺研究资料。

（5）变更后连续生产的 3 批样品的自检报告书。

（6）稳定性研究资料。

（7）修订完善的说明书、标签。

（二）中等变更

1. 变更情况

此类变更包括但不限于以下情形：

（1）普通口服中药复方或单方制剂中除填充剂、稀释剂、润湿剂、润滑剂、助流剂外，其他辅料种类或用量的变更（不包括增加或减少可能影响药物溶解、释放的辅料种类）；普通口服中药复方和单方固体制剂变更胃溶型薄膜包衣材料、糖衣片变更为胃溶型薄膜包衣片等。

（2）变更普通口服固体制剂辅料的级别，不影响药品质量的。

（3）增加或改变涉及儿童用药的香精、色素、矫味剂的种类或用量，不影响药品质量的。

（4）增加挥发性成份的包合材料，如：β- 环糊精。

（5）变更起局部作用（用于严重溃疡、烧伤等除外）的外用制剂辅料（不包括渗透促进剂）种类或用量，如：蜂蜡替代石蜡等。

此类变更一般应符合以下要求：不属于缓释/控释等特殊剂型；辅料变更幅度应符合各辅料允许使用范围，应尽量减少辅料用量，筛选最佳辅料用量。此类变更情况较为复杂，无论何种情形，如果可能对药品的安全性、有效性和质量可控性有重大影响，应按照重大变更要求。

2. 研究验证工作

（1）变更的原因、具体情况，说明变更的必要性和合理性。

（2）变更前后辅料相关情况说明及其质量标准。

（3）制剂处方研究资料。

（4）变更所涉及的生产工艺研究与验证资料、批生产记录等。

（5）变更前后质量对比研究资料，质量研究工作的试验资料及文献资料，质量标准。

（6）变更后连续 3 批样品的自检报告书。

（7）稳定性研究资料，包括与变更前药品稳定性情况的比较。

（8）用于儿童的矫味剂、香精、色素等药用辅料，必要时应提供安全性研究资料。

（9）外用制剂等必要时应根据制剂特点进行非临床刺激性、过敏性等研究。

（10）修订完善的说明书、标签。

（三）重大变更

1. 变更情况

此类变更包括但不限于以下情形：

（1）提取的单一成份或提取物制成的制剂以及含大毒（剧毒）药味或现代研究发现有严重毒性药味的普通口服制剂中辅料种类及用量的改变。

（2）起局部作用（用于严重溃疡、烧伤等除外）的外用制剂中渗透促进剂的种类或用量改变；起局部作用且用于严重溃疡、烧伤等，及起全身作用的外用制剂的辅料（渗透促进剂除外）种类或用量的改变等。

（3）所用辅料未在相同给药途径上市品种中使用过的。

（4）变更纳入登记管理的辅料，且变更后的辅料尚未登记或登记状态为"I"。

2. 研究验证工作

除中等变更项下研究工作外，必要时还应提供以下研究资料：

（1）提取的单一成份或提取物制成的口服固体制剂应提供溶出度研究资料，必要时应开展生物等效性研究。

（2）提取的单一成份或提取物制成的制剂、眼用制剂、吸入制剂、外用制剂（如：气雾剂等）、缓释/控释等特殊剂型制剂必要时应提供吸收利用相关的研究资料。

（3）根据制剂特点提供非临床刺激性、过敏性等研究资料。

六、变更规格或包装规格

变更规格应遵循科学、合理、必要及方便临床用药的原则，根据药品用法用量合理确定。研究工作需关注变更规格后的药品与原规格药品处方、工艺、日服/用药量等方面的一致性。变更药品规格不得引起药用物质基础的变化，不得改变药品原批准的用法用量或者适用人群。可能会引起药用物质基础的明显改变或对吸收、利用可能产生明显影响的改变，应进行安全性、有效性全面评价。涉及辅料变更的应参照辅料变更的相关要求进行。

（一）微小变更

1. 变更情况

此类变更包括但不限于以下情形：

变更药品包装中最小单位药品的数量，如：颗粒剂每盒装 A 袋变更为每盒装 B 袋，片剂每板 A 片变更为每板 B 片等。

2. 研究验证工作

（1）变更的原因、具体情况，说明变更的必要性和合理性。

（2）修订完善的说明书、标签。

（二）中等变更

1. 变更情况

此类变更包括但不限于以下情形：

颗粒剂、煎膏剂、糖浆剂等最小包装药品装量的变更。

2. 研究验证工作

（1）变更的原因、具体情况，说明变更的必要性和合理性。

（2）变更所涉及的生产工艺研究与验证资料、批生产记录等（如适用）。

（3）变更前后质量对比研究资料，质量研究工作的试验资料及文献资料，质量标准（如适用）。

（4）变更后连续生产的 3 批样品的自检报告书。

（5）稳定性研究资料，包括与变更前药品稳定性情况的对比研究资料。如不涉及包装材质等的改变，一般可不提供；但如涉及包装容器空间大小等影响药品稳定性的因素，应提供稳定性研究资料。

（6）修订完善的说明书、标签。

（三）重大变更

1. 变更情况

此类变更包括但不限于以下情形：

（1）规范药品规格表述，应参照《中成药规格表述技术指导原则》规范规格表述，并相应修改质量标准、说明书、标签等。

（2）药品规格实际发生变更，如：片剂片重大小、胶囊剂装量的改变，液体制剂药物浓度（单位体积所含饮片量）的改变等。

2. 研究验证工作（规范规格表述的除外）

（1）变更的原因、具体情况，说明变更的必要性和合理性。

（2）变更所涉及的生产工艺研究与验证资料、批生产记录等。

（3）变更前后质量对比研究资料，质量研究工作的试验资料及文献资料，质量标准。

（4）变更后连续生产的3批样品的自检报告书。

（5）稳定性研究资料，包括与变更前药品稳定性情况的对比研究资料。

（6）修订完善的说明书、标签。

七、变更注册标准

本技术指导原则所指变更注册标准主要是指注册标准中检查、鉴别、含量测定等检验项目及其方法或限度/范围的修订。修改的药品注册标准应不低于国家药品标准。

中药上市后，持有人应根据对药品认知的不断丰富，结合检测技术、方法和手段的最新进展，持续提升、完善质量标准，以增加其可控性。变更注册标准不应引起药品质量控制水平的降低，对药品质量保证不应产生负面影响。通常情况下，在现有注册标准基础上增加检验项目、严格限度范围或提高检验方法的专属性等可以更好地控制和保证药品质量。检验项目变更研究的工作重点在于检验方法的方法学研究和验证，以及限度/范围的确定等。

变更注册标准需考虑是否会影响到药品的有效期，如对注册标准进行了提高（例如：缩小限度、增加检验项目等），应考察药品在原定的有效期内是否符合修订后质量标准的要求。

（一）中等变更

1. 变更情况

此类变更包括但不限于以下情形：

（1）在原标准规定范围内收紧限度

这类变更是指在原标准规定范围内收紧控制限度。由于药品的生产工艺等方面的重大变更而引起限度范围缩小不属于此类变更范畴。

（2）注册标准中文字描述的变更，此类变更不应涉及检验方法、限度等的变更。

（3）根据已批准事项对注册标准进行相应修改，如：变更贮藏条件或规格的申请获批后，对注册标准中相应的内容进行修订。

（4）新增检验项目。

新增检验项目应可以更有效地控制产品质量，新增检测项目的方法学验证和拟定的控制限度，均应符合相关技术指导原则的要求。该变更不包括因安全性或质量原因导致的增加检验项目。因生产工艺改变导致药学方面特性发生变化，而在标准中增加检验项目也不属于此类变更范畴。

2. 研究验证工作

（1）注册标准变更的原因及详细变更情况。

（2）注册标准变更相关的研究资料，以及变更前后的对比研究资料。若增加或改变分析方法，应提供方法学研究资料以及变更前后比较研究资料。若变更检查项中相关物质的规定限度或变更含量限度或范围，应提供变更的依据，如：临床研究用样品的测定数据、上市以来药品的检测数据等，必要时应提供相关的安全性研究资料或文献资料等。

（3）变更前后的质量标准。

（4）连续 3 批样品的自检及复核检验报告书（如适用）。

（5）稳定性研究资料。

（二）重大变更

1. 变更情况

此类变更包括但不限于以下情形：

（1）变更检验方法，不包括随国家药品标准变更而引起的注册标准变更。

（2）放宽控制限度。

（3）删除注册标准中的任何项目。

2. 研究验证工作

此类变更可参照中等变更提供相关研究资料。

八、变更包装材料和容器

包装材料和容器是药品的组成部分，本技术指导原则涉及的包装材料和容器主要指直接接触药品的包装。包装材料和容器的变更可能对涉及到药品的安全性、有效性及质量可控性的相关因素产生影响，其风险取决于制剂的给药途径、包装材料和容器的性能以及包装和制剂之间的相容性等。

总体上，变更药品的包装材料和容器应能对保证药品的质量和稳定性起到有益的作用，或至少不降低药品包装材料和容器的保护作用，药品和包装材料之间不得发生不良相互作用。

研究工作需根据药品包装材料的适用范围、包装容器系统的特性、剂型的特点、药品的给药途径等综合进行。研究工作中重点关注药品和包装材料、容器之间是否发生相互作用，变更前后药品的稳定性是否受到影响。

与药品生产过程中的中间体直接接触的包装材料和容器的变更，应按照品种相关要求对变更类别进行评估，并进行相关研究。

（一）微小变更

1. 变更情况

此类变更包括但不限于以下情形：

（1）本技术指导原则中未规定的非无菌固体制剂包装材料和容器的材质和/或类型的变更。变更后的包装材料和容器已在具有相同给药途径的已上市药品中使用，并且具有相同或更好适用性能。

（2）本技术指导原则中未规定的包装材料和容器的供应商、尺寸和/或形状的变更。

2. 研究验证工作

（1）说明包装材料和容器变更的原因，并详细描述变更后的包装材料和容器情况。列出变更后包装材料和容器的质量标准。

（2）变更前后包装材料和容器相关特性的对比研究。

（3）变更后连续3批样品的自检报告书。

（4）稳定性研究资料（如适用）。

（二）中等变更

1. 变更情况

此类变更包括但不限于以下情形：

（1）变更液体/半固体制剂（注射剂、眼用制剂、吸入制剂除外）的包装材料和容器的材质和/或类型。如：口服液体药用聚丙烯瓶变更为口服液体药用聚酯瓶等。

（2）变更非无菌固体制剂的包装材料和容器的材质和/或类型的下列情形：泡罩包装、瓶装、袋装等之间的变更，双铝泡罩变更为铝塑泡罩等。

（3）变更注射剂的包装材料和容器的供应商、尺寸和/或形状。

2. 研究验证工作

（1）说明包装材料和容器变更的原因，并详细描述变更后的包装材料和容器情况。列出变更后包装材料和容器的质量标准。

（2）变更前后包装材料和容器相关特性的对比研究，进行包材的等同性/可替代性研究。

（3）根据品种情况进行包材相容性研究。对于密封件的变更还应开展包装密封性研究。

（4）进行包装工艺验证。

（5）变更后连续 3 批样品的自检报告书。

（6）稳定性研究资料，并与变更前药品的稳定性情况进行比较。

（7）修订完善的说明书、标签。

（三）重大变更

1. 变更情况

此类变更包括但不限于以下情形：

（1）变更吸入制剂、注射剂、眼用制剂的包装材料和容器的材质和/或类型。

（2）变更吸入制剂定量给药装置的供应商、尺寸和/或形状。

（3）去除对药品提供额外保护的次级包装（如：高阻隔性外袋）。

（4）变更为全新材料、全新结构、风险度提高的新用途的包装材料和容器。

（5）变更纳入登记管理的包装材料和容器，且变更后的包装材料和容器尚未登记或登记状态为"I"。

2. 研究验证工作

（1）说明包装材料和容器变更的原因，并详细描述变更后的包装材料和容器情况。列出变更后包装材料和容器的质量标准。

（2）变更前后包装材料和容器相关特性的对比研究，进行包材的等同性/可替代性研究。

（3）根据品种情况进行包材相容性研究。对于密封件的变更还应开展包装密封性研究。对于定量给药装置发生变更，需根据给药装置的特点进行相应的研究，证明变更后给药剂量准确性不低于变更前。

（4）进行包装工艺验证。对于无菌制剂，必要时进行无菌/灭菌工艺验证。

（5）变更后连续 3 批样品的自检报告书。

（6）稳定性研究资料，并与变更前药品的稳定性情况进行比较。

（7）修订完善的说明书、标签。

九、变更有效期或贮藏条件

药品有效期和/或贮藏条件变更可能包含以下几种情况：①延长有效期；②缩短有效期；③严格贮藏条件；④放宽贮藏条件。变更可能只涉及上述某一种情况的变更，也可能涉及上述多种情况的变更。此种情况下，需注意进行各自相应的研究工作。如果稳定性试验方案与药品上市注册时不一致，质量控制项目和实验方法发生改变，或者生产工艺或制剂处方发生变更等，应根据相应的变更情况对有效期或贮藏条件进行相应的研究工作。拟变更的药品有效期应不超过所进行的长期稳定性试验考察时间。应关注生产过程中中间体的贮藏时间和贮藏条件的变更。

（一）中等变更

1. 变更情况

此类变更包括但不限于以下情形：

（1）延长药品有效期

此种变更仅指药品生产工艺及生产质控方法、处方、质量标准、直接接触药品的包装材料和容器、贮藏条件等情况没有发生任何变化情形下的药品有效期延长。

（2）缩短药品有效期或严格药品贮藏条件。

一般而言，通过缩短药品有效期和严格药品贮藏条件，可以更好地保证药品质量。包括根据药品使用区域的变更和相应的稳定性试验结果，要求缩短有效期等情况。

2. 研究验证工作

（1）变更的原因、具体情况，说明变更的必要性和合理性。

（2）按照确定的稳定性试验方案对 3 批药品进行稳定性研究。

（3）修订完善的说明书、标签。

（二）重大变更

1. 变更情况

此类变更包括放宽贮藏条件等。

2. 研究验证工作

（1）变更的原因、具体情况，说明变更的必要性和合理性。

（2）按照确定的稳定性试验方案对 3 批药品进行稳定性研究，包括与变更前条件下的稳定性情况进行的对比研究。

（3）修订完善的说明书、标签。

十、变更制剂生产场地

中药制剂生产场地（包括前处理、提取纯化、浓缩干燥、制剂成型、包装的地址）变更，包括制剂实际生产地址的改变或新增，或同一生产地址内的生产场地的改建、重建和新建。同一生产地址，是指负责实际生产的新旧厂房拥有同一物理地址，应当在药品批准证明文件中标明。制剂的生产场地包括持有人自有的或是受托生产企业相关的生产场地。

变更制剂生产场地，一般需进行全面的研究和验证工作，重点关注生产场地变更前后生产全过程的质量控制一致性情况，通过对变更前后药品关键工艺控制参数、药用物质基础的对比研究和分析，判定变更前后药品质量是否存在明显差异。持有人应确保药品生产技术转移至新生产场地后能持续稳定地生产出符合预定用途和注册要求的药品。制剂生产场地的变更不应改变药品的处方、工艺、直接接触药品的包装材料和容器，不应降低质量过程控制水平及药品标准。提取物生产场地变更的技术要求同制剂生产场地变更。

变更制剂生产场地应执行《药品生产监督管理办法》《药品上市后变更管理办法（试行）》相关规定，研究验证工作可以参考下述内容：

（1）变更的具体情况和原因。

（2）比较新旧场地生产工艺情况。对变更前后生产设备的性能、工作原理、生产能力、生产厂家及型号进行比较，进行质量风险评估并说明变更情况。

（3）变更所涉及的生产工艺研究与验证资料、批生产记录（如适用）。

（4）变更前后质量对比研究资料（如适用）。

（5）变更后连续生产的3批样品的自检报告书（如适用）。

（6）稳定性研究资料，包括与变更前药品稳定性情况的比较（如适用）。

Guideline for Study on Samples for Toxicology Studies on New Traditional Chinese Medicines (TCMs) (Trial)

I. Overview

Toxicology studies run through the whole process of new TCMs research and development. These studies play a crucial role in researching and evaluating the safety of TCMs and in lifecycle management. Therefore, the test substances used in toxicology studies should be representative of the quality attributes and safety of samples for clinical trials and samples applying for marketing authorization. They play a crucial role in ensuring the reliability of toxicology study results and the safety of clinical applications. Generally, the composition of TCMs is complex, with many unknown components. In addition, there is insufficient understanding of the active and/or toxic components, and the correlation between the exposure of components in the body and toxicity is unclear. That leads to the specificity of the study and management of samples for toxicology studies on new TCMs.

This guideline aims to provide guidance and standardization for the studies and process management of preparation, quality control, formulation, and other parts related to the samples used in toxicology studies for the application of new TCMs. The goal is to minimize factors that may interfere with study results and scientific evaluation, ensuring an objective and accurate evaluation of the non-clinical safety of medicines. By doing so, reliable non-clinical safety data can be obtained for use in clinical trials and marketing authorization applications. Samples for toxicology studies on natural medicines can refer to this guideline for relevant references.

II. Basic Principles

(I) The test substances should be representative

The quality of the test substances for toxicology studies should be stable, uniform, and controllable. It should also reflect the quality attributes and safety of the samples for clinical trials and samples applying for marketing authorization. The studies on TCM crude drugs and prepared slices/decoction pieces for test substances research, manufacturing process, quality control and stability, etc. can refer to relevant guidelines for TCMs.

(II) Strengthen quality control during the study process

During the toxicology studies, it is important to strengthen the quality control and process management of the samples. Additionally, complete original records should be maintained to ensure quality control and traceability of the study samples.

(III) Compliance with relevant regulations in the *Good Laboratory Practice* (GLP)

The *Good Laboratory Practice* (GLP) is the basis for guaranteeing the quality of non-clinical drug studies. The samples for toxicology studies in the registration application should comply with the relevant requirements of GLP and this guideline for sample management and use.

(IV) Carry out targeted studies based on the product characteristics

Due to the complexity of TCMs, different dosage forms, routes of administration, and experimental purposes may have different requirements for samples used in toxicology studies. Therefore, to meet the specific requirements of studies and ensure the scientific validity and reliability of the study process and results, the study on samples for toxicology studies should adhere to the principle of "specific analysis of specific problems" based on the general requirements outlined in this guideline.

III. Main Contents

(I) General requirements for Pharmacognosy, Chemistry, Manufacturing and Controls (PCMC) studies on test substances

1. Preparation of test substances

The test substances should be prepared in accordance with the determined prescription and manufacturing process, and additionally should be produced in pilot or larger scale.

For toxicology studies of new TCMs, the test substances may be preparations. Considering the limitations of administration volume or method, intermediates such as extracts or extract powders can also be used as test substances, but their representativeness should be explained. In cases where excipients and dosage forms significantly affect the absorption and utilization of medicines, or when special administration routes are involved, to ensure that toxicology studies are adequate for evaluating the safety of the test substances, toxicology studies should be conducted using test substances that contain excipients. In such cases, it is important to consider the impact of factors such as the ratio between extracts and excipients in the test substances on the study results. If the test substances are preparations, then the composition of the excipient control should be consistent with that of the excipients used in the preparations.

To improve the administration dose/system exposure in toxicology studies, and meet the needs for administration compliance and other study requirements, specially prepared test substances such as those made by adjusting the amount of excipients to prepare test substances with different amounts of decoction pieces should have a manufacturing process and category of excipients as consistent as possible with the preparations, except for cases where the drug loading quantity needs to be changed to accommodate the needs of toxicology studies. In cases where the study requirements are met, such as by adding treatment steps that are not present in the original manufacturing process, or adjusting the treatment methods (such as concentrating the liquid preparation to increase the drug loading quantity), or modifying the category of excipients, etc., these changes should not cause significant changes in medicinal substances and their absorption & utilization. In such cases, comparative studies on manufacturing process, quality, stability, etc. with the preparations should be conducted to evaluate the impact of the changes.

2. Quality studies and quality standards

Quality studies should be conducted taking into consideration the physical and chemical properties, stability, and other characteristics of the test substances. Additionally, the study results of the chemical composition of ingredients should be considered, and the quality standards for the test substances should be developed in conjunction with the quality standards for intermediates or preparations. From the perspective of risk assessment, test items related to safety in the quality standards for the test substances for toxicology studies should be as comprehensive as possible. The test markers should be able to reflect the quality attributes and safety of the test substances. Furthermore, markers that have significant impacts on the safety and efficacy of medicines should be studied with emphasis.

3. Stability

The stability study results of the test substances should ensure the quality stability of the test substances throughout the duration of the toxicology studies. Storage conditions, packaging, and expiry date of the test substances should be specified.

(II) General requirements for administration preparations for toxicology studies

Toxicology studies typically utilize the test substances as the administration preparations for toxicology studies (referred to as the administration preparations hereinafter) after being prepared using suitable solvents. There are also instances where the test substances are directly used as the administration preparations. The specific requirements for the formulation of administration preparations using solvents are as follows:

1. Formulation of administration preparations

The selection of suitable solvents and formulation methods should be based on the physical and chemical properties of the test substances, the administration regimens (usage and dosage in the studies), and the characteristics of the experimental system. The formulation regimens for administration preparations should be studied, and the complete formulation process and key parameters should be documented. Considering the complexity of TCM components, real-time formulation of the administration preparations is recommended.

2. Analysis of administration preparations

The analysis of administration preparations involves developing analytical methods and testing the administration preparations. The main objective is to study the stability and uniformity of the quality of administration preparations throughout the administration period. A reasonable number of tests should be prescribed, and for toxicology studies with extended administration, the number of tests should be increased accordingly. If different batch numbers of test substances are used during the toxicology studies the new batch should be re-analyzed.

For the analysis of administration preparations, appropriate test markers should be selected in connection with the quality study results of the test substances. Additionally, the analytical methods should be validated to ensure their feasibility before they can be utilized. Analytical method validation should simulate the concentration of the administration preparations to be used in the studies. This should cover at least the maximum and minimum concentrations in the administration regimens, and study the possible formulation volumes for the studies. Homogeneity analysis should be conducted for non-true solution systems to ensure that the samples are thoroughly mixed. The acceptable limits or ranges of various test markers for administration preparations should be specified based on the characteristics of the administration preparations and the specific requirements of toxicology studies.

Quality control content of the administration preparations should be developed based on the proposed test markers, test methods, and limit requirements. These content will then be used to test the administration preparations. If necessary, the test results may be compared with those of the test substances.

3. Stability of administrative preparations

For administration preparations that need to be stored, their stability should be examined. The time frame for stability studies should encompass the period from the start of formulation of the administration preparations to the completion of administration. Additionally, the concentration range should include all concentrations of the administration preparations used in the toxicology studies. The samples for stability studies should be tested in accordance with the quality control requirements for administration preparations. Additionally, the expiry dates and storage conditions of the preparations should be determined based on the results of the stability studies.

(III) Sample files

To ensure the traceability of samples for toxicology studies and provide data and materials to support the application for marketing authorization, applicants or toxicology study institutions should establish sample files for the test substances and administration preparations. These files should include, but are not limited to, the following information:

1. Regarding test substances

(1) The sources, batch numbers, quality standards, and test reports, etc. of the TCM crude drugs, prepared slices/decoction pieces, as well as the excipients.

(2) The batch numbers, feeding amounts, batch sizes, and batch production records of the test substances, as well as the relevant study data and instructions for the test substances specially prepared to meet the study requirements.

(3) Quality standards, methodology validation data, test reports, and relevant data atlas, etc.

(4) Methods and data for stability studies, expiry dates, storage conditions, and packaging materials, etc.

(5) The labels should include sample names or codes, batch numbers, packaging specification , specifications, contents, production dates, expiry dates,

storage conditions, and applicants/manufacturers, etc.

2. Regarding administration preparations

Formulation methods and concentrations of the administration preparations, essential information about the solvents used for formulation (such as sources, batch numbers, and specifications, etc.), quality control contents and methodology validation, test reports and relevant atlas, stability study data, and expiry dates of administration preparations, etc.

(Ⅳ) Management of samples during toxicology studies

1. PCMC information on the test substances that need to be provided

It is necessary to provide the batch numbers, quality standards/quality test methods, test reports, stability study results, expiry dates, packaging, storage conditions, and other relevant information about the test substances to the toxicology study institutions.

2. Transfer and reception of samples

According to the physical and chemical properties(e.g., hygroscopicity and stability, etc.) of the test substances and the formulation requirements of the administration preparations, appropriate packaging materials and packaging specification should be selected to ensure no leakage, contamination, or deterioration during delivery to the toxicology study institutions and throughout the study process. The package of the test substances should be clearly labeled, including at least the names or codes, batch number, specifications, packaging specification, contents, storage conditions, production dates, expiry dates, applicants/manufacturers, and other relevant information. Attention should be paid to the influence of temperature, humidity, and illumination on the quality of the test substances during the transfer process. When receiving the samples, a complete record of the reception should be maintained, and relevant information about the samples should be checked.

3. Storage of samples

Storage conditions(such as temperature, humidity, and illumination, etc.) should meet the stability requirements of the research samples.

4. Retention of samples

The test substances should be retained and stored under appropriate conditions in accordance with the provisions of GLP, study requirements, and file management requirements.

中药新药毒理研究用样品
研究技术指导原则（试行）

一、概述

中药新药的毒理研究贯穿于中药新药研发的整个过程，是研究和评价中药安全性以及药品全生命周期管理的重要环节，因此毒理学试验受试物能代表临床试验样品及申请上市样品的质量属性和安全性，对于毒理学试验结果的可靠性、临床应用的安全性具有重要意义。通常，中药成份复杂，存在较多未知成份，对有效成份和/或毒性成份的认识不充分，成份的体内暴露与毒性的相关性不明确，导致中药新药毒理研究用样品的研究和管理具有其特殊性。

本指导原则旨在指导和规范用于注册申报的中药新药毒理研究用样品制备、质量控制、配制等环节的研究和过程管理，尽量减少干扰试验结果与科学评价的因素，以保障客观、准确地评价药物非临床安全性，为药物进入临床试验和上市提供可靠的非临床安全性信息。天然药物的毒理研究用样品可参考本指导原则进行相关研究。

二、基本原则

（一）受试物应具有代表性

毒理研究用受试物质量应稳定、均一、可控，能体现临床试验用样品及申请上市样品的质量属性和安全性。受试物所用药材/饮片、生产工艺、质量控制、稳定性等的研究可参照中药相关指导原则。

（二）加强研究过程的质量控制

在毒理研究过程中应加强对研究用样品的质量控制和过程管理，并有完整的原始记录，以保证研究用样品的质量可控和可追溯。

（三）应符合 GLP 相关规定

药物非临床研究质量管理规范（GLP）是药物非临床研究质量保证的基础，用于支持注册申报的毒理研究用样品需遵循 GLP 及本指导原则中关于样品管理和使用的相关要求。

（四）根据品种特点开展针对性研究

由于中药的复杂性，不同剂型、不同给药途径、不同试验目的对毒理研究用样品的要求可能存在差异，为满足具体试验的要求，保证试验过程和结果科学、可靠，毒理研究用样品的研究应在本指导原则一般要求的基础上遵循具体问题具体分析的原则。

三、主要内容

（一）受试物药学研究一般要求

1.受试物的制备

应以确定的处方、工艺制备受试物，受试物应为中试及以上规模的样品。

对于中药新药毒理学试验，可选择制剂作为受试物，考虑到给药容量或给药方法等的限制，也可采用浸膏、浸膏粉等中间体作为受试物，但应说明其代表性。如果辅料、剂型对药物的吸收利用影响较大或为特殊给药途径的，为保证毒理学试验足以评估受试物的安全性，应采用含辅料制备的受试物进行毒理学试验，此种情况下应考虑受试物中浸膏与辅料比例等因素可能对试验结果的影响。如果受试物采用制剂，则辅料对照的组成应与制剂所用辅料保持一致。

为提高毒理学试验的给药剂量/系统暴露量、满足给药顺应性等试验需要而特殊制备的受试物，如通过调整辅料用量制成含饮片量不同的受试物，除可根据毒理学试验需要而改变载药量外，其生产工艺、辅料种类应尽量与制剂一致。若为满足试验需要，制备受试物时需要增加原制剂工艺中没有的处理步骤或调整处理方法（如将液体制剂进行浓缩作为受试物，以增加载药量），或需要调整辅料种类等，其改变不应引起药用物质基础、吸收利用的明显变化。这种情况下，应与制剂进行工艺、质量、稳定性等方面的对比研究，以评价改变的影响程度。

2.质量研究及质量标准

应根据受试物的理化性质、稳定性等方面的特点以及处方药味化学成份研究结果进行质量研究，并结合中间体或制剂质量标准建立受试物的质量标准。从风险评估的角度考虑，毒理研究用受试物质量标准中与安全性相关的检测项目应尽可能全面，检测指标应能反映受试物的质量属性和安全性，并应重点考察对药物安全性、有效性有较大影响的指标。

3.稳定性

受试物的稳定性研究结果应能保证受试物在毒理学试验给药期限内质量稳

定。应明确受试物的贮藏条件、包装和有效期。

（二）毒理试验用给药制剂一般要求

毒理学试验一般将受试物经适当溶媒配制后作为毒理试验用给药制剂（以下简称给药制剂），也存在受试物直接作为给药制剂的情况。经溶媒配制的给药制剂具体要求如下：

1. 给药制剂的配制

应结合受试物的理化性质、给药方案（试验中的用法和用量）及实验系统特点等选择合适的溶媒并采用合适的配制方法。应研究建立给药制剂的配制方案，并记录完整的配制过程及关键参数。鉴于中药成份的复杂性，给药制剂建议采用现用现配的方式。

2. 给药制剂的分析

给药制剂分析包括分析方法的建立以及给药制剂的检测，其主要目的是考察给药期间内给药制剂质量的稳定、均一。应规定合理的检测次数，对于给药期限较长的毒理学试验应适当增加检测次数。如毒理学试验过程中更换不同批号的受试物，应对新批号受试物制备的给药制剂重新进行分析。

给药制剂分析应结合受试物的质量研究结果选择合适的检测指标，并应进行分析方法的方法学验证，证明方法可行后方可应用于给药制剂的检测。分析方法验证需模拟试验中将会采用的给药制剂浓度，至少涵盖试验方案中的最高、最低浓度，并考察试验中可能的配制体积。对非真溶液体系需开展均一性分析，以保证样品混合均匀。应根据给药制剂的特点以及具体毒理学试验的要求明确给药制剂各检测指标的可接受限度或限度范围。

根据拟定的检测指标、检测方法、限度要求制定给药制剂的质量控制内容，并对给药制剂进行检测，必要时与受试物检测结果进行对比分析。

3. 给药制剂的稳定性

对于确需放置的给药制剂应考察其稳定性。稳定性考察的时间范围应涵盖从给药制剂配制完成至给药结束，浓度范围应覆盖毒理学试验的全部浓度。应按给药制剂质量控制要求对稳定性试验样品进行检测，并根据稳定性试验结果确定给药制剂的使用期限、贮藏条件等。

（三）样品档案

为保证毒理研究过程中研究用样品的可溯源性，并为注册申报提供数据和资料支持，申请人或毒理研究机构应对受试物、给药制剂建立相应的样品档案，包括但不限于以下内容：

1. 受试物

（1）药材/饮片和辅料等的来源、批号、质量标准、检验报告等。

（2）样品的批号、投料量、批量、批生产记录等，为满足试验需要而特殊制备受试物的相关研究资料及说明。

（3）质量标准、方法学验证数据、检验报告及相关数据图谱等。

（4）稳定性研究方法及数据、有效期、贮藏条件、包装材料等。

（5）标签应包括样品名称或代号、批号、装量、规格、含量、生产日期、有效期、贮藏条件、申请人/生产单位等。

2. 给药制剂

给药制剂的配制方法、浓度、配制用溶媒基本信息（来源、批号、规格等），质量控制内容及方法学验证，检验报告及相关图谱，稳定性研究数据及给药制剂使用期限等。

（四）毒理研究过程中样品的管理

1. 需提供的受试物药学信息

需提供给毒理研究机构受试物批号、质量标准/质量检验方法、检验报告、稳定性研究结果及有效期、包装、贮藏条件等样品相关信息。

2. 样品的转运及接收

应根据受试物的理化性质（如吸潮性、稳定性等）、给药制剂的配制需求，采用适宜的包装材料、装量，确保在送达毒理研究机构及试验过程中不会泄露、受污染或变质。受试物的包装应有明确的标识，至少包括名称或代号、批号、规格、装量、含量、贮藏条件、生产日期、有效期、申请人/生产单位等信息。应在运送过程中注意温度、湿度、光照等对受试物质量的影响。样品接收时应有完整的接收记录，并核对样品的相关信息。

3. 样品的贮藏

样品的贮藏条件（如温度、湿度、光照等）应满足研究用样品稳定性的要求。

4. 留样

应按照 GLP 的规定，根据试验需求及档案管理要求在适宜的条件下对受试物进行留样。

Guidance on Safety Pharmacology Studies for Pharmaceuticals

I. Overview

The safety pharmacology is mainly to study potential adverse effects of pharmaceuticals on physiological functions (central nervous system (CNS), cardiovascular system and respiratory system) in relation to exposure in the therapeutic range and above. Supplemental and follow-up safety pharmacology studies are required as appropriate.

Follow-up safety pharmacology studies: Adverse effects may be suspected based on the pharmacodynamic properties or chemical structure of the test substance. Additionally, concerns may arise from animal studies and/or clinical trials. When such potential adverse effects raise concern for human safety, these should be explored in follow-up safety pharmacology studies which provide a greater depth of understanding of the effects on CNS, cardiovascular system and respiratory system.

Supplemental safety pharmacology studies: These studies aim to evaluate potential adverse effects of pharmaceuticals on organ system functions besides CNS, cardiovascular system and respiratory system, including studies on urinary system, autonomic nervous system, gastrointestinal system and other organ tissues.

The objectives of safety pharmacology studies are: to identify undesirable pharmacological properties of a substance that may have relevance to human safety; to evaluate adverse pharmacodynamic and/or pathophysiological effects of a substance observed in toxicology and/or clinical studies; and to study the mechanism of the adverse pharmacodynamic effects observed and/or suspected.

This Guideline is applicable to traditional Chinese medicines (TCMs), natural medicines and chemical drugs.

II. Basic Principles

(I) Test methods

Studies should be designed rationally according to the individual properties and clinical uses of the medicines. Appropriate validated methods should be used, including those scientific and valid new technologies and new methodologies. Methods for certain safety pharmacology studies may be selected according to the pharmacodynamic responsiveness of the model, pharmacokinetic profile, and species, strain of the experimental animals, etc. Both *in vivo* and/or *in vitro* methodologies can be adopted for testing.

(II) Study phases

Safety pharmacology studies run through the whole process of studies on new-registered pharmaceuticals and can be conducted in the phased manner. Core battery studies on CNS, cardiovascular system and respiratory system should be completed prior to clinical trials. Follow-up and/or supplemental safety pharmacology studies can be completed as appropriate during clinical development or before product approval.

(III) Implementation of GLP requirements

Drug safety assessment studies should be conducted in compliance with *Good Laboratory Practice* (GLP), and safety pharmacology studies are in principle conducted in compliance with GLP. When studies are not conducted in compliance with GLP in some circumstances, appropriate test management and data archiving should be ensured. The safety pharmacology core battery should ordinarily be conducted in compliance with GLP. Follow-up and/or supplemental safety pharmacology studies should be conducted in compliance with GLP to the greatest extent feasible.

(IV) Test substances

TCMs and natural medicines: Test substances should be selected from those that sufficiently represent the quality and safety of the proposed samples for clinical trials and/or marketed products. The preparation of the test substance should be carried out using techniques with determined process route and key process parameters. Generally, they should be samples produced in pilot or larger scale, or otherwise, sufficient reasons should be provided. Information on test substances such as name, source, batch number, content (or specification), storage condition, expiry date and preparation method should be noted and the certificate of analysis (COA) should be provided. Due to the special characteristics of TCMs, freshly prepared test substance is recommended; otherwise, data should be provided to support quality stability and uniformity of the test substance after preparation. When the administration lasts for a long time, it should be considered whether there is any inaccuracy in the final concentration due to expansion of the prepared volume after prolonged storage time. Studies can be performed using active pharmaceutical ingredients (APIs) under limitations of administration dose or administration method. The name, standard, batch number, expiry date, specification and manufacturer of solvent and/or excipients used in the study should be noted.

Chemical drugs: Test substances should be samples that are process-stable and have purity and impurity level reflecting the quality and safety of samples for clinical trials and/or marketed samples. Information of test substances such as name, source, batch number, content (or specification), storage condition, expiry date and preparation method should be noted and the COA should be provided. The name, standard, batch number, expiry date, specification and manufacturer of solvent and/or excipients used in the study should be noted and they should meet the requirements of the study.

If there are changes in the manufacturing processes of a test substance that may affect its safety during R&D of pharmaceuticals, the corresponding safety study should be conducted.

For chemical drugs, samples of the test substance should be analyzed during the studies and the analysis report should be provided. For TCMs and natural medicines with basically clear ingredients, sample analysis for test substance should also be performed.

III. Basic Contents

(I) Basic requirements of test design

1. Biological materials

Biological materials include: integral animals, isolated organs and tissues, *in vitro* cultured cells, cellular fragments, subcellular organelles, receptors, ion channels and enzymes, etc. Integral animals used are commonly mice, rats, guinea pigs, rabbits, dogs, and non-human primates, etc. Selected animals should match the study methods and factors such as species, gender and age should also be noticed. Sensitivity, reproducibility and feasibility, as well as correlation with humans should also be noticed when selecting biological materials. Unanesthetized animals are suggested to be used in conducting *in vivo* studies. If anesthetized animals are used, the selection of anesthetics and the control of anesthesia depth should be noticed.

Laboratory animals should meet the national quality requirements for animals of corresponding classes and the Laboratory Animal Quality Certificate should be provided.

2. Sample size

The size and number of the groups should be sufficient to allow meaningful and scientific interpretation of the data generated, properly reflect the biologically significant effects and comply with the requirements of statistics. Generally, rodents are not less than 10 per group, and non-rodents are not less than 6 per group, with half male and half female.

3. Dose

In vivo safety pharmacology studies should be designed to define the dose-response relationship of the adverse effects observed. The time-effect relationship of adverse effect (s) should be studied, when feasible. In general, 3 groups of doses should be designed for safety pharmacology studies, and doses eliciting adverse effect (s) should be compared with doses eliciting the primary pharmacodynamic effect in animals or the proposed effective dose in humans.

As there are species differences in pharmacodynamic sensitivity, doses in safety pharmacology studies should include or exceed the primary pharmacodynamic or therapeutic range. In the absence of an adverse effect on the safety pharmacology parameter (s) evaluated in the study, the highest tested dose should be a dose that produces toxic reaction in other toxicology studies of similar administration route and duration. *In vitro* studies should be designed to establish a concentration-effect relationship. In the absence of an effect, the range of concentrations selected should be justified.

4. Control

Vehicles and/or excipients can be generally selected as a negative control. Positive controls may also be used if it is intended to illustrate the similarities and differences between properties of the test substance and the known drug.

5. Route of Administration

For integral animal tests, the expected clinical route of administration should be considered first, and the route that allows adequate exposure should be considered secondly. For special clinical administration route that is difficult to perform in animal tests, an alternative route can be selected and justified according to characteristics of the test substance.

6. Administration times

Safety pharmacology studies are generally performed by single dose administration. When the primary pharmacodynamic studies show that pharmacodynamic effects occur only after a certain duration of treatment, or when results from non-clinical studies with repeated doses or those from clinical studies give rise to concerns about safety, the administration times of safety pharmacology studies should be rationally designed as the case may be.

7. Observation time

The observation time points and duration of observation should be determined in conjunction with pharmacokinetics (PK)/pharmacodynamics (PD) characteristics of test substances, test animals and clinical study protocols, etc.

(II) Main study contents

1. **Core battery studies**: The purpose of the safety pharmacology core battery is to investigate the effects of the test substance on vital functions. In this regard, the CNS, cardiovascular system and respiratory system are usually considered the vital organ systems that should be studied in the core battery. In some instances, based on scientific rationale, the core battery should be supplemented or need not be implemented. The supplement or exclusion of certain test (s) should be scientifically justified.

1.1 Central nervous system

Effects of the test substance on the CNS should be assessed appropriately. Motor activity, behavioral changes, coordination, sensory/motor reflex responses and body temperature changes should be evaluated qualitatively and quantitatively on animals after administration. For example, a functional observation battery (FOB) can be used.

1.2 Cardiovascular system

The changes in blood pressure (e.g., systolic blood pressure, diastolic blood pressure and mean pressure), ECG (e.g., QT interval, PR interval and QRS wave) and heart rate should be detected at pre- and post-administration. Unanesthetized animals are suggested to be used to measure cardiovascular parameters (e.g., telemetry technology).

Consideration should be given to whether the test substance belongs to a class of compounds in which some members have been shown to induce QT interval prolongation in humans in terms of indications, pharmacological effects or chemical structure (e.g., antipsychotics, antihistamines, antiarrhythmics and fluoroquinolones), and further studies should be performed to assess the effects of the test substance on QT interval. Studies on QT can be conducted according to relevant guidelines.

1.3 Respiratory system

The changes in respiratory function (e.g., respiratory rate, tidal volume and respiratory depth) on animals should be evaluated at pre- and post-administration.

2. Follow-up and/or supplemental safety pharmacology studies

Adverse effects may be suspected based on the safety pharmacology core battery studies, clinical trials, epidemiology, experimental *in vitro* or *in vivo* studies, or literature reports. When such potential adverse effects raise concern for human safety, these should be explored in follow-up and/or supplemental safety pharmacology studies, as appropriate. Follow-up safety pharmacology studies are meant to provide a greater depth of understanding than, or additional knowledge to, that provided by the core battery studies on CNS, cardiovascular system and respiratory system. The follow-up studies should be selected on a case-by-case basis according to previous information. Supplemental safety pharmacology studies should be performed with concern for safety when relevant functions of urinary/kidney system, autonomic nervous system, and gastrointestinal system are not observed in core battery studies or repeated-dose toxicity studies.

2.1 Follow-up safety pharmacology studies

Central nervous system: Behavioral pharmacology, learning and memory, neurobiochemistry, visual, auditory and/or electrophysiology examinations, etc.

Cardiovascular system: Cardiac output, ventricular contractility, and vascular resistance, etc.

Respiratory system: Airway resistance, pulmonary arterial pressure, and blood gases, etc.

2.2 Supplemental safety pharmacology studies

Urinary/kidney system: Effects of the test substance on renal parameters should be assessed. For example, urine volume, specific gravity, osmolality, pH, electrolyte balance, proteins, cytology and blood biochemistry (e.g., blood urea nitrogen, creatinine and protein).

Autonomic nervous system: Effects of the test substance on the autonomic nervous system should be assessed. For example, binding to receptors relevant to the autonomic nervous system, functional responses to agonists or antagonists *in vivo* or *in vitro*, direct stimulation on autonomic nerves and measurement of cardiovascular responses, baroreflex testing and heart rate variability can be used.

Gastrointestinal system: Effects of the test substance on the gastrointestinal system should be assessed. For example, gastric secretion, pH, gastrointestinal injury, bile secretion, gastric emptying time, transit time *in vivo* and ileal contraction *in vitro* can be used.

2.3 Other studies

Effects of the test substance on organ systems not studied elsewhere should be assessed when there is a reason for concern. For example, dependency potential, skeletal muscle, immune and endocrine functions can be studied.

IV. Analysis and Evaluation of Results

Qualitative and quantitative analysis of data should be performed based on detailed test records by appropriate statistical methods.

Comprehensive evaluation should be made in combination with pharmacodynamic, toxicological, pharmacokinetic and other study data to provide recommendations on the design of clinical studies.

V. References

1. ICH. ICH Guidance for Industry ICH S7A: Safety Pharmacology Studies for Human Pharmaceuticals. 2001.

2. ICH. ICH Guidance for Industry ICH S7B: Safety Pharmacology Studies for Assessing the Potential for Delayed Ventricular Repolarization (QT Interval Prolongation) by Human Pharmaceuticals. 2005.

3. China Food and Drug Administration (CFDA). *Technical Guidelines for General Pharmacology Studies of Traditional Chinese Medicines and Natural Medicines*, 2005.

4. China Food and Drug Administration (CFDA). *Technical Guidelines for General Pharmacology Studies of Chemical Drugs*, 2004.

药物安全药理学研究技术指导原则

一、概述

安全药理学（Safety Pharmacology）主要是研究药物在治疗范围内或治疗范围以上的剂量时，潜在的不期望出现的对生理功能的不良影响，即观察药物对中枢神经系统、心血管系统和呼吸系统的影响。根据需要进行追加和/或补充的安全药理学研究。

追加的安全药理学研究（Follow-up Safety Pharmacology Studies）：根据药物的药理作用、化学结构，预期可能出现的不良反应。如果对已有的动物和/或临床试验结果产生怀疑，可能影响人的安全性时，应进行追加的安全药理学研究，即对中枢神经系统、心血管系统和呼吸系统进行深入的研究。

补充的安全药理学研究（Supplemental Safety Pharmacology Studies）：评价药物对中枢神经系统、心血管系统和呼吸系统以外的器官功能的影响，包括对泌尿系统、自主神经系统、胃肠道系统和其他器官组织的研究。

安全药理学的研究目的包括以下几个方面：确定药物可能关系到人安全性的非期望药理作用；评价药物在毒理学和/或临床研究中所观察到的药物不良反应和/或病理生理作用；研究所观察到的和/或推测的药物不良反应机制。

本指导原则适用于中药、天然药物和化学药物。

二、基本原则

（一）试验方法

应根据药物的特点和临床使用的目的，合理地进行试验设计。选用适当的经验证的方法，包括科学而有效的新技术和新方法。某些安全药理学研究可根据药效反应的模型、药代动力学的特征、实验动物的种属等来选择试验方法。试验可采用体内和/或体外的方法。

（二）研究的阶段性

安全药理学研究贯穿在新药研究全过程中，可分阶段进行。在药物进入临床试验前，应完成对中枢神经系统、心血管系统和呼吸系统影响的核心组合（Core Battery）试验的研究。追加和/或补充的安全药理学研究视具体情况，可在申报临床前或生产前完成。

（三）执行 GLP 的要求

药物的安全性评价研究必须执行《药物非临床研究质量管理规范》（GLP）。安全药理学研究原则上须执行 GLP。对一些难以满足 GLP 要求的特殊情况，也要保证适当的试验管理和数据保存。核心组合试验应执行 GLP。追加的或/和补充的安全药理学研究应尽可能地最大限度遵循 GLP 规范。

（四）受试物

中药、天然药物：受试物应采用能充分代表临床试验拟用样品和/或上市样品质量和安全性的样品。应采用工艺路线及关键工艺参数确定后的工艺制备，一般应为中试或中试以上规模的样品，否则应有充分的理由。应注明受试物的名称、来源、批号、含量（或规格）、保存条件、有效期及配制方法等，并提供质量检验报告。由于中药的特殊性，建议现用现配，否则应提供数据支持配制后受试物的质量稳定性及均匀性。当给药时间较长时，应考察配制后体积是否存在随放置时间延长而膨胀造成终浓度不准的因素。如果由于给药容量或给药方法限制，可采用原料药进行试验。试验中所用溶媒和/或辅料应标明名称、标准、批号、有效期、规格及生产单位。

化学药物：受试物应采用工艺相对稳定、纯度和杂质含量能反映临床试验拟用样品和/或上市样品质量和安全性的样品。受试物应注明名称、来源、批号、含量（或规格）、保存条件、有效期及配制方法等，并提供质量检验报告。试验中所用溶媒和/或辅料应标明名称、标准、批号、有效期、规格和生产单位等，并符合试验要求。

在药物研发的过程中，若受试物的工艺发生可能影响其安全性的变化，应进行相应的安全性研究。

化学药物试验过程中应进行受试物样品分析，并提供样品分析报告。成分基本清楚的中药、天然药物也应进行受试物样品分析。

三、基本内容

（一）试验设计的基本要求

1. 生物材料

生物材料有以下几种：整体动物，离体器官及组织，体外培养的细胞、细胞片段、细胞器、受体、离子通道和酶等。整体动物常用小鼠、大鼠、豚鼠、家兔、犬、非人灵长类等。动物选择应与试验方法相匹配，同时还应注意品系、性别及年龄等因素。生物材料选择应注意敏感性、重现性和可行性，以及与人的相关性等因素。体内研究建议尽量采用清醒动物。如果使用麻醉动物，应注意麻醉药物的选择和麻醉深度的控制。

实验动物应符合国家对相应等级动物的质量规定要求，并具有实验动物质量合格证明。

2. 样本量

试验组的组数及每组动物数的设定，应以能够科学合理地解释所获得的试验结果，恰当地反映有生物学意义的作用，并符合统计学要求为原则。小动物每组一般不少于 10 只，大动物每组一般不少于 6 只。动物一般雌雄各半。

3. 剂量

体内安全药理学试验要对所观察到的不良反应的剂量反应关系进行研究，如果可能也应对时间效应关系进行研究。一般情况下，安全药理学试验应设计 3 个剂量，产生不良反应的剂量应与动物产生主要药效学的剂量或人拟用的有效剂量进行比较。由于不同种属的动物对药效学反应的敏感性存在种属差异，因此安全药理学试验的剂量应包括或超过主要药效学的有效剂量或治疗范围。如果安全药理学研究中缺乏不良反应的结果，试验的最高剂量应设定为相似给药途径和给药时间的其他毒理试验中产生毒性反应的剂量。体外研究应确定受试物的浓度–效应关系。若无明显效应时，应对浓度选择的范围进行说明。

4. 对照

一般可选用溶媒和/或辅料进行阴性对照。如为了说明受试物的特性与已知药物的异同，也可选用阳性对照药。

5. 给药途径

整体动物试验，首先应考虑与临床拟用途径一致，可以考虑充分暴露的给药途径。对于在动物试验中难以实施的特殊的临床给药途径，可根据受试物的特点选择，并说明理由。

6. 给药次数

一般采用单次给药。但是若主要药效学研究表明该受试物在给药一段时间后才能起效，或者重复给药的非临床研究和/或临床研究结果出现令人关注的安全性问题时，应根据具体情况合理设计给药次数。

7. 观察时间

结合受试物的药效学和药代动力学特性、受试动物、临床研究方案等因素选择观察时间点和观察时间。

（二）主要研究内容

1. 核心组合试验：安全药理学的核心组合试验的目的是研究受试物对重要生命功能的影响。中枢神经系统、心血管系统、呼吸系统通常作为重要器官系统考虑，也就是核心组合试验要研究的内容。根据科学合理的原则，在某些情况下，可增加或减少部分试验内容，但应说明理由。

1.1 中枢神经系统

定性和定量评价给药后动物的运动功能、行为改变、协调功能、感觉/运动反射和体温的变化等，以确定药物对中枢神经系统的影响。可进行动物的功能组合试验。

1.2 心血管系统

测定给药前后血压（包括收缩压、舒张压和平均压等）、心电图（包括 QT 间期、PR 间期、QRS 波等）和心率等的变化。建议采用清醒动物进行心血管系统指标的测定（如遥测技术等）。

如药物从适应症、药理作用或化学结构上属于易于引起人类 QT 间期延长类的化合物，例如：抗精神病类药物、抗组织胺类药物、抗心律失常类药物和氟喹诺酮类药物等，应进行深入的试验研究，观察药物对 QT 间期的影响。对 QT 的研究见相关指导原则。

1.3 呼吸系统

测定给药前后动物的各种呼吸功能指标的变化，如呼吸频率、潮气量、呼吸深度等。

2. 追加和/或补充的安全药理学试验

当核心组合试验、临床试验、流行病学、体内外试验以及文献报道提示药物存在潜在的与人体安全性有关的不良反应时，应进行追加和/或补充的安全药理学研究。追加的安全药理学试验是除了核心组合试验外，反映受试物对中枢神经系统、心血管系统和呼吸系统的深入研究。追加的安全药理学试验根据已有的信息，具体情况具体分析选择追加的试验内容。补充的安全药理学试验是，出于对安全性的关注，在核心组合试验或重复给药毒性试验中未观察泌尿/肾脏系统、自主神经系统、胃肠系统等相关功能时，需要进行的研究。

2.1 追加的安全药理学试验

中枢神经系统：对行为、学习记忆、神经生化、视觉、听觉和/或电生理等指标的检测。

心血管系统：对心输出量、心肌收缩作用、血管阻力等指标的检测。

呼吸系统：对气道阻力、肺动脉压力、血气分析等指标的检测。

2.2 补充的安全药理学试验

泌尿/肾脏系统：观察药物对肾功能的影响，如对尿量、比重、渗透压、pH、电解质平衡、蛋白质、细胞和血生化（如尿素、肌酐、蛋白质）等指标的检测。

自主神经系统：观察药物对自主神经系统的影响，如与自主神经系统有关受体的结合，体内或体外对激动剂或拮抗剂的功能反应，对自主神经的直接刺激作用和对心血管反应、压力反射和心率等指标的检测。

胃肠系统：观察药物对胃肠系统的影响，如胃液分泌量和 pH、胃肠损伤、胆汁分泌、胃排空时间、体内转运时间、体外回肠收缩等指标的测定。

2.3 其他研究

在其他相关研究中，尚未研究药物对下列器官系统的作用但怀疑有影响的可能性时，如潜在的药物依赖性、骨骼肌、免疫和内分泌功能等的影响，则应考虑药物对这方面的作用，并作出相应的评价。

四、结果分析与评价

根据详细的试验记录，选用合适的统计方法，对数据进行定性和定量分析。应结合药效、毒理、药代以及其他研究资料进行综合评价，为临床研究设计提出建议。

五、参考文献

1. ICH.ICH Guidance for Industry ICH S7A：Safety Pharmacology Studies for Human Pharmaceuticals.2001.

2. ICH.ICH Guidance for Industry ICH S7B：Safety Pharmacology Studies for assessing the potential for delayed ventricular repolarization（QT interval prolongation）by Human Pharmaceuticals.2005.

3. 国家食品药品监督管理局. 中药、天然药物一般药理研究学研究技术指导原则，2005.

4. 国家食品药品监督管理局. 化学药物一般药理研究学研究技术指导原则，2004.

Guidance on Single Dose Toxicity Studies for Pharmaceuticals

I. Overview

Acute toxicity is the toxic effects occurring within a period of administration of a single dose of a test substance or multiple doses given within 24 hours [1,2]. The narrow definition of "Single dose toxicity study" refers to the study of acute toxic effects that arise following the administration of a test substance in a single dose [2]. The studies referred to in this guideline are single dose toxicity studies in a broad sense, which allow for the administration of a test substance either as a single dose or multiple doses given within 24 hours to obtain information on the acute toxicity of the test substance.

Single dose toxicity studies are typically conducted for test substances intended for use in humans (Annotation 1). These studies play a crucial role in providing preliminary insights into the toxic effects of a test substance and understanding its target organs for toxicity. The information obtained from single dose toxicity studies is valuable for dose selection in repeated dose toxicity studies and determining the starting dose for certain clinical trials of drugs. Additionally, these studies can provide relevant information related to acute toxicity caused by overdose in humans [1].

This guideline is applicable to traditional Chinese medicines (TCMs), natural medicines and chemical drugs.

II. Basic Principles

(I) Test management

The single dose toxicity studies conducted to support drug registration must comply with the *Good Laboratory Practice* (GLP).

(II) Case-by-case basis

When designing a single dose toxicity study, it is important to follow the principle of "Case-by-case" based on the understanding of the test substance.

For chemical drugs, the selection of appropriate test methods and the design of suitable study protocols should be based on various factors, including the structural characteristics, physicochemical properties, information on homogeneous compounds, indications, characteristics of the target population, and the purpose of the study. Additionally, it is important to comprehensively evaluate the study results by considering other available pharmacology and toxicology study data.

For TCMs and natural medicines, it is also important to consider their unique characteristics, which may differ from those of chemical drugs. When designing a single dose toxicity study for these medicines, it is essential to take into account their specific properties and adjust the study design accordingly.

(III) Randomization, control, and repetition

Single dose toxicity studies should adhere to the general principles of animal studies, namely randomization, control, and repetition.

III. Basic Contents

(I) Test substance

TCMs and natural medicines: The test substances should be representative of the quality and safety of the samples for clinical trials and/or marketed products. The test substances should be prepared using the manufacturing process and key process parameters that have been established. Typically, they should be produced in pilot or larger scale, unless there are adequate justifications for using a smaller scale. The test substance should be clearly labeled with its name, source, batch number, content (or specification), storage conditions, expiry date, and preparation method. Additionally, a certificate of analysis should be provided for the test substance. Due to the unique nature of TCMs, it is recommended to prepare the test substance at the time of use. Alternatively, if the test substance is prepared in advance, it is required to provide data supporting the quality stability and uniformity of the prepared test substance. When administering a test substance over a prolonged period, it is important to study whether the volume of the prepared test substance expands with prolonged storage time, leading to inaccuracies in the final concentration. If there are limitations in terms of administration dose or methods, it is permissible to use active pharmaceutical ingredients (APIs) for the study. The solvents and/or excipients used in the study should be clearly labeled with their names, standards, batch numbers, expiry dates, specifications, and the name of the manufacturer.

Chemical drugs: The test substance should be representative of the quality and safety of the samples for clinical trials and/or marketed products. It should be prepared using the manufacturing process that is relatively stable, ensuring consistency in purity and impurity content. The test substance should be clearly labeled with its name, source, batch number, content (or specification), storage conditions, expiry date, and preparation method. Additionally, a certificate of analysis should be provided for the test substance. The solvents and/or excipients used in the study should be clearly labeled with their names, standards, batch numbers, expiry dates, specifications, and the name of the manufacturer. These materials should also meet the requirements of the study.

During the R&D process of pharmaceuticals, if there are potential changes in the manufacturing process of the test substance that may affect its safety, corresponding safety studies should be conducted.

In the process of chemical drug testing, analysis of the test substance samples should be conducted, and analysis reports should be provided. This applies not only to chemical drugs but also to TCMs and natural medicines with clearly identified ingredients.

(II) Laboratory animals [1,3,4]

1. Species: Different species of animals have their own characteristics, and their responses to the same test substance may vary. In order to provide a comprehensive evaluation of the toxicity of a test substance, conducting studies using different species of animals can provide more safety information. Therefore, for chemical drugs, single dose toxicity studies should be conducted

using at least two mammalian species, typically one rodent species and one non-rodent species. If no non-rodent species is used in the study, the rationale for this decision should be provided. For TCMs and natural medicines, the choice of rodent and/or non-rodent species in studies should base on specific circumstances (Appendix Ⅱ).

Laboratory animals should comply with the national quality regulations for the corresponding animal grades and possess a quality certificate for laboratory animals.

2. **Gender**: Typically, studies are conducted using both male and female animals, with an equal number in each gender. While if studies are conducted using only one gender of animals, the rationale for this approach should be clearly explained.

3. **Age**: Typically, studies are conducted using healthy adult animals. However, if the test substance is intended for or may be used in children, it may be necessary to conduct studies using juvenile animals.

4. **Number of animals**: The required number of animals should be determined based on the animal species and study objectives. The number of animals should be in accordance with the requirements of the experimental methods and the analysis and evaluation of results.

5. **Body weight**: The body weight difference among animals should not be excessively large at each initial dosing in the experiment. For rodents, the body weight at the initial dosing should not be over or lower than 20% of the average weight.

(Ⅲ) Route of administration

The absorption rate, extent of absorption, and exposure level of the test substance can vary depending on the route of administration. Generally, the routes of administration should include at least the intended clinical route(s). If the clinical routes are not used, a justification should be provided.

(Ⅳ) Experimental method and dose level [1,3,4]

The focus of single dose toxicity studies is to observe the toxic effects in animals. There are various methods available for conducting single dose toxicity studies, including the approximate lethal dose method, maximal feasible dose method, maximal tolerance dose method, fixed-dose method, up-and-down method (sequential method), cumulative dose method (pyramid method), and median lethal dose method, etc. The selection of an appropriate method should be based on the characteristics of the test substance, and suitable doses should be chosen according to the specific method (Annotation 2).

In principle, the administration dose should cover a range from doses that do not elicit any toxic effects to doses that induce severe toxic effects, or reach the maximal feasible dose.

The maximal administration dose volume for different animals and routes of administration can be determined by referring to relevant literature and considering the specific experimental conditions.

According to the selected experimental methods, it may be necessary to include blank and/or vehcile (excipient) control group.

The stomach contents can affect the administration dose volume of the test substance, and the duration of fasting in rodents can affect the absorption in the gastrointestinal tract and the activity of drug-metabolizing enzymes, thereby influencing the manifestation of toxicity. Therefore, animals are generally subjected to a period of fasting before oral administration, while access to water is typically not restricted.

(V) Observation period and indicators [1,3-5]

After administration, it is generally recommended to observe the animals continuously for at least 14 days. The intervals and frequency of observations should be appropriate to allow for detection of the onset and recovery time of toxic effects, as well as the time to death. If toxic effects occur slowly or the recovery takes longer, the observation period should be extended accordingly.

The observation indicators include clinical symptoms (such as appearance, behavior, food and water intake, response to stimuli, secretions, and excretions, etc.), mortality (time to death and moribund reactions, etc.), and body weight changes (weighing once before administration and once at the end of the observation period, with multiple weighing during the observation period. The animals should also be weighed when they are dead or in a moribund state). It is important to record all cases of mortality, symptoms, including the onset time, severity, and duration, as well as body weight changes.

All laboratory animals should undergo gross anatomical examination. Animals that are euthanized due to moribund conditions or found dead during the experiment should be promptly subjected to gross anatomical examination. Other animals should be euthanized and undergo gross anatomical examination at the end of the observation period. When there are changes in the size, color, and texture of organs or tissues, histopathological examination should be conducted.

In certain circumstances, in order to acquire more comprehensive information on acute toxicity, multiple dose groups can be designed to observe additional indicators such as hematological indicators, blood biochemistry indicators, and histopathological examination, etc., to better determine target organs of toxicity or dose-response relationship[2,5].

IV. Analysis and Evaluation of Results

(I) Based on the onset time, duration, and severity of various effects, it is important to analyze the incidence and severity of these effects at different doses. By analyzing the data, it is possible to determine the dose-response relationship and the time-response relationship.

(II) To determine the tissues, organs, or systems that might be involved in the observed effects, reference can be made to Appendix (I).

(III) Based on results from gross pathological examination and histopathological examination, the potential target organs of toxicity can be preliminarily identified. A comprehensive histopathological examination report should be provided, which includes detailed descriptions of all tissues, particularly those showing abnormal changes. In cases where abnormal changes are observed, corresponding histopathological images should be included.

(Ⅳ) The description of the calculation methods and statistical methods used in the study is essential. It is important to provide a clear explanation of the specific methods employed and their basis.

(Ⅴ) Assess the correlation between observed effects and the pharmaceutical based on factors such as time, incidence, dose-response relationship, different species of animals, laboratory history, pathological findings, and characteristics of similar pharmaceuticals. It is important to determine the nature, severity, recoverability, and safety range of the toxic effects caused by the test substance. Based on the potential sites affected by toxicity, it is required to integrate gross anatomy and histopathological examination results to preliminarily identify the target organs of toxicity.

Results from single dose toxicity studies can serve as a reference for dose selection of subsequent toxicity studies, and can identify indicators to be closely observed in subsequent toxicity studies.

V. Glossary

Maximum feasible dose (MFD): the maximum dose to be administered to animals in a single dose or multiple doses (2-3 times) within 24 hours.

Maximum tolerance dose (MTD): the highest dose that animals can tolerate without causing death.

Median lethal dose (LD$_{50}$): the dose that is expected to cause death in 50% of the animals tested. This value is calculated through statistical analysis.

VI. References

1. CDER, FDA. Guidance for industry: single dose acute toxicity testing for pharmaceuticals (Final). 1996.

2. CHMP, EMA. Questions and answers on the withdrawal of the "Note for guidance on single dose toxicity". 2010.

3. Cordier A. Single dose toxicity: Industry perspectives. In: P.F. D'Arcy and D.W.G. Harron edited, Proceedings of the First International Conference on

Harmonization. Brussels: 1991, 189-191.

4. Outcome-Single dose toxicity. In: P.F. D'Arcy and D.W.G. Harron edited, Proceedings of the First International Conference on Harmonization. Brussels: 1991, 184.

5. ICH M3 (R2). Nonclinical Safety Studies for the Conduct of Human Clinical Trials and Marketing Authorization for Pharmaceuticals.2009.

6. Blazka ME, Hayes A W. Acute toxicity and eye irritancy. In: Hayes A W edited, Principles and methods of toxicology. Fifth edition, 2007:1132-1150.

VII. Annotations

Annotation 1: Sufficient information on acute toxicity could also be obtained from other sources [2,5]. It should be noted that the information should be obtained from studies in compliance with *Good Laboratory Practice* (GLP).

Annotation 2: The administration dose can be different due to different study methods used. Studies may be designed based on relevant literature. However, it should be noted that since the anticipated clinical dose of TCMs or natural medicines is usually high, the dose limits specified in single dose toxicity study methods (e.g., the dose limit of 2,000 mg/kg or 5,000 mg/kg in the up-and-down method) are only applicable to chemical drugs. Dose selection for TCMs or natural medicines should be determined by considering multiple factors.

Because the acute toxicity of most TCMs and natural medicines may be relatively low, an MFD (or MTD) is commonly used in the acute toxicity studies.

VIII. Appendixes

(I) General observations and signs [6]

Below is a list of common observational signs and the potentially involved tissues, organs, or systems. In single dose toxicity studies, it might be necessary to collect all or parts of these signs listed in the table. This table is only used as reference when performing result analysis and evaluation, and other scientific and reasonable analyses are also acceptable.

Observation		Signs	Tissues, organs, or systems most likely to be involved
I. Respiratory blockage in the nostril, changes in rate and depth of breathing, changes in color of body surface		Dyspnea: difficult or labored breathing, essentially gasping for air, respiration rate usually slow	
	A	1. Abdominal breathing: breathing by diaphragm, greater deflection of abdomen upon inspiration	Central nervous system (CNS) respiratory center, paralysis of costal muscles, cholinergic
		2. Gasping: deep labored inspiration, accompanied by a wheezing sound	CNS respiratory center, pulmonary edema, secretion accumulation in airways, increased cholinergic
	B	Apnea: a transient cessation of breathing following a forced respiration	CNS respiratory center, pulmonary-cardiac insufficiency
	C	Cyanosis: bluish appearance of tail, mouth, foot pads	Pulmonary-cardiac insufficiency, pulmonary edema
	D	Tachypnea: quick and usually shallow respiration	Stimulation of respiratory center, pulmonarycardiac insufficiency
	E	Nostril discharges: red or colorless	Pulmonary edema, hemorrhage
II. Motor activities: changes in frequency and nature of movements	A	Decrease or increase in spontaneous motor activities, curiosity, preening, or locomotions	Somatomotor, CNS
	B	Somnolence: animal appears drowsy, but can be aroused by prodding and resumes normal activities	CNS sleep center
	C	Loss of righting reflex, loss of reflex to maintain normal upright posture when placed on the back	CNS, sensory, neuromuscular
	D	Anesthesia: loss of righting reflex and pain response (animal will not respond to tail and toe pinch)	CNS, sensory

continued

Observation		Signs	Tissues, organs, or systems most likely to be involved
II. Motor activities: changes in frequency and nature of movements	E	Catalepsy: animal tends to remain in any position in which it is placed	CNS, sensory, neuromuscular, autonomic
	F	Ataxia: Inability to control and coordinate movement while animal is walking with no spasticity, epraxia, paresis, or rigidity	CNS, sensory, autonomic
	G	Unusual locomotion: Spastic, toe walking, pedaling, hopping, and low body posture	CNS, sensory, neuromuscular
	H	Prostration: immobile and rests on belly	CNS, sensory, neuromuscular
	I	Tremors: involving trembling and quivering of the limbs or entire body	Neuromuscular, CNS
	J	Fasciculation: involving movements of muscles, seen on the back, shoulders, hind limbs, and digits of the paws	Neuromuscular, CNS, autonomic
III. Convulsion (seizure): marked involuntary contraction or seizures of contraction of voluntary muscle	A	Clonic convulsion: convulsive alternating contraction and relaxation of muscles	CNS, respiratory failure, neuromuscular, autonomic
	B	Tonic convulsion: persistent contraction of muscles, attended by rigid extension of hind limbs	CNS, respiratory failure, neuromuscular, autonomic
	C	Tonic-clonic convulsion: both types may appear consecutively	CNS, respiratory failure, neuromuscular, autonomic
	D	Asphyxial convulsion: usually of clonic type but accompanied by gasping and cyanosis	CNS, respiratory failure, neuromuscular, autonomic
	E	Opisthotonos: tetanic spasm in which the back is arched and the head is pulled toward the dorsal position	CNS, respiratory failure, neuromuscular, autonomic
IV. Reflexes	A	Corneal eyelid closure: touching of the cornea causes eyelids to close	Sensory, neuromuscular
	B	Primal: twitch of external ear elicited by light stroking of inside surface of ear	Sensory, neuromuscular

continued

Observation		Signs	Tissues, organs, or systems most likely to be involved
IV. Reflexes	C	Righting: ability of animal to recover when placed dorsal side down	CNS, sensory, neuromuscular
	D	Myotact: ability of animal to retract its hind limb when limb is pulled down over the edge of a surface	Sensory, neuromuscular
	E	Light (pupillary): constriction of pupil in presence of light	Sensory, neuromuscular, autonomic
	F	Startle reflex: response to external stimuli such as touch, noise	Sensory, neuromuscular
V. Ocular signs	A	Lacrimation: excessive tearing, clear or colored	Autonomic
	B	Miosis: constriction of pupil regardless of the presence or absence of light	Autonomic
	C	Mydriasis: dilation of pupils regardless of the presence or absence of light	Autonomic
	D	Exophthalmos: abnormal protrusion of eye in orbit	Autonomic
	E	Ptosis: dropping of upper eyelids, not reversed by prodding animal	Autonomic
	F	Chromodacryorrhea: red lacrimation	Autonomic, hemorrhage, infection
	G	Relaxation of nictitating membrane	Autonomic
	H	Corneal opacity, iritis, conjunctivitis	Irritation of the eye
VI. Cardiovascular signs	A	Bradycardia: decreased heart rate	Autonomic, pulmonary-cardiac insufficiency
	B	Tachycardia: increased heart rate	Autonomic, pulmonary-cardiac insufficiency
	C	Vasodilation: redness of skin, tail, tongue, ear, foot pad, conjunctivae, sac, and warm body	Autonomic, CNS, increased cardiac output, hot environment
	D	Vasoconstriction: blanching or whitening of skin, cold body	Autonomic, CNS, decreased cardiac output, cold environment

Observation		Signs	Tissues, organs, or systems most likely to be involved
VI. Cardiovascular signs	E	Arrhythmia: abnormal cardiac rhythm	CNS, autonomic, pulmonarycardiac insufficiency, myocardiac infraction
VII. Salivation	A	Excessive secretion of saliva: hair around mouth becomes wet	Autonomic
VIII. Piloerection	A	Contraction of erectile tissue of hair follicles resulting in rough hair	Autonomic
IX. Analgesia	A	Decrease in reaction to induce pain (e.g., hot plate)	Sensory, CNS
X. Muscular tone	A	Hypotonia: generalized decrease in muscle tone	Autonomic
	B	Hypertonia: generalized increase in muscle tension	Autonomic
XI. GI signs			
Droppings (feces)	A	Solid, dried and scant	Autonomic, constipation, GI motility
	B	Loss of fluid, watery stool	Autonomic, diarrhea, GI motility
Emesis	A	Vomiting and retching	Sensory, CNS, autonomic (in rat, emesis absent)
Diuresis	A	Red urine	Damage in kidney
	B	Involuntary urination	Autonomic sensory
XII. Skin	A	Edema: swelling of tissue filled with fluid	Irritation, renal failure, tissue damage, long-term immobility
	B	Erythema: redness of skin	Irritation, inflammation, sensitization

(II) Special requirements for single dose toxicity studies of TCMs and natural medicines in different situations

Due to the special characteristics of TCMs and natural medicines, the following requirements should be considered in conducting studies; if the following requirements are not followed, the basis should be provided.

1. Active ingredients extracted from TCMs, animals, or minerals, and preparations containing such active ingredients which have not been marketed in China, new raw TCM materials and their preparations, new substitutes of raw TCM materials, new medicinal parts of raw TCM materials and their preparations, preparations made from active ingredients extracted from TCMs, animals, or minerals which have not been marketed in China, and injection preparations of TCMs and natural medicines which have not been marketed in China.

Because the formula composition of the above materials has changed significantly from those of TCMs, or their clinical application experience is very limited, both rodent and non-rodent animals are generally required in order to comprehensively study the acute toxic effects of test substances. If this requirement is not met, the basis should be provided.

2. Non-injectable compound preparations of TCMs and natural medicines which have not been marketed in China.

If the formula composition of such compound preparations is consistent with the TCM theories and there is certain clinical application experience, one animal species may be used, and acute toxic effects should be observed according to the proposed clinical route of administration.

If such compound preparations are originated from natural medicines, both rodent and non-rodent species should be used, and acute toxic effects should be observed according to the proposed clinical route of administration. If this requirement is not met, the basis should be provided.

If formulas of the above preparations contain natural medicines or their active ingredients, or chemical drugs, acute toxic interaction of the above test substances should be studied.

3. Preparations where changes are made to the route of administration of the domestically marketed TCMs and natural medicines (excluding the change from non-injection to injection).

One animal species may be used to characterize the acute toxic effects of these two different routes of administration.

4. Compound preparations of TCMs and natural medicines where changes are made to the dosage form and manufacturing process of domestically marketed medicines without changing the route of administration.

If the change of manufacturing process may significantly change the formula composition, or change the absorption or utilization of the medicine, one animal species may be used with the proposed clinical route of administration to characterize the acute toxic effects under the current and proposed manufacturing processes.

5. Varieties with new indications or functions and indications

If administration duration is to be prolonged or dose is to be increased, a review of the existing toxicology data and the formula composition of the medicine should be conducted to determine if single dose toxicity studies are needed and if so, the corresponding study contents.

药物单次给药毒性研究技术指导原则

一、概述

急性毒性（Acute toxicity）是指药物在单次或 24 小时内多次给予后一定时间内所产生的毒性反应[1, 2]。狭义的单次给药毒性研究（Single dose toxicity study）是考察单次给予受试物后所产生的急性毒性反应[2]。本指导原则所指为广义的单次给药毒性研究，可采用单次或 24 小时内多次给药的方式获得药物急性毒性信息。

拟用于人体的药物通常需要进行单次给药毒性试验（见注释 1）。单次给药毒性试验对初步阐明药物的毒性作用和了解其毒性靶器官具有重要意义。单次给药毒性试验所获得的信息对重复给药毒性试验的剂量设计和某些药物临床试验起始剂量的选择具有重要参考价值，并能提供一些与人类药物过量所致急性中毒相关的信息[1]。

本指导原则适用于中药、天然药物和化学药物。

二、基本原则

（一）试验管理

用于支持药品注册的单次给药毒性试验必须执行《药物非临床研究质量管理规范》（GLP）。

（二）具体问题具体分析

单次给药毒性试验的设计，应该在对受试物认知的基础上，遵循"具体问题具体分析"的原则。

对于化学药，应根据受试物的结构特点、理化性质、同类化合物情况、适应症和用药人群特点、试验目的等选择合适的试验方法，设计适宜的试验方案，并结合其他药理毒理研究信息对试验结果进行全面的评价。

对于中药和天然药物，还应考虑到其与化学药的不同特点，试验时应根据各自不同的情况进行针对性设计。

（三）随机、对照、重复

单次给药毒性试验应符合动物试验的一般基本原则，即随机、对照和重复。

三、基本内容

（一）受试物

中药、天然药物：受试物应采用能充分代表临床试验拟用样品和/或上市样品质量和安全性的样品。应采用工艺路线及关键工艺参数确定后的工艺制备，一般应为中试或中试以上规模的样品，否则应有充分的理由。应注明受试物的名称、来源、批号、含量（或规格）、保存条件、有效期及配制方法等，并提供质量检验报告。由于中药的特殊性，建议现用现配，否则应提供数据支持配制后受试物的质量稳定性及均匀性。当给药时间较长时，应考察配制后体积是否存在随放置时间延长而膨胀造成终浓度不准的因素。如果由于给药容量或给药方法限制，可采用原料药进行试验。试验中所用溶媒和/或辅料应标明名称、标准、批号、有效期、规格及生产单位。

化学药物：受试物应采用工艺相对稳定、纯度和杂质含量能反映临床试验拟用样品和/或上市样品质量和安全性的样品。受试物应注明名称、来源、批号、含量（或规格）、保存条件、有效期及配制方法等，并提供质量检验报告。试验中所用溶媒和/或辅料应标明名称、标准、批号、有效期、规格和生产单位等，并符合试验要求。

在药物研发的过程中，若受试物的工艺发生可能影响其安全性的变化，应进行相应的安全性研究。

化学药物试验过程中应进行受试物样品分析，并提供样品分析报告。成分基本清楚的中药、天然药物也应进行受试物样品分析。

（二）实验动物 [1, 3, 4]

1. 种属：不同种属的动物各有其特点，对同一受试物的反应可能会有所不同。从充分暴露受试物毒性的角度考虑，采用不同种属的动物进行试验可获得较为充分的安全性信息。因此，对于化学药，单次给药毒性试验应采用至少两种哺乳动物进行试验，一般应选用一种啮齿类动物和一种非啮齿类动物。若未采用非啮齿类动物进行试验，应阐明其合理性。对于中药、天然药物，根据具体情况，可选择啮齿类和/或非啮齿类动物进行试验［参见附录（二）］。

实验动物应符合国家对相应等级动物的质量规定要求，并具有实验动物质量合格证明。

2. 性别：通常采用两种性别的动物进行试验，雌雄各半。若采用单性别动物进行试验，应阐明其合理性。

3. 年龄：通常采用健康成年动物进行试验。如果受试物拟用于或可能用于儿童，必要时应采用幼年动物进行试验。

4. 动物数：应根据动物种属和研究目的确定所需的动物数。动物数应符合试验方法及结果分析评价的需要。

5. 体重：试验中的每批动物初始给药时的体重差异不宜过大，啮齿类动物初始给药时体重不应超过或低于平均体重的20%。

（三）给药途径

给药途径不同，受试物的吸收速度、吸收率和暴露量会有所不同。通常情况下给药途径应至少包括临床拟用途径。如不采用临床拟用途径，应说明理由。

（四）试验方法与给药剂量[1, 3, 4]

单次给药毒性试验的重点在于观察动物出现的毒性反应。单次给药毒性试验的试验方法较多，常用的试验方法有近似致死量法、最大给药量法、最大耐受量法、固定剂量法、上下法（序贯法）、累积剂量法（金字塔法）、半数致死量法等。应根据受试物的特点选择合适的方法，根据不同的试验方法选择合适的剂量（注释2）。

原则上，给药剂量应包括从未见毒性反应的剂量到出现严重毒性反应的剂量，或达到最大给药量。

不同动物和给药途径下的最大给药容量可参考相关文献及根据实际情况来确定。

根据所选择的试验方法，必要时应设置空白和/或溶媒（辅料）对照组。

考虑到胃内容物会影响受试物的给药容量，而啮齿类动物禁食时间的长短会影响到受试物的肠道内吸收和药物代谢酶活性，从而影响毒性的暴露。因此，动物经口给药前一般应进行一段时间的禁食，不禁水。

（五）观察时间与指标[1, 3-5]

给药后，一般连续观察至少14天，观察的间隔和频率应适当，以便能观察到毒性反应的出现时间及恢复时间、动物死亡时间等。如果毒性反应出现较慢或恢复较慢，应适当延长观察时间。

观察指标包括临床症状（如动物外观、行为、饮食、对刺激的反应、分泌物、排泄物等）、死亡情况（死亡时间、濒死前反应等）、体重变化（给药前、观察期结束时各称重一次，观察期间可多次称重，动物死亡或濒死时应称重）等。记录所有的死亡情况，出现的症状以及症状的起始时间、严重程度、持续时间，体重变化等。

所有的试验动物应进行大体解剖。试验过程中因濒死而安乐死的动物、死亡动物应及时进行大体解剖，其他动物在观察期结束后安乐死并进行大体解剖。当组织器官出现体积、颜色、质地等改变时，应进行组织病理学检查。

在一些情况下，为获得更为全面的急性毒性信息，可设计多个剂量组，观察更多的指标，如血液学指标、血液生化学指标、组织病理学检查等，以更好地确定毒性靶器官或剂量反应关系[2, 5]。

四、结果分析与评价

（一）根据所观察到的各种反应出现的时间、持续时间及严重程度等，分析各种反应在不同剂量时的发生率、严重程度。对观察结果进行归纳分析，判断每种反应的剂量-反应及时间-反应关系。

（二）判断出现的各种反应可能涉及的组织、器官或系统［参考附录（一）］等。

（三）根据大体解剖中肉眼可见的病变和组织病理学检查的结果，初步判断可能的毒性靶器官。应出具完整的组织病理学检查报告，检查报告应详细描述，尤其是有异常变化的组织。对于有异常变化者，应附有相应的组织病理学照片。

（四）说明所使用的计算方法和统计学方法，必要时提供所选用方法合理性的依据。

（五）根据各种反应在不同剂量下出现的时间、发生率、剂量-反应关系、不同种属动物及实验室的历史背景数据、病理学检查结果以及同类药物的特点，判断所出现的反应与药物的相关性。判断受试物引起的毒性反应性质、严重程度、可恢复性以及安全范围；根据毒性可能涉及的部位，综合大体解剖和组织病理学检查的结果，初步判断毒性靶器官。

单次给药毒性试验的结果可作为后续毒理试验剂量选择的参考，也可提示一些后续毒性试验需要重点观察的指标。

五、名词解释

最大给药量（Maximal feasible dose，MFD）：指动物单次或24小时内多次（2-3次）给药所采用的最大给药剂量。

最大耐受量（Maximal tolerance dose，MTD）：是指动物能够耐受的而不引起动物死亡的最高剂量。

半数致死量（Median lethal dose，LD_{50}）：预期引起50%动物死亡的剂量，该值是经统计学处理所推算出的结果。

六、参考文献

1. CDER，FDA.Guidance for industry：single dose acute toxicity testing for pharmaceuticals（Final）.1996.

2. CHMP，EMA.Questions and answers on the withdrawal of the "Note for guidance on single dose toxicity".2010.

3. Cordier A.Single dose toxicity：Industry perspectives.In：P.F.D' Arcy and D.W.G.Harron edited，Proceedings of the First International Conference on Harmonization.Brussels：1991，189–191.

4. Outcome – Single dose toxicity.In：P.F.D' Arcy and D.W.G.Harron edited，Proceedings of the First International Conference on Harmonization.Brussels：1991，184.

5. ICH M3（R2）.Nonclinical Safety Studies for the Conduct of Human Clinical Trials and Marketing Authorization for Pharmaceuticals.2009.

6. Blazka ME，Hayes A W.Acute toxicity and eye irritancy.In：Hayes A W edited，Principles and methods of toxicology.Fifth edition，2007：1132–1150.

七、注释

注释1：急性毒性的充分信息也可从其他来源获得[2, 5]，需要说明的是，这些信息应是从执行《药物非临床研究质量管理规范》（GLP）的试验中获得。

注释2：试验方法不同，所采用的给药剂量不同。可参考相关的文献进行试验设计。但应注意，由于中药、天然药物的预期临床用药剂量通常较大，因此单次给药毒性试验方法中所规定的剂量限度（如上下法中的2000mg/kg或5000mg/kg的剂量限度）仅适用于化学药，中药、天然药物的剂量设计应综合考虑多方面因素进行确定。

由于大多数中药、天然药物的急性毒性可能相对较低，中药、天然药物常常采用最大给药量（或最大耐受量法）进行急性毒性研究。

八、附录

（一）一般观察与指征[6]

以下列出了一些常见的观察指征及其可能涉及的组织、器官和系统。单次给药毒性试验中，可能需要对该表格中列出的全部或部分指征进行观察。该表格仅作为结果分析评价的参考，其他科学、合理的分析均是可以接受的。

观察		指征	可能涉及的组织、器官或系统
Ⅰ.鼻孔呼吸阻塞，呼吸频率和深度改变，体表颜色改变	A	呼吸困难：呼吸困难或费力，喘息，通常呼吸频率减慢	
		1.腹式呼吸：膈膜呼吸，吸气时膈膜向腹部偏移	CNS 呼吸中枢，肋间肌麻痹，胆碱能神经麻痹
		2.喘息：吸气很困难，伴随有喘息声	CNS 呼吸中枢，肺水肿，呼吸道分泌物蓄积，胆碱能功能增强
	B	呼吸暂停：用力呼吸后出现短暂的呼吸停止	CNS 呼吸中枢，肺心功能不全
	C	紫绀：尾部、口和足垫呈现青紫色	肺心功能不全，肺水肿
	D	呼吸急促：呼吸快而浅	呼吸中枢刺激，肺心功能不全
	E	鼻分泌物：红色或无色	肺水肿，出血
Ⅱ.运动功能：运动频率和特征的改变	A	自发活动、探究、梳理、运动增加或减少	躯体运动，CNS
	B	嗜睡：动物嗜睡，但可被针刺唤醒而恢复正常活动	CNS 睡眠中枢
	C	正位反射（翻正反射）消失：动物体处于异常体位时所产生的恢复正常体位的反射消失	CNS，感觉，神经肌肉
	D	麻痹：正位反射和疼痛反应消失	CNS，感觉
	E	僵住：保持原姿势不变	CNS，感觉，神经肌肉，自主神经
	F	共济失调：动物行走时无法控制和协调运动，但无痉挛、局部麻痹、轻瘫或僵直	CNS，感觉，自主神经
	G	异常运动：痉挛，足尖步态，踏步，忙碌，低伏	CNS，感觉，神经肌肉
	H	俯卧：不移动，腹部贴地	CNS，感觉，神经肌肉
	I	震颤：包括四肢和全身的颤抖和震颤	神经肌肉，CNS
	J	肌束震颤：包括背部、肩部、后肢和足趾肌肉的运动	神经肌肉，CNS，自主神经

观察		指征	可能涉及的组织、器官或系统
Ⅲ.惊厥（癫痫发作）：随意肌明显的不自主收缩或痉挛性收缩	A	阵挛性惊厥：肌肉收缩和松弛交替性痉挛	CNS，呼吸衰竭，神经肌肉，自主神经
	B	强直性惊厥：肌肉持续性收缩，后肢僵硬性伸展	CNS，呼吸衰竭，神经肌肉，自主神经
	C	强直性-阵挛性惊厥：两种惊厥类型交替出现	CNS，呼吸衰竭，神经肌肉，自主神经
	D	窒息性惊厥：通常是阵挛性惊厥并伴有喘息和紫绀	CNS，呼吸衰竭，神经肌肉，自主神经
	E	角弓反张：背部弓起、头向背部抬起的强直性痉挛	CNS，呼吸衰竭，神经肌肉，自主神经
Ⅳ.反射	A	角膜性眼睑闭合反射：接触角膜导致眼睑闭合	感觉，神经肌肉
	B	基本条件反射：轻轻敲击耳内表面，引起外耳抽搐	感觉，神经肌肉
	C	正位反射：翻正反射的能力	CNS，感觉，神经肌肉
	D	牵张反射：后肢被牵拉至从某一表面边缘掉下时缩回的能力	感觉，神经肌肉
	E	对光反射：瞳孔反射；见光瞳孔收缩	感觉，神经肌肉，自主神经
	F	惊跳反射：对外部刺激（如触摸、噪声）的反应	感觉，神经肌肉
Ⅴ.眼检指征	A	流泪：眼泪过多，泪液清澈或有色	自主神经
	B	缩瞳：无论有无光线，瞳孔缩小	自主神经
	C	散瞳：无论有无光线，瞳孔扩大	自主神经
	D	眼球突出：眼眶内眼球异常突出	自主神经
	E	上睑下垂：上睑下垂，针刺后不能恢复正常	自主神经

观察		指征	可能涉及的组织、器官或系统
V. 眼检指征	F	血泪症：眼泪呈红色	自主神经，出血，感染
	G	瞬膜松弛	自主神经
	H	角膜浑浊，虹膜炎，结膜炎	眼睛刺激
VI. 心血管指征	A	心动过缓：心率减慢	自主神经，肺心功能不全
	B	心动过速：心率加快	自主神经，肺心功能不全
	C	血管舒张：皮肤、尾、舌、耳、足垫、结膜、阴囊发红，体热	自主神经、CNS、心输出量增加，环境温度高
	D	血管收缩：皮肤苍白，体凉	自主神经、CNS、心输出量降低，环境温度低
	E	心律不齐：心律异常	CNS、自主神经、肺心功能不全，心肌梗塞
VII. 流涎	A	唾液分泌过多：口周毛发潮湿	自主神经
VIII. 竖毛	A	毛囊竖毛组织收缩导致毛发蓬乱	自主神经
IX. 痛觉缺失	A	对痛觉刺激（如热板）反应性降低	感觉，CNS
X. 肌张力	A	张力低下：肌张力全身性降低	自主神经
	B	张力过高：肌张力全身性增高	自主神经
XI. 胃肠指征			
排便（粪）	A	干硬固体，干燥，量少	自主神经，便秘，胃肠动力
	B	体液丢失，水样便	自主神经，腹泻，胃肠动力
呕吐	A	呕吐或干呕	感觉，CNS，自主神经（大鼠无呕吐）
多尿	A	红色尿	肾脏损伤
	B	尿失禁	自主感觉神经
XII. 皮肤	A	水肿：液体充盈组织所致肿胀	刺激性，肾功能衰竭，组织损伤，长时间静止不动
	B	红斑：皮肤发红	刺激性，炎症，过敏

（二）不同情况的中药、天然药物单次给药毒性试验的要求

由于中药、天然药物的特殊性，在具体进行试验时可参照以下要求进行；如不按以下要求进行，应充分说明理由。

1.未在国内上市销售的从中药、动物、矿物等物质中提取的有效成分及其制剂，新发现的药材及其制剂，新的中药材代用品、药材新的药用部位及其制剂，未在国内上市销售的从中药、动物、矿物等物质中提取的有效部位制成的制剂，未在国内上市销售的中药、天然药物注射剂。

以上情况，由于其物质基础较传统中药发生了明显改变，或应用经验较少，一般采用啮齿类和非啮齿类两种动物，全面考察受试物的急性毒性反应情况。如不按以上要求进行，应说明理由。

2.未在国内上市销售的非注射给药的中药、天然药物复方制剂。

如该复方制剂处方组成符合中医药理论，有一定的临床应用经验，一般情况下，可采用一种动物、按临床拟用途径进行急性毒性反应的观察。

如该复方制剂为天然药物复方制剂，建议采用啮齿类和非啮齿类两种动物，按临床拟用途径进行急性毒性反应的观察；如不按以上要求进行，应阐明其合理性。

如以上制剂处方中含有天然药物、有效成分或化学药品，则应当对上述药用物质进行急性毒性的相互作用研究。

3.改变国内已上市销售中药、天然药物给药途径（不包括由非注射剂改为注射剂）的制剂。

可仅采用一种动物，比较改变前后两种不同给药途径的急性毒性反应。

4.改变国内已上市销售药品剂型或改变生产工艺但不改变给药途径的中药、天然药物复方制剂。

如生产工艺的改变会引起物质基础的明显改变，或对药物的吸收、利用可能产生明显影响，建议采用一种动物，按临床拟用途径比较改变前后的急性毒性反应。

5.增加新的适应症或者功能主治的品种。

如需延长用药周期或增加剂量者，应结合原有毒理学资料及处方组成等情况确定是否还需要进行单次给药毒性试验以及相应的试验内容。

Guidance for Repeated-Dose Toxicity Study of Pharmaceuticals

I. Overview

The objective of the repeated-dose toxicity study is to describe the toxicity profiles after repeated dose of the test article to animals, and it is regarded as an important part of non-clinical safety evaluation. Repeated-dose toxicity studies are conducted to: 1) predict the potential adverse effects induced by the test article in clinical trials, including the nature, degree, dose-effect and time-effect relationship, reversibility, etc. of adverse effects; 2) identify the target organs or tissues of toxicity following repeated administration of the test article; 3) determine the no observed adverse effect level (NOAEL), if possible; 4) speculate the starting dose for First-in-human (FIH) clinical trials and provide a safe dose range for subsequent clinical trials; and 5) provide information for clinical monitoring, prevention, and treatment of adverse effects.

This guideline is applicable to traditional Chinese medicines (TCMs), natural medicines and chemical drugs.

II. Basic Principles

The safety evaluation studies of pharmaceuticals should comply with *Good Laboratory Practices* (GLPs). The repeated-dose toxicity study is an integral part of the R&D system of pharmaceuticals. In the study design, the correlation with the designs and results of other pharmacology and toxicology studies, the clinical use, clinical indications and target population, and clinical dosage regimen of pharmaceuticals of the same kind, and the physicochemical properties and action characteristics of the test article should be focused so that the results of the repeated-dose toxicity study and other pharmacology and toxicology studies are mutually illustrative, complementary, or/and supportive.

III. Basic Contents

(I) Test article

TCMs and natural medicines: The test articles should be representative of the quality and safety of the samples for clinical trials and/or marketed products. The test articles should be prepared using the process route and key process parameters that have been established. Typically, they should be produced on a pilot or larger scale, unless there are adequate justifications for using a smaller scale. The name, source, batch number, assay (or specification), storage conditions, expiration date, preparation method, etc. of the test article should be clearly indicated, with a certificate of analysis provided. Due to the particularity of TCMs, they are recommended to be freshly prepared before use. Otherwise, the data supporting the quality stability and homogeneity of the prepared test article should be provided. If the administration lasts for a long time, whether the volume of the prepared substance will increase with prolonged storage time, leading to inaccuracy in the final concentration, should be assessed. Due to limitations in terms of dose volume or administration methods, active pharmaceutical ingredients (APIs) are allowed for the study. The names, standards, batch numbers, expiration dates, specifications, and manufacturers of vehicles and/or excipients used in the study should be indicated.

Chemical drugs: The test articles should be representative of the quality and safety of the samples for clinical trials and/or marketed products in purity and impurity content, with a stable manufacturing process. The name, source, batch number, assay (or specification), storage conditions, expiration date, preparation method, etc. should be clearly indicated, with a certificate of analysis provided. The names, standards, batch numbers, expiration dates, specifications, and manufacturers of vehicles and/or excipients used in the study should be indicated. These materials should also meet the requirements of the study.

During the R&D process of pharmaceuticals, if potential changes in the manufacturing process of the test article may affect its safety, corresponding safety studies should be conducted.

In studies of chemical drugs, the test article samples should be analyzed, with sample analysis reports provided. This applies not only to chemical drugs but also to TCMs or natural medicines with clearly identified ingredients.

(II) Laboratory animals

There are two kinds of laboratory animals commonly used for repeated-dose toxicity studies, namely rodents and non-rodents. Ideal laboratory animals should have the following features: 1) Its metabolism of the test article is similar to that of humans; 2) It is sensitive to the test article; 3) There is a large amount of background data, with a clear source, strain, and genetic background. The laboratory animal species or strains should be selected using appropriate test methods before the repeated-dose toxicity study. In general, rats are preferred as rodents and Beagle dogs as non-rodents. In some special cases, animals of other species or strains can be used for repeated-dose toxicity studies. When necessary, disease model animals can be used for study.

Laboratory animals should comply with the national quality regulations for animals at the corresponding grades, and a quality certificate for laboratory animals should be provided.

In general, normal and healthy animals with sexual maturation are selected, and individual body weight should be within 20% of mean body weight of each sex.

The animal age is generally determined based on the duration of the study and the clinically intended population. In general, the rats, Beagle dogs, and monkeys are 6-9 weeks, 6-12 months, and 3-5 years old, respectively. Ages of animals should be close to each other as much as possible, and the animal age at the beginning of administration should be indicated.

The number of animals in each dose group should be no less than 15 animals/sex (10 main study animals and 5 recovery animals) for rodents and no less than 5 animals/sex for non-rodents (3 main study animals and 2 recovery animals).

(III) Administration regimen

1. Dose groups: In principle, at least three dose groups of the test article, namely low, middle, and high dose groups, and one vehicle (or excipient) control group should be used in the repeated-dose toxicity study. When necessary, a blank control group and/or a positive control group can also be included. In principle, the high dose can cause obvious toxic effects in animals, while the low dose is equal to or higher than the effective dose in animals or the equivalent dose in clinical trials. The middle dose is set between the high dose and the low dose based on toxicity mechanism and characteristics to assess the dose-response relationship of toxicity.

2. Route of administration: In principle, the proposed clinical route of administration should be used. A justification should be provided when other routes are used.

3. Frequency of administration: In principle, animals should be exposed to the test article daily in the repeated-dose toxicity study. For a special type, the frequency of administration can be designed based on the characteristics, toxicity profiles, and clinical dose regimen, etc. of the test article.

4. Duration of testing: It is recommended to conduct the repeated-dose toxicity study in a phased manner to support clinical trials with different duration. The study duration can be determined according to the proposed clinical treatment course, indications, target population, etc. The duration of the repeated-dose toxicity study to support the conduct of clinical trials and marketing authorizationis detailed in Appendix (I).

(IV) Endpoints

Endpoints that should be tested in the repeated-dose toxicity study are shown in Appendix (II). Additional parameters can be assessed based on the characteristics of the test article and changes observed or background information revealed in other studies (such as literature reports on the toxicity of components of formula), without affecting regular toxicity observation and evaluation. Historical background data of relevant parameters in laboratory animals provide important information for the repeated-dose toxicity study.

A comprehensive examination should be conducted on animals after euthanasia. When the study duration is relatively long, proper time points are selected for staged examination on the basis of characteristics and relevant information of the test article. During the study period, specimens should be collected in time from any moribund or dead animals for testing and identifying causes. A comprehensive examination should also be conducted at the end of recovery period.

Prior to administration, rodent species should have an acclimation period of at least 5 days, while non-rodent species should have an acclimation period of at least 2 weeks. During the acclimation period, the appearance, behavioral activity, food intake and body weight of laboratory animals should be monitored. Body temperature, hematology and blood chemistry of non-rodent animals are tested at least twice, and the ECG is tested at least once.

During the administration period, examination time and frequency are determined on the basis of study duration and characteristics of the test article. In principle, they should be selected to ensure the earlier observation of toxic effects and reveal the relationship between parameter changes and the study duration.

At the end of the administration period, a systematic gross anatomy should be conducted on the animals of main study groups, with the major organs weighed and organ coefficients calculated. Histopathological examinations should be conducted, and an individual pathology report should be issued. For any abnormal findings, corresponding histopathological images should be attached. For non-rodent animals, the major organs and tissues collected from the control group and treatment groups should be examined histopathologically. For rodent animals, the collected organs/tissues from the control and high dose groups and the tissues with any gross pathological changes at necrospy should be examined thoroughly. If there is any pathological changes in certain tissues of animals in the high dose group, the same tissues of animals in other dose groups will undergo histopathological examination. Bone marrow smears should usually be prepared for bone marrow examination when the test article may affect the hematopoietic system of animals.

After the completion of administration, animals are observed continuously during the recovery period to evaluate the potential reversibility and delayed occurrence of any toxic changes. The duration of a recovery period is determined according to pharmacokinetic characteristics of the test article, target organ toxicity, and recovery conditions, which should generally be not less than 4 weeks.

(V) Concomitant toxicokinetics

Toxicokinetic measurements should be integrated within the repeated-dose toxicity studies. Please refer to corresponding guidelines for specific contents.

IV. Analysis and Evaluation of Results

The repeated-dose toxicity study is mainly to predict the potential toxicity in the human body. The toxicities in animals should be clearly described based on the scientific analysis and comprehensive evaluation of the study results, so as to extrapolate toxicity information from animals to humans. The analysis and evaluation of results are an essential part of the repeated-dose toxicity study.

(I) Analysis of study results

Analyses of the results of a repeated-dose toxicity study include judging whether there is any toxicity in animals, identifying the target organ of toxicity, and describing the nature and severity of toxicity (including the starting time, severity, change patterns, and elimination time). If any animal dies, the cause of its death should be analyzed, the safe dose range should be determined, and the possible toxicity mechanism should also be explored.

1. Correct understanding of the significance of study data

When the results of a repeated-dose toxicity study are analyzed, the significance of mean data and individual data should be understood correctly. In a repeated-dose toxicity study of rodent animals, the significance of group mean values is generally greater than that of individual animal data. Laboratory historical background data and literature data provide information for the analysis of results. For non-rodent animals, individual data are of important toxicological significance given the limited number of laboratory animals and large individual differences. In addition, study results of non-rodent animals must be subject to multiple comparisons with pre-administration data, control group data, and laboratory historical background data, and the limited reference value of literature data should also be taken into consideration. When the results of repeated-dose toxicity study are analyzed, both statistical significance and biological significance of data should be considered comprehensively. Proper use of statistical hypothesis testing can help determine the biological significance of study results. It should be noted that the presence of statistical significance does not mean presence of biological significance. In the judgment of biological significance, factors such as the dose-response relationship of parameter changes, changes in other associated parameters, and comparison with historical background data must be taken into account. When study results are analyzed, any abnormal data must be scientifically explained whether caused by the toxicity of the test article or not.

2. Correct assessment of toxic reactions

Differences in study results between the administration groups and control group can be possibly attributed to the toxicity related to the test article, adaptive change of animals to medicines or normal physiological fluctuation, or misoperation and animal stress. When study results are analyzed, attention should be paid to the dose-response relationship of parameter changes and the amplitude of parameter changes and the gender difference within the groups. Meanwhile, a comprehensive consideration of the test results of multiple toxicological parameters and analysis of the inherent correlation and toxicity mechanism of the test article is required for correct judgment of toxicities. The changes of a single parameter may not be sufficient to assess the potential toxicity induced by the test article, and further related studies may be needed. Furthermore, toxicokinetic studies provide important data for assessing the toxicity and target organs of toxicity.

(II) Significance of animal toxic reactions for clinical trials

When the results of the repeated-dose toxicity study are extrapolated to humans, differences in toxicity of the test article between animals and humans may be unavoidably involved. Firstly, there may be differences in toxic reactions to a certain test article between different species and different strains or individuals of the same species. Secondly, as relatively high doses are used in the repeated-dose toxicity study, the test article may be metabolized in animals following non-linear kinetics, inducing toxic effects irrelevant to the human body. Thirdly, it is difficult to predict some toxicities with low incidence in the human body or idiosyncratic reactions only occurring in the small portion of populations in the repeated-dose toxicity study. In addition, some toxic reactions, such as headache, wooziness, dizziness, skin pruritus and blurred vision, are difficultly observed in animals. Given the above-mentioned reasons, the results of repeated-dose toxicity study in animals will not be fully reproduced in the human clinical trials. However, if there is no experimental or literature-based evidence proving that the toxic reactions of a test article in animals are not relevant to humans, it must be primarily assumed in drug evaluation that humans are the most sensitive and the toxic reactions observed in animals in repeated-dose toxicity studies will occur in clinical trials. An in-depth study on toxicity mechanism will help judge the correlation of toxic reactions between animals and humans.

(III) Comprehensive evaluation

As an integral part of non-clinical safety assessment of pharmaceuticals, the repeated-dose toxicity study is the most comprehensive, informative, and clinically significant one in the non-clinical toxicology studies. Study results should be comprehensively evaluated in combination with pharmaceutical characteristics of the test article, pharmacodynamics, pharmacokinetics and other toxicology study results, as well as the clinical trial results obtained. Eventually, the evaluation of repeated-dose toxicity study results should help to confirm adverse effects of the test article, target organ or tissue of toxicity, safety range, critical parameters to be monitored, and necessary monitoring or rescue measures in clinical trials.

V. References

1. *Technical Guidelines for Long-term Toxicity Study of Chemical Drugs,* National Medical Products Administration, 2005.3.

2. *Technical Guidelines for Long-term Toxicity Study of Traditional Chinese Medicines and Natural Medicines.* National Medical Products Administration, 2005.3.

3. Zhou Zongcan. Toxicology Basis. Second Edition. Beijing Medical University Press, 2000.

4. Qin Boyi. Introduction to the Evaluation of New Drugs. Second Edition. People's Medical Publishing House, 1998.

5. Guidance on nonclinical safety studies for the conduct of human clinical trials and marketing authorization for pharmaceuticals, ICH/M3 (R2) 2009.6.

6. Guideline on repeated dose toxicity, EMA 2010.3.

7. Redbook 2000 Ⅳ.C, FDA 2003, 2007.

8. Note for guidance on toxicokinetics: The assessment of systemic exposure in toxicity studies, ICH/S3A 2007.

Ⅵ. Annotations

(Ⅰ) Considerations for Study Duration

he study duration should match with the proposed clinical trial duration and marketing authorization requirements. The information from toxicity studies with relatively short duration can provide references for toxicity studies with relatively long duration in the aspects of dose levels, frequency of administration, observations, etc. At the same time, the information from clinical trials may help design the protocol of animal toxicity studies with relatively long duration and reduce risks of drug development. When repeated-dose toxicity studies with different study durations are used to support clinical trials with different durations of dosing and the marketing authorization evaluation, the contents of the repeated-dose toxicity studies should be complete and standardized, and the analysis and evaluation of results should be objective and scientific.

If there are several clinical indications to be studied, the duration of repeated-dose toxicity studies should be determined according to the clinical indication with the longest course of treatment.

(Ⅱ) Considerations for dose selection

Endpoints evaluated, physicochemical properties, and bioavailability of the test substance in the studies conducted previously should be considered for dose selection. Sufficient contact time should be guaranteed for local administration. High doses should result in obvious toxicities or reach the maximum feasible dose (MFD), or systemic exposure should reach 50-fold the clinical systemic exposure (based on AUC). If it is necessary to change the dose levels in the course of study, the reasons for dose adjustment should be provided and the process of dose adjustment should be fully recorded.

(III) Study requirements of TCMs and natural medicines under different conditions

In consideration of differences in the prescription source and the project basis of TCMs and natural medicines, the following requirements can be referred to in practice. These requirements are only general requirements. Following the objective law of development of new drugs, individualized tests for a certain study should be designed based on characteristics of the test substance.

1. Active ingredients extracted from TCMs, animals, or minerals, and formulations containing such active ingredients which have not been marketed in China, new raw TCM materials and their formulations, new substitutes of raw TCM materials, new medicinal parts of raw TCM materials and their formulations, formulations prepared from active ingredients extracted from TCMs, animals, or minerals which have not been marketed in China, and injection of TCMs and natural medicines which have not been marketed in China. Given the above situations, because its material basis has changed significantly compared with TCMs, or there is less application experience, the repeated-dose toxicity study should be conducted using both rodent and non-rodent animals to comprehensively evaluate the toxicity of repeated administration of the test substance.

2. Non-injection compound formulations composed of TCMs and natural medicines that are not marketed in China can first be used for the repeated-dose toxicity study in one species (rodent), and when obvious toxic effect is observed, the second species (non-rodent) can be used for further toxicity study. If such formulas contain raw TCM materials that have toxicity [Annotation (IV)], or no statutory standards, or contraindications of "eighteen antagonisms" and "nineteen incompatibilities", the repeated-dose toxicity study should be conducted in two

species of animals (both rodent and non-rodent). For non-injection compound formulations of natural medicines, the repeated-dose toxicity study should be conducted in both rodent and non-rodent animals before clinical trial.

3. For the formulations where changes are made to the route of administration of the domestically marketed drugs (excluding the change from non-injection to injection), and formulations where changes are made to the dosage form and manufacturing process of non-injection formulations without changing the route of administration, it is recommended to add a high dose control group of original administration route, original dosage form, or original manufacturing process and conduct the repeated-dose toxicity study in one species (rodent) first. If obvious toxic effects or more severe toxic effects different from those of original administration route, original dosage form, or original manufacturing process are observed, the repeated-dose toxicity study in the other species (non-rodent) should be conducted.

4. For varieties with new indications or functions and indications, if it is necessary to prolong the administration duration or increase dose, it is required to determine whether the repeated-dose toxicity study should be conducted in combination with application dossiers and formula composition of the original variety.

(IV) Varieties of toxic raw TCM materials

Toxic raw TCM materials: TCMs listed in the *Administrative Measures for Toxic Drugs for Medical Use* released by the State Council, namely Arsenolite, Arsenic sublimate, Mercury, Raw semen strychnia, Raw radix aconite, Raw radix aconite kusn, Raw rhizoma typhoid, Raw radix aconite lateralis, Raw pinellia ternate, Raw rhizoma arisaematis, Raw Croton tiglium, Mylabris, Lytta caraganae Pallas, Huechys, Raw Euphorbia kansui, Raw Euphorbia ebracteolata Hayata, Raw Garcinia hanburyi, Raw Euphorbiae Semen, Raw Hyoscyamus niger L., Rhododendron Mollis Flos, Aconitum brachypodum Diels, Hongsheng Dan, Baijiang Dan, Bufonis Venenum, Daturae Flos, Hydrargyri Oxydum Rubrum, Calomelas, Realgar.

In addition, all raw TCM materials (or medicinal substances) with toxicity found in recent years or those containing obvious toxic components in the formula are treated as toxic raw TCM materials.

VII. Appendixes

(I) Study Duration

Support the Conduct of Clinical Trials of Drugs

Maximum Duration of Clinical Trial	Minimum Duration of Repeated-Dose Toxicity Studies	
	Rodents	Non-rodents
Up to 2 weeks	2 weeks	2 weeks
Between 2 weeks and 6 months	Same as clinical trial	Same as clinical trial
> 6 months	6 months	9 months [1,2]

Support Marketing Authorization of Drugs

PDuration of Indicated Treatment	Rodent	Non-rodent
Up to 2 weeks	1 month	1 month
> 2 weeks to 1 month	3 months	3 months
> 1 month to 3 months	6 months	6 months
> 3 months	6 months	9 months [1,2]

Notes:

1. Studies of less than 6 months duration in non-rodents are considered acceptable:

    When immunogenicity or intolerance confounds conduct of longer term studies;

    Repeated short-term administration even if clinical trial duration exceeds 6 months, such as intermittent treatment of migraine, erectile dysfunction, or herpes simplex;

    When it is proposed to be used for life-threatening diseases (such as progressive diseases or tumor chemotherapy drugs).

2. A long-term juvenile animal toxicity study can be appropriate if a pediatric population is the primary proposed population and existing toxicology or pharmacology studies suggest potential developmental toxicity. A study initiated in the appropriate age and species with the relevant end points to address the developmental toxicity (e.g., 12 months duration in dog or 6 months in rat) can be appropriate. A 12-month study should cover the full development period in the dog. These long-term studies in juvenile animals can be adapted to replace the standard chronic study and separate juvenile animal study.

(II) Endpoints

Item		Endpoint
1. Clinical observation		Appearance, sign, behavioral activity, glandular secretion, respiration, feces characteristics, local response after administration, mortality, etc.
2. Food intake, body weight and ophthalmology		
3. Body temperature and ECG (non-rodent)		
4. Hematology		RBC count, hemoglobin, corpuscular volume, mean corpuscular volume, mean corpuscular hemoglobin, mean corpuscular-hemoglobin concentration, reticulocyte count, WBC count and its classification, blood platelet count, prothrombin time, activated partial thromboplastin time, etc.
5. Blood biochemistry		Aspartate Aminotransferase (AST), Alanine Aminotransferase (ALT), Alkaline Phosphatase (ALP), creatine phosphokinase, urea nitrogen (urea), creatinine, total protein, albumin, blood glucose, total bilirubin, total cholesterol, triglyceride, gamma-glutamyltransferase, potassium (K^+), chloride (Cl^-), and sodium (Na^+)
6. Urine observation and analysis		Urine appearance, specific gravity, pH value, urine glucose, urine protein, urine bilirubin, urobilinogen, acetone body, occult blood, and WBC
7. Organs and tissues subject to histopathological examination	(1) Organs needing weighing and calculation of organ coefficient	Brain, heart, liver, kidney, adrenal glands, thymus, spleen, testis, epididymis, ovary, uterus, and thyroid gland (including parathyroid glands) [1]
	(2) Tissues or organs needing histopathological examination	Adrenal glands, aorta, bone (femur), bone marrow (sternum), brain (at least three levels), cecum, colon, uterus and cervix uteri, duodenum, epididymis, esophagus, eye, gallbladder (if any), Harderian gland (if any), heart, ileum, jejunum, kidney, liver, lung (with main-stem bronchus), lymph nodes (one is related to route of administration while the other is at remote

continued

Item		Endpoint
7. Organs and tissues subject to histopathological examination	(2) Tissues or organs needing histopathological examination	distance), mammary glands, conchae nasals[2], ovary and fallopian tubes, pancreas, pituitary, prostate, rectum, salivary gland, sciatic nerve, seminal vesicles (if any), skeletal muscle, skin, spinal cord (3 sites: cervical vertebra, middle thoracic vertebra, and lumbar vertebra), spleen, stomach, testis, thymus (or thymus region), thyroid gland (including parathyroid glands), trachea, urinary bladder, vagina, tissues with gross lesions, tissue masses, and administration sites

Notes:

1. Only weigh the non-rodent animals.

2. Specific to dose formulations with route of administration of inhalation.

药物重复给药毒性研究技术指导原则

一、概述

重复给药毒性试验是描述动物重复接受受试物后的毒性特征，它是非临床安全性评价的重要内容。重复给药毒性试验可以：①预测受试物可能引起的临床不良反应，包括不良反应的性质、程度、量效和时效关系，以及可逆性等；②判断受试物重复给药的毒性靶器官或靶组织；③如果可能，确定未观察到临床不良反应的剂量水平（No Observed Adverse Effect Level，NOAEL）；④推测第一次临床试验（First in Human，FIH）的起始剂量，为后续临床试验提供安全剂量范围；⑤为临床不良反应监测及防治提供参考。

本指导原则适用于中药、天然药物和化学药物。

二、基本原则

药物安全性评价试验必须执行《药物非临床研究质量管理规范》（GLP），药物重复给药毒性试验是药物研发体系的有机组成部分，试验设计要重视与其他药理毒理试验设计和研究结果的关联性，要关注同类药物临床使用情况、临床适应症和用药人群、临床用药方案，还要结合受试物理化性质和作用特点，使得重复给药毒性试验结果与其他药理毒理试验研究互为说明、补充或/和印证。

三、基本内容

（一）受试物

中药、天然药物：受试物应采用能充分代表临床试验拟用样品和/或上市样品质量和安全性的样品。应采用工艺路线及关键工艺参数确定后的工艺制备，一般应为中试或中试以上规模的样品，否则应有充分的理由。应注明受试物的名称、来源、批号、含量（或规格）、保存条件、有效期及配制方法等，并提供质量检验报告。由于中药的特殊性，建议现用现配，否则应提供数据支持配制后受试物的质量稳定性及均匀性。当给药时间较长时，应考察配制后体积是否存在随放置时间延长而膨胀造成终浓度不准的因素。如果由于给药容量或给药方法限制，可采用原料药进行试验。试验中所用溶媒和/或辅料应标明名称、标准、批号、有效期、规格及生产单位。

化学药物：受试物应采用工艺相对稳定、纯度和杂质含量能反映临床试验拟用样品和/或上市样品质量和安全性的样品。受试物应注明名称、来源、批号、含量（或规格）、保存条件、有效期及配制方法等，并提供质量检验报告。试验中所用溶媒和/或辅料应标明名称、标准、批号、有效期、规格和生产单位等，并符合试验要求。

在药物研发的过程中，若受试物的工艺发生可能影响其安全性的变化，应进行相应的安全性试验。

化学药物试验过程中应进行受试物样品分析，并提供样品分析报告。成分基本清楚的中药、天然药物也应进行受试物样品分析。

（二）实验动物

重复给药毒性试验通常采用两种实验动物，一种为啮齿类，另一种为非啮齿类。理想的动物应具有以下特点：①对受试物的代谢与人体相近；②对受试物敏感；③已有大量历史对照数据，来源、品系、遗传背景清楚。在重复给药毒性试验前应采用合适的试验方法对实验动物种属或品系进行选择。通常，啮齿类动物首选大鼠、非啮齿类动物首选 Beagle 犬，特殊情况下可选用其他种属或品系动物进行重复给药毒性试验，必要时选用疾病模型动物进行试验。

实验动物应符合国家对相应等级动物的质量规定要求，具有实验动物质量合格证明。

一般选择正常、健康、性成熟动物，同性别体重差异应在平均体重的20%之内。

应根据试验期限和临床拟用人群确定动物年龄，一般大鼠为6-9周龄，Beagle 犬 6-12 月龄，猴 3-5 岁，动物年龄应尽量接近，应注明开始给药时动物年龄。

每个剂量组动物数，啮齿类一般不少于15只/性别（主试验组10只，恢复组5只），非啮齿类一般不少于5只/性别（主试验组3只，恢复组2只）。

（三）给药方案

1. 给药剂量：重复给药毒性试验原则上至少应设低、中、高3个剂量组，以及1个溶媒（或辅料）对照组，必要时设立空白对照组和/或阳性对照组；高剂量原则上使动物产生明显的毒性反应，低剂量原则上相当或高于动物药效剂量或临床使用剂量的等效剂量，中剂量应结合毒性作用机制和特点在高剂量和低剂量之间设立，以考察毒性的剂量-反应关系。

2. 给药途径：原则上应与临床拟用途径一致，如不一致则应说明理由。

3. 给药频率：原则上重复给药毒性试验中动物应每天给药，特殊类型的受试物就其毒性特点和临床给药方案等原因，可根据具体药物的特点设计给药频率。

4. 试验期限：建议分阶段进行重复给药毒性试验以支持不同期限的临床试验。试验期限的选定可以根据拟定的临床疗程、适应症、用药人群等进行设计。一般重复给药毒性试验的试验期限与所支持的临床试验及上市申请的关系详见附录（一）。

（四）检测指标

重复给药毒性试验应检测指标详见附录（二）。此外，还应结合受试物的特点及其他试验中已观察到的改变或背景信息（如关于处方组成成分毒性的文献报道等），在不影响正常毒性观察和检测的前提下增加合理的指标。实验动物相关指标的历史背景数据在重复给药毒性试验中具有重要的参考意义。

在结束动物安乐死时进行一次全面检测；当试验期限较长时，应根据受试物的特点及相关信息选择合适的时间点进行阶段性检测；试验期间对濒死或死亡动物应及时采集标本进行检测，分析濒死或死亡的原因；恢复期结束时进行一次全面的检测。

给药前应对动物进行适应性饲养，啮齿类动物应不少于 5 天，非啮齿类动物不少于 2 周。在适应性饲养时，对实验动物进行外观体征、行为活动、摄食情况和体重检查，非啮齿类动物至少应进行 2 次体温、血液学、血液生化学和至少 1 次心电图检测。

给药期间，根据试验期限的长短和受试物的特点确定检测时间和检测次数。原则上应尽早发现毒性反应，并反映出观测指标或参数变化与试验期限的关系。

给药结束，对主试验组动物进行系统的大体解剖，称重主要脏器并计算脏器系数；进行组织病理学检查并出具完整的病理学检查报告，如发现有异常变化，应附有相应的组织病理学照片。非啮齿类动物对照组和各给药组主要脏器组织均应进行组织病理学检查；啮齿类动物对照组、高剂量组、尸检异常动物应进行详细检查，如高剂量组动物某一组织发生病理改变，需要对其他剂量组动物的相同组织进行组织病理学检查；通常需要制备骨髓涂片，以便当受试物可能对动物造血系统有影响时进行骨髓检查。

给药结束后，继续观察恢复期动物，以了解毒性反应的可逆性和可能出现的迟发毒性；应根据受试物代谢动力学特点、靶器官毒性反应和恢复情况确定恢复期的长短，一般情况下应不少于 4 周。

（五）伴随毒代动力学

重复给药毒性试验应伴随进行药物毒代动力学试验，具体内容参照相应指导原则。

四、结果分析与评价

重复给药毒性试验的最终目的在于预测人体可能出现的毒性反应。只有通过对试验结果的科学分析和全面评价才能够清楚描述动物的毒性反应，并推断其与人体的相关性。重复给药毒性试验结果的分析和评价是重复给药毒性试验的必要组成部分。

（一）试验结果的分析

分析重复给药毒性试验结果，判断动物是否发生毒性反应及毒性靶器官，描述毒性反应的性质和程度（包括毒性反应的起始时间、程度、变化规律和消除时间），如果有动物死亡应分析死亡原因，确定安全范围，并探讨可能的毒性作用机制。

1. 正确理解试验数据的意义

在对重复给药毒性试验结果进行分析时，应正确理解均值数据和个体数据的意义。啮齿类动物重复给药毒性试验中组均值的意义通常大于个体动物数据的意义，实验室历史背景数据和文献数据可以为结果的分析提供参考；非啮齿类动物单个动物的试验数据往往具有重要的毒理学意义，是试验动物数量较少、个体差异较大的原因。此外，非啮齿类动物试验结果必须与给药前数据、对照组数据和实验室历史背景数据进行多重比较，要考虑文献数据参考价值有局限性。在分析重复给药毒性试验结果时应综合考虑数据的统计学意义和生物学意义，正确利用统计学假设检验有助于确定试验结果的生物学意义，要考虑具有统计学意义并不一定代表具有生物学意义；在判断生物学意义时要考虑参数变化的剂量–反应关系、其他关联参数的改变、与历史背景数据的比较等因素；分析试验结果时，须对出现的异常数据应判断是否由受试物毒性引起并给予科学解释。

2. 正确判断毒性反应

给药组和对照组之间检测结果的差异可能来源于受试物有关的毒性、动物对药物的适应性改变或正常的生理波动，也可能源于试验操作失误和动物应激。在分析试验结果时，应关注参数变化的剂量—反应关系、组内动物的参数变化幅度和性别差异，同时综合考虑多项毒理学指标的检测结果，分析其中的关联和受试物作用机制，以正确判断药物的毒性反应。单个参数的变化往往并不足以判断化合物是否引起毒性反应，可能需要进一步进行相关的试验。此外，毒代动力学试验可以为毒性反应和毒性靶器官的判断提供重要的参考依据。

（二）动物毒性反应对于临床试验的意义

将重复给药毒性试验结果外推至人体时，不可避免地会涉及到受试物在动物和人体内毒性反应之间的差异。首先，不同物种、同物种不同种属或个体之间对于某一受试物的毒性反应可能存在差异；其次，由于在重复给药毒性试验中通常采用较高的给药剂量，受试物可能在动物体内呈非线性动力学代谢过程，从而导致与人体无关的毒性反应；另外，重复给药毒性试验难以预测一些在人体中发生率较低的毒性反应或仅在小部分人群中出现的特异质反应；同时有些毒性反应目前在动物中难以观察，如头痛、头昏、头晕、皮肤瘙痒、视物模糊等。鉴于以上原因，动物重复给药毒性试验的结果不一定完全再现于人体临床试验。但如果没有试验或文献依据证明受试物对动物的毒性反应与人体无关，在进行药物评价时必须首先假设人为最敏感，重复给药毒性试验中动物的毒性反应将会在临床试验中出现。进行深入的作用机制研究将有助于判断动物和人体毒性反应的相关性。

（三）综合评价

重复给药毒性试验是药物非临床安全性研究的有机组成部分，是药物非临床毒理学研究中综合性最强、获得信息最多和对临床指导意义最大的一项毒理学试验。对其结果进行评价时，应结合受试物的药学特点，药效学、药代动力学和其他毒理学的试验结果，以及已取得的临床试验结果，进行综合评价。对于重复给药毒性试验结果的评价最终应落实到受试物的临床不良反应、临床毒性靶器官或靶组织、安全范围、临床需重点检测的指标，以及必要的临床监护或解救措施。

五、参考文献

1. 化学药物长期毒性试验技术指导原则. 国家药品监督管理局，2005.3.

2. 中药、天然药物长期毒性试验技术指导原则. 国家药品监督管理局，2005.3.

3. 周宗灿. 毒理学基础. 第二版. 北京医科大学出版社，2000.

4. 秦伯益. 新药评价概论. 第二版. 人民卫生出版社，1998.

5. Guidance on nonclinical safety studies for the conduct of human clinical trials and marketing authorization for pharmaceuticals，ICH/M3（R2）2009.6.

6. Guideline on repeated dose toxicity，EMA 2010.3.

7. Redbook 2000 Ⅳ.C，FDA 2003，2007.

8. Note for guidance on toxicokinetics：The assessment of systemic exposure in toxicity studies，ICH/S3A 2007.

六、注释

（一）试验期限的考虑

试验期限应与拟开展的临床试验期限和上市要求相匹配；通过较短试验期限的毒性试验获得的信息，可以为较长试验期限的毒性试验设计提供给药剂量、给药频率、观察指标等方面的参考；同时，临床试验中获得的信息有助于设计较长试验期限的动物毒性试验方案，降低药物开发的风险。以不同试验期限的重复给药毒性试验支持不同用药期限的临床试验及上市评价时，重复给药毒性试验内容都应完整、规范，结果分析评价强调客观性、注重科学性。

拟试验的临床适应症如有若干项，应按最长疗程的临床适应症来确定重复给药毒性试验的试验期限。

（二）剂量设计的考虑

剂量设计应考虑之前进行的各项试验所评价的终点、受试物的理化性质和生物利用度等；局部给药应保证充分的接触时间。高剂量应出现明显毒性反应，或达到最大给药量（Maximum Feasible Dose，MFD），或系统暴露量达到临床系统暴露量的 50 倍（基于 AUC）。如需要在试验中途改变给药剂量，应说明剂量调整理由，完整记录剂量调整过程。

（三）不同情况中药、天然药物的试验要求

考虑到中药、天然药物各类药物处方来源、立题依据等差别，在具体进行试验时可参照以下要求进行。这些要求仅是一般要求，应遵循新药开发的客观规律，具体试验结合受试物特点考虑需开展的试验，进行个性化的设计。

1. 未在国内上市销售的从中药、动物、矿物等物质中提取的有效成分及其制剂，新发现的药材及其制剂，新的中药材代用品、药材新的药用部位及其制剂，未在国内上市销售的从中药、动物、矿物等物质中提取的有效部位制成的制剂，未在国内上市销售的中药、天然药物注射剂。以上情况，由于其物质基础较传统中药发生了明显改变，或应用经验较少，为全面考察受试物的重复给药毒性反应情况，应采用啮齿类和非啮齿类两种动物进行重复给药毒性试验。

2. 未在国内上市销售的由中药、天然药物组成的非注射给药的复方制剂可先进行一种动物（啮齿类）的重复给药毒性试验，当发现有明显毒性时，为进

一步研究毒性情况，再采用第二种动物（非啮齿类）进行试验。若该类处方中含有毒性药材［见注释（四）］、无法定标准药材或有十八反、十九畏等配伍禁忌时，则应进行两种动物（啮齿类和非啮齿类）的重复给药毒性试验。天然药物组成的非注射给药的复方制剂临床试验前采用啮齿类和非啮齿类两种动物进行重复给药毒性试验。

3.改变国内已上市销售药品给药途径（不包括由非注射剂改为注射剂）的制剂、不改变给药途径的非注射给药改剂型制剂和改工艺制剂，建议增设一个原给药途径、原剂型或原工艺的高剂量对照组，先进行一种动物（啮齿类）的重复给药毒性试验。如发现与原给药途径、原剂型或原工艺制剂不同的明显毒性反应或更严重的毒性反应，应进行另一种动物（非啮齿类）的重复给药毒性试验。

4.增加新的适应症或者功能主治的品种如需延长用药期限或增加剂量者，应结合原品种的申报资料及处方组成的情况，确定是否需进行重复给药毒性试验。

（四）中药毒性药材品种

毒性药材：系指收入国务院《医疗用毒性药品管理办法》的中药品种。即：砒石、砒霜、水银、生马钱子、生川乌、生草乌、生白附子、生附子、生半夏、生南星、生巴豆、斑蝥、青娘虫、红娘虫、生甘遂、生狼毒、生藤黄、生千金子、生天仙子、闹羊花、雪上一枝蒿、红升丹、白降丹、蟾酥、洋金花、红粉、轻粉、雄黄。

另外，凡在近年来发现的有毒性作用的药材（原材料）或在复方中含有明显有毒组分的，均按毒性药材处理。

七、附录

（一）试验期限

支持药物临床试验

最长临床试验期限	重复给药毒性试验的最短期限	
	啮齿类动物	非啮齿类动物
≤2周	2周	2周
2周–6个月	同临床试验	同临床试验
>6个月	6个月	9个月[1, 2]

支持药物上市申请

临床拟用期限	啮齿类动物	非啮齿类动物
≤ 2 周	1 个月	1 个月
2 周 –1 个月	3 个月	3 个月
1 个月 –3 个月	6 个月	6 个月
> 3 个月	6 个月	9 个月 [1, 2]

注：1. 非啮齿类动物不超过 6 个月期限的试验可接受情况：

当免疫原性或耐受性问题使更长期限的试验难以进行时；

重复、短期用药（即便临床试验期限 6 个月以上）的疾病，如偏头痛、勃起障碍、单纯性疱疹等的反复间歇给药时；

拟用于危及生命的疾病（如进展性疾病、辅助使用的肿瘤化疗药）时。

2. 如果儿童为主要拟用药人群，而已有毒理学或药理学研究结果提示可能发生发育毒性，应考虑在幼年动物上进行长期毒性试验。该试验应采用合适年龄和种系的动物，试验观察指标应针对发育方面的毒性，试验期限犬 12 个月、大鼠 6 个月。12 个月的犬试验期限应涵盖其发育的全过程。这些幼年动物的长期试验可用于替代标准的长期毒性试验和单独的幼年动物试验。

（二）检测指标

项目类别	指标
1. 临床观察	外观、体征、行为活动、腺体分泌、呼吸、粪便性状、给药局部反应、死亡情况等。
2. 摄食量、体重、眼科检查	
3. 体温和心电图检测（非啮齿动物）	
4. 血液学检测	红细胞计数、血红蛋白、红细胞容积、平均红细胞容积、平均红细胞血红蛋白、平均红细胞血红蛋白浓度、网织红细胞计数、白细胞计数及其分类、血小板计数、凝血酶原时间、活化部分凝血活酶时间等。
5. 血液生化学检测	天门冬氨酸氨基转换酶、丙氨酸氨基转换酶、碱性磷酸酶、肌酸磷酸激酶、尿素氮（尿素）、肌酐、总蛋白、白蛋白、血糖、总胆红素、总胆固醇、甘油三酯、γ- 谷氨酰转移酶、钾离子浓度、氯离子浓度、钠离子浓度。

项目类别		指标
6. 尿液观察和分析		尿液外观、比重、pH 值、尿糖、尿蛋白、尿胆红素、尿胆原、酮体、潜血、白细胞。
7. 组织病理学检查的脏器组织	（1）需称重并计算脏器系数的器官	脑、心脏、肝脏、肾脏、肾上腺、胸腺、脾脏、睾丸、附睾、卵巢、子宫、甲状腺（含甲状旁腺）[1]。
	（2）需进行组织病理学检查的组织或器官	肾上腺、主动脉、骨（股骨）、骨髓（胸骨）、脑（至少 3 个水平）、盲肠、结肠、子宫和子宫颈、十二指肠、附睾、食管、眼、胆囊（如果有）、哈氏腺（如果有）、心脏、回肠、空肠、肾脏、肝脏、肺脏（附主支气管）、淋巴结（一个与给药途径相关，另一个在较远距离）、乳腺、鼻甲 [2]、卵巢和输卵管、胰腺、垂体、前列腺、直肠、唾液腺、坐骨神经、精囊（如果有）、骨骼肌、皮肤、脊髓（3 个部位：颈椎、中段胸椎、腰椎）、脾脏、胃、睾丸、胸腺（或胸腺区域）、甲状腺（含甲状旁腺）、气管、膀胱、阴道、所有大体观察到异常的组织、组织肿块和给药部位。

注：1. 仅在非啮齿类动物称重。

2. 针对吸入给药的给药制剂。

The Guideline for Drafting of Application Dossiers for Traditional Chinese Medicine (TCM) Theories of Compound Preparations of New TCMs (Trial)

The *Guideline for Drafting of Application Dossiers for Traditional Chinese Medicine (TCM) Theories of Compound Preparations of New TCMs (Trial)* is drafted in accordance with the relevant requirements for TCM theories involved in the application dossiers of clinical trials as specified in the *Registration Classifications and Requirements for Application Dossiers of Traditional Chinese Medicines (TCMs)* to accelerate the construction of a registration evaluation evidence system for TCMs integrating TCM theories, application experience in humans, and clinical trials.

The Guideline is applicable to the explanation of TCM theories involved in the registration application of compound preparations of new TCMs. The Guideline can be referenced if other TCM registration applications involve the explanation of TCM theories.

I. Brief Description of Formula Composition, Functions and Indications

The formula composition, functions and indications should be expressed in a standardized manner.

The names of ingredients contained in the formulas should be consistent with those standard names included in the national drug standards, drug registration standards, or standards of provinces, autonomous regions and municipalities directly under the Central Government for TCM crude drugs, prepared slices/ decoction pieces, or the specifications for processing. The daily dosage of each ingredient should be clearly defined. The arrangement of ingredients of TCM compound preparations should comply with the principles of TCM formulas.

In terms of indications, clinical positioning of formulas should be described. It is necessary to distinguish treatment of disease, syndrome treatment and symptom treatment. Characteristics of the action of medicines should be described, e.g., treatment of disease, symptom relief or alleviation, and effects on medicines for combination, etc.

For compound preparations of TCMs of ancient classic formulas, their functions and indications should be expressed with TCM terms.

II. Basic Understanding of Indications Based on TCM Theories

The sources of TCM theories related to indications should be described.

The causes, development process, prognosis, stage and type of the diseases should be addressed.

TCM theories should be used to describe the characteristics of syndromes/patterns, treatment principles and methods, and advantages and characteristics of corresponding causes and mechanisms.

The source of the basis for TCM theories used should be indicated. If it is from ancient medical books, relevant sections, volumes and books should be marked, and the original text can be provided. If it is from modern TCM theory researches or medical treatises, relevant literatures or other related materials should be provided, and the basis of TCM theories should be demonstrated.

III. TCM Theories for Proposed Formulas

(I) Formula source and historical development

The formula source should be clearly identified, and it's necessary to briefly describe the evolution of ingredients, dosage of ingredients, dosage form, target population (indications and population scope), usage and dosage, course of treatment of formulas as well as the basis. Changes in a formula can be described using either text or tables (Table 1).

Table 1 Summary of formula changes

Formula	Change					Basis for change
	Ingredients and dosage	Dosage form	Target population	Usage and dosage	Course of treatment	
Formula 1						
Formula 2						
...						

For other compound preparations of TCMs originated from ancient classic formulas the origin and development of the formula (usage in history and related medical evaluations) should be briefly described in text or tables (Table 2) according to relevant contents of the original text. Comparative data about causes and mechanisms, treatment principles and methods, indications, ingredients, and dosage of ingredients between the formula under application and the original formula should be provided in text or tables (Tables 3, 4 and 5). In addition, relevant textual research contents should be described, and the basis for determining the dosage of each ingredient contained in the formula should be addressed. Changes in the origin of ingredients and processing for the formula under application should be described in this section, if any. If modification of TCMs is made based on the ancient classic formulas, the specific reasons for such modification should be addressed. If it is from several classic formulas, the reasons for the combination should be explained, so as to provide basis for the confirmation of classic formulas and support of application experience in humans.

Table 2 Analysis of the origin and development of formulas

No.	Dynasty	Source	Author	Contents discussed
1				
2				
...				

Table 3 Analysis of the causes and mechanisms, treatment principles and methods for formulas

	Original formula	Formula under application	Consistent or not?(If "Not" , please describe the reasons)
Causes and mechanisms			
Treatment principles and methods			
Indications			

Note: If related information about the formula is missing in the original text, other arguments or studies can be provided as evidence.

Table 4 Comparison of names of ingredients contained in formulas

	Name of ingredient contained in the original formula	Name of ingredient contained in the current formula	Textual research results
Ingredient 1			
Ingredient 2			
...			

Note: If there is no difference in the names between ancient and current ingredients, this item may not be listed. If any, changes in the origin and processing of an ingredient should be described in this section.

Table 5 Comparison of dosage of ingredients contained in formulas

	Dosage of ingredient contained in the original formula	Ingredient dosage conversion	Dosage of ingredient selected for the current formula	Selection basis of dosage of ingredient
Ingredient 1				
Ingredient 2				
...				

(II) Formula explanation

The principles of forming a formula should be clearly explained under the guidance of TCM theories based on indications, causes and mechanisms, as well as the treatment principles and methods to show the consistency between the formula and indications. The order of ingredients should be consistent with the order in the "formula".

Generally, analysis can be performed based on the formula analysis theory of "Sovereign, Minister, Adjuvant and Courier". For those containing sovereign, minister, adjuvant and courier medicines, the sovereign, minister, adjuvant and courier medicines should be identified and the principle of compatibility should be clarified, and in addition, the function of a single ingredient or the function of combination of multiple ingredients should be described. If not all sovereign, minister, adjuvant and courier medicines are contained or it is difficult to confirm, the sovereign medicine and its function should be identified. Other ingredients should be at least classified by their functions in the formula. It is necessary to distinguish between the sovereign medicines and other medicines, and describe the principle of compatibility and efficacy.

If it is difficult to explain the formula based on "Sovereign, Minister, Adjuvant and Courier", other formula compatibility analysis methods meeting TCM theories can be adopted.

Formula explanation should summarize the functions and compatibility characteristics of the whole formula.

(III) Usage and dosage

The basis for determining usage and dosage should be described based on indications, target population, and theory of drug properties as well as application experience in humans or clinical practice. For special usages of TCM, such as medication guided administration and acupoint administration, the referenced TCM theories should be addressed with emphasis.

For other compound preparations of TCMs originated from ancient classic formulas, the basis for usage and dosage can be described in conjunction with records in ancient books of classic formulas.

IV. Theoretical Basis for Functions and Indications of Formulas

Formulas should be comprehensively reviewed in combination with common understanding of the indications based on TCM theories as well as specific information of formulas. The theoretical basis for determining functions and indications of formulas should be analyzed and described from the aspects of ingredient compatibility principle, extent of agreement between causes and mechanisms of the treated disease, and whether the origin and inheritance of the formula is clear, etc.

V. Safety Analysis of Formulas

(I) Dosage of ingredients

There is a need to list the daily dosage of each ingredient contained in the formula as well as its dosage range in the national drug standards, drug registration standards, or standards of provinces, autonomous regions, and municipalities directly under the Central Government for TCM crude drugs, prepared slices /decoction pieces, or the specifications for processing. If an ingredient is beyond the range, relevant materials can be submitted to illustrate the corresponding basis. The table below can be referenced:

Name of ingredient	Daily dosage	Dosage specified in the standard	Source of the reference standard
Ingredient 1			
Ingredient 2			

(II) Contraindicated combinations and toxic ingredients

Whether the formula contains traditional contraindicated TCM combinations (eighteen antagonisms and nineteen incompatibilities) should be described. Whether the formula contains toxic ingredients marked in existing standards should be specified. At the same time, the ingredients found to have safety risks upon modern pharmacology and toxicology studies or clinical application should also be presented.

(III) Contraindications and precautions for use of formulas

Based on TCM theories and formula characteristics, it is necessary to standardize the expression of patients who should use the formula with caution and those who should not use the formula based on TCM indications or constitutions; contraindications in pregnancy and lactating period; and precautions when taking the medicine together with food or other medicines. Post-administration care, if any, should also be specified.

VI. Comparison with Similar variety of TCMs

Comparison with the marketed variety of TCMs with similar ingredients and consistent functions and indications is required to clarify the characteristics and advantages of the formula.

VII. Other Matters Requiring Explanation

Other necessary contents to be supplemented may be provided in this section.

VIII. References

References should be presented in the standard format.

IX. Annexes

In case of any available literatures or materials supporting the TCM theories used, relevant annexes should be provided here. If the TCM theories used are supported by ancient medical books, the original text can be provided here.

中药新药复方制剂中医药理论申报资料撰写指导原则（试行）

为加快构建中医药理论、人用经验和临床试验相结合的中药注册审评证据体系，按照《中药注册分类及申报资料要求》中临床研究申报资料涉及的中医药理论相关要求，撰写了《中药新药复方制剂中医药理论申报资料撰写指导原则》（试行）。

本指导原则适用于中药新药复方制剂注册申请涉及的中医药理论阐述。其他中药注册申请涉及中医药理论阐述的，可参照执行。

一、处方组成及功能主治简述

应当规范表述处方组成，功能主治。

处方组成药味名称应当与国家药品标准、药品注册标准或省、自治区、直辖市药材/饮片标准或炮制规范中收载的规范名称一致，应当明确每日用各药味药量。中药复方制剂药味的排列顺序需符合中医药的组方原则。

主治需说明处方的具体临床定位，注意区别疾病治疗、对证治疗和症状治疗的表述；说明药物作用特点，如疾病治疗、症状缓解或减轻、对联合用药物的影响等。

古代经典名方中药复方制剂，其功能主治采用中医药术语表述。

二、中医药理论对主治的基本认识

应当说明与主治相关的中医药理论来源。

阐述主治病证的发病原因、疾病发展过程及转归、病证的分期分型等。

运用中医药理论说明与病因病机对应的证候特点、治则治法，以及治疗优势和特点。

使用的中医药理论依据应标明出处，来源于古代医籍的，应标明所属的篇、卷、册，可提供原文；来源于现代中医药理论研究或医家论述的，应当提供文献或其他相关成果等资料，并且论证中医药理论的合理性。

三、拟定处方的中医药理论

（一）处方来源及历史沿革

应当明确处方来源，并简要说明处方药味、处方药量、剂型、适用人群

（主治及人群范围）、用法用量及疗程等的演变情况及依据。可使用文字或表格（见表1）描述处方变化情况。

表1 处方变化情况梳理

处方	变化情况					变化依据
	药味及药量	剂型	适用人群	用法用量	疗程	
处方1						
处方2						
……						

其他来源于古代经典名方的中药复方制剂，应当依据原文中相关内容，通过文字或表格（见表2）简述处方源流（各朝代使用情况、历代医评）。应当通过文字或表格（见表3、表4、表5）列明申报处方与原处方在病因病机、治则治法、主治、药味、药量等方面的对比资料，并给出相应的考证内容，说明处方各药味药量确定的依据。如申报处方在药味基原和炮制方面有变化，应当在此处说明。基于古代经典名方加减化裁的，还应当阐述加减化裁的具体理由，其中源于多个经典名方的，应当阐述其组合使用的缘由，以便为经典名方的确认及人用经验的支持提供依据。

表2 处方源流分析

序号	朝代	出处	作者	论述内容
1				
2				
…				

表3 处方病因病机及治则治法分析

	原方	申报处方	是否一致（否，请说明理由）
病因病机			
治则治法			
主治			

注：如原文中处方相关信息有缺失，可提供其他论述或研究作为佐证。

表 4　处方药味名对比

	原方药味名	现处方药味名	考据情况
药味 1			
药味 2			
…			

注：若无古今药味名差异的，可不列此项。如药味基原和炮制有变化的，应当在此处说明。

表 5　处方各药味药量对比

	原方药量	药量换算	现处方选择药量	药量选择依据
药味 1				
药味 2				
…				

（二）方解

应当以中医药理论为指导，围绕主治病证的病因病机和治则治法，清晰阐释组方原理，体现方证一致。药味出现顺序应与"处方"中顺序一致。

一般可以采用"君臣佐使"的组方分析理论进行分析：对于君药、臣药、佐药和使药齐备者，方解中应当明确君药、臣药、佐药和使药及其配伍原理，说明单味药的功效或多味药相合的功效；对于君药、臣药、佐药和使药难以齐备或确定者，应当明确君药及其功效，其他药味至少按其方药作用归类，分清主次，说明配伍原理和功效。

难以采用"君臣佐使"的方式进行方解的，可以采用其他符合中医药理论的组方配伍分析方法。

方解应当归纳全方的功能和配伍特点。

（三）用法用量

应当结合主治病证、用药人群、药性理论等特点和人用经验或临床实践的结果，说明用法用量确定的依据。对于中医特色的用法（如药引、穴位给药等），应当着重阐述其所依据的中医药理论。

其他来源于古代经典名方的中药复方制剂，可结合经典名方古籍中的记载，说明用法用量确定的依据。

四、处方功能主治确定的理论依据

结合中医药理论对主治的普遍认识及处方情况，对处方进行综合评述，分析说明处方功能主治确定的理论依据，可依据组方配伍法则与所治疗疾病病因病机契合度、处方传承来源是否清晰等方面进行阐述。

五、处方安全性分析

（一）用药剂量

列明处方中各药味的日用量，及其在国家药品标准、药品注册标准或省、自治区、直辖市药材/饮片标准或炮制规范中的用量范围。如有超出范围的情况，可提交相关资料以说明合理性。可参考下表：

药味名	日用量	标准中用量	引用标准出处
处方药味 1			
处方药味 2			

（二）配伍禁忌及毒性药味

说明处方中是否含有中药传统配伍禁忌（十八反、十九畏）。明确处方是否含已有标准中标注具有毒性的药味。同时，如涉及现代药理毒理研究或临床应用发现有安全性风险的药味，应当一并列出。

（三）使用处方的禁忌与注意

根据中医药理论及处方特点，规范表述基于中医病证或体质等因素需要慎用、禁用者；妊娠、哺乳期等特殊情况下的禁忌；在饮食以及与其他药物同时应用等方面的注意。如有药后调护，应当予以明确。

六、和同类品种的比较

与已上市组方类同、功能主治一致的品种进行对比，以说明处方的特点和优势。

七、其他需要说明的事项

如有其他需补充的内容，可在此项下提供。

八、参考文献

应当以参考文献标准格式列明参考文献。

九、附件

所依据的中医药理论如有文献或成果支持，应在此处提供相关附件；如有古代医籍支持，可在此处提供原文。

The Guideline for Clinical Trials of New Traditional Chinese Medicines (TCMs) for Patterns

Patterns (synonym: syndromes) highly generalize the causes, nature, location, and tendency of a disease (unhealthy condition in general) which has been developed to a certain stage, manifested by a group of symptoms and signs with internal correlation, and is also the basis for TCM clinical diagnosis and treatment. In order to better inherit and develop the characteristics and advantages of TCM, the National Medical Products Administration (NMPA) has formulated the *Guideline for Clinical Trials of New Traditional Chinese Medicines (TCMs) for Patterns* (hereinafter referred to as the Guideline) according to relevant regulations on the registration of medicines.

New TCMs for patterns refer to new TCM compound preparations whose indications are TCM patterns. The Guideline is intended to provide fundamental guidance for the conduct of clinical trials and the evaluation of efficacy and safety of new TCMs for patterns. Each principle requirement in the text will be further enriched and developed to detailed technical standards with subsequent in-depth research.

I. Formula Sources and Basic Requirements for New TCMs for Patterns

The formulas of new TCMs for patterns should be derived from clinical practice, meet TCM theories, and reflect the principle of consistency among theory, method, formula and medicine. In order to apply for clinical trials of new TCMs for patterns, there should be adequate supporting documentation on the history of human use, including the formula source, basis of formula composition, clinical application (including the evolution process of clinical practice to improve formulas), functions and indications, usage and dosage, and other relevant details. If the new TCMs for patterns to be developed is based on the accumulation of clinical TCM experience and intended for common patterns in clinical settings, relevant evidence should be provided. If it is from a relatively mature and effective formula found during comparative analysis and study of medical case reports, the typical medical case reports and serial medical case reports should be provided. If it is a mature and effective formula with certain clinical study bases and available supporting data, relevant clinical study summary reports should be provided, which should clarify TCM patterns, efficacy characteristics, and safety information. If it is from clinical study achievements supported by national scientific and technological programs, summary materials of clinical studies and relevant achievement appraisal materials should be provided.

When developing new TCMs for patterns, it is necessary to evaluate the difference in clinical value from similar marketed medicines to clarify whether they have clinical development value.

II. Possible Targets of New TCMs for Patterns

New TCMs for patterns should be positioned clinically to eliminate, improve, or control the main clinical symptoms and signs of a group of diseases with inherent correlations. They can also be positioned to treat diseases by improving patterns.

III. Diagnosis of Patterns of New TCMs for Patterns

TCM patterns identification for the development of new TCMs should be based on relevant clinical practices and adhere to TCM theories.

The diagnostic criteria for TCM patterns can be developed based on relevant national standards, industry standards, and association standards, etc. If there are no applicable diagnostic criteria, they can be self-developed and agreed upon to reach expert consensus through expert argumentation. The elements of pattern diagnosis can be determined in a qualitative or semi-quantitative manner or using the method of primary and secondary symptoms. It is encouraged to develop pattern diagnosis scales with TCM characteristics supplemented with objective diagnostic indicators depending on the specific study contents.

IV. Basic Study Categories and Clinical Trial Design for New TCMs for Patterns

(I) Basic study categories

There are multiple modes for clinical studies of new TCMs for patterns, such as simple TCM pattern study, study on the combination of TCM diseases and patterns, or study on TCM patterns that integrate diseases. Regardless of the study mode, studies of new TCMs for patterns should clearly define the dynamic change laws of the studied pattern and the specific stage of relevant disease.

1. Simple TCM pattern study

The study can be performed by selecting the applicable population meeting certain TCM pattern diagnostic criteria to observe the improvement of symptoms, signs, and relevant indicators involved in the TCM pattern with the medicine.

2. TCM disease and pattern study

In the context of meeting the diagnostic criteria of a certain TCM disease, a specific pattern of the TCM disease should be selected for study to observe the improvement of symptoms, signs, and relevant indicators of the pattern with the medicine.

3. Study on the combination of disease and pattern

Under the guidance of TCM diagnosis and treatment mode of "same treatment for different diseases" and "integrating diseases based on pattern", if different diseases have the same mechanism characteristics and similar pattern elements at a certain stage during the occurrence and development of the diseases, at least 3 diseases that belong to the same pattern can be selected for study to highlight the pattern-centered design concept and observe the efficacy of the medicine on TCM patterns and diseases.

(II) Design considerations

1. Inclusion criteria

The inclusion criteria should be developed by taking into account the objective and implementation process of the clinical trial, including the requirements for adherence to relevant diagnostic criteria and baseline consistency in terms of subjects' conditions and disease progression. It is recommended to include patients stable on basic treatment and pattern manifestations, and patients whose basic treatment is in a dynamic adjustment stage should not be included. When incorporating diseases, attention should be paid to understanding the relationship between the pattern and western medical treatment. Clinical trial designers can develop reasonable inclusion criteria according to the needs of the clinical trial. Subjects should voluntarily participate in clinical trials with full informed consent.

2. Exclusion criteria

The population with other patterns that may affect the diagnosis of the target pattern or the judgment of efficacy should be excluded. The exclusion criteria should be developed based on considerations for subject safety. The circumstances where disease progression is covered by symptom improvement should be ruled out. Specific populations that may experience serious consequences or accelerated disease progression after taking the medicine should be excluded.

3. Clinical trial design

Various clinical trial designs can be applied to exploratory studies depending on the objective of the clinical trial. Confirmatory studies should follow the principles of being randomized, double-blind, controlled, and reproducible, and it is required to estimate the sample size based on the preliminary results of exploratory studies.

If the add-on design is used, the basic treatment must be predetermined, such as indications of medicines, types of medicines, dosage, usage and time of administration for the basic treatment.

4. Comparator

Placebo is preferred as the control drug. If Chinese proprietary medicines for the same pattern have been commercially available, industry-recognized Chinese proprietary medicines can be chosen as a positive control, but its efficacy must be confirmed through placebo-control trials.

The placebos should be as close as possible to the investigational drug in terms of the dosage form, appearance, flavor, taste, texture and other characteristics to ensure that the clinical study is conducted with investigators and subjects blinded. When a positive drug with a different dosage form is used as a control, double-blind, double-dummy techniques must be used to ensure that the study is conducted under blinded conditions.

If a clinical study involves multiple diseases, stratified randomization should be used based on the included diseases to ensure that the baseline between groups is comparable and to avoid affecting efficacy evaluation of the medicine.

V. Course of Treatment and Follow-up

Observation time points and the course of treatment should be set reasonably based on the characteristics of the medicine and pre-study information. Moreover, the follow-up methods, time points, and contents should be scientifically designed according to different study objectives.

VI. Efficacy Evaluation

New TCMs for patterns should adopt scientifically recognized standards for evaluating the efficacy in TCM patterns. The primary and secondary efficacy outcomes should be determined based on the study objective, and the evaluation of the clinical value of efficacy in the pattern should be emphasized. The selection of efficacy outcomes are as follows:

1. For those intended to improve target symptoms or signs, the disappearance rate/normalization rate or clinical control rate of the target symptoms or signs should be used as the efficacy endpoint. However, attention should also be paid to evaluating the recovery time and/or the onset time of target symptoms or signs.

2. It is suggested to include patient-reported outcome measures and integrate "self-evaluation" by patients with "other evaluation" by doctors.

3. It is encouraged to use objective response indicators that can reflect the efficacy in the pattern for efficacy evaluation. Objective indicators of efficacy in

the pattern include physiological and biochemical parameters and biomarkers in modern medicine. During clinical trials, it is necessary to observe and evaluate the onset time, remission time, or disappearance time of the TCM pattern.

4. Based on considerations of improving the quality of life, activities of daily living, and adaptive capacity, it is recommended to use recognized universal or specific scales for quality of life, activities of daily living, and adaptive capacity in the evaluation of efficacy. The efficacy can also be evaluated using evaluation tools for efficacy in TCM patterns developed based on scientific principles.

5. It is encouraged to evaluate the efficacy using outcome measures or surrogate measures reflecting the disease progression.

VII. Safety Evaluation

Safety evaluation can be performed in conjunction with disease-related examinations of subjects, such as some physiological and biochemical parameters that can reflect the progression of the disease; in addition, safety evaluation must reflect the safety of the investigational drug through parallel control with placebo or positive drugs. During the clinical trial, investigators need to pay attention to changes in TCM patterns and disease progression, and timely evaluate possible risks of the medicine.

VIII. Quality Control and Data Management of Clinical Trials

(I) Information collection

The collection of information from the four diagnostic methods in TCM is necessary for modern studies on TCM patterns. The collection of information about TCM data is beneficial for controlling the quality of clinical trials. It is suggested that the information collection from the four diagnostic methods of TCM be based on the latest *Operation Specifications for Four Diagnostic Methods in Traditional Chinese Medicine* (TCM Diagnosis Society of China Association of Chinese Medicine), and that investigators develop the "Standard Operating Procedure (SOP) for Information Collection from Four Diagnostic Methods" according to the Specifications and strictly adhere to it. Before the clinical trial, staff of study sites should receive training in the standardization of information collection from four diagnostic methods in TCM, and the consistency in information collection from four diagnostic methods in TCM of the investigators of study sites should be evaluated.

Information collection from four diagnostic methods in TCM should comply with the principle of objectivity. The information collection tools can be paper versions of collection forms, graphic collection systems based on computer software, or even applications of TCM artificial intelligence and cloud computing in the future. The information collection form/system for four diagnostic methods in TCM can be universal or specific, and presented in the form of quantitative evaluation. It is encouraged to introduce nationally approved and relatively mature information collection devices for four diagnostic methods in TCM, such as tongue diagnostic instrument and pulse diagnostic instrument, which should have functions of real-time display, storage and repetition conducive to the traceability of clinical trial data.

(II) Data management

Sponsors and investigators should strengthen data management. It is recommended that an independent data monitoring committee be established for clinical study projects of new TCMs for patterns. Investigators are encouraged to use an electronic data collection system to ensure the authenticity and reliability of the collected study data. In addition, clinical trial risk control plans and measures, clinical trial data management plans and reports, data verification plans and reports, as well as statistical analysis plans and reports, should be developed for clinical study projects so as to promote the overall quality control of clinical trials for new TCMs for patterns.

(III) Study personnel

The principal investigator (PI) should hold senior and above technical titles in TCM or integrative medicine. Investigators should hold deputy senior technical titles in TCM or integrative medicine.

IX. Principles for Drafting of Package Inserts

The [Functions and Indications] of the package inserts for new TCMs for patterns should be expressed using TCM terms. The [Clinical Trials] should briefly summarize the clinical trials that support the marketing of the medicine. Other contents of the package insert can be written in reference to the *Provisions for Drug Package Inserts and Labels* and relevant TCM guidelines.

References

[1] Kou Guanjun, Tang Jianyuan. Current Status of Research on Patterns in Traditional Chinese Medicine and Keys to Research on TCMs for Patterns [J]. Pharmacology and Clinics of Chinese Materia Medica, 2017, 33(04):213-214.

[2] Guo Jie, Dong Yu, Tang Jianyuan. Discussion on Clinical Problems about Bases of New Drugs of Traditional Chinese Medicine Development[J]. China Journal of Chinese Materia Medica, 2017, 42(05):844-847.

[3] Gao Ying, Wu Shengxian, Wang Shaoqing, Wang Zhong, Wang Yongyan. Thinking on Chinese Medicine Diagnosis Model in Clinical Trials of Syndrome Class New Drug[J]. Chinese Journal of Integrative Medicine on Cardio-Cerebrovascular Disease, 2014, 12(08):1010-1012.

[4] Li Bing, Wang Zhong, Zhang Yingying, et al. Overview of Common Methods and Applications in the Study of TCM Patterns Classification[J]. Journal of Basic Chinese Medicine, 2014, 20(01):30-33+36.

[5] Li Bing, Wang Zhong, Zhang Yingying, et al. Clinical Literature Based Statistical Analysis of Common Chinese Medical Syndrome Types[J]. Chinese Journal of Integrated Traditional and Western Medicine, 2014, 34(08):1013-1016.

[6] Wu Wenbin, An Na, Pei Xiaojing, et al. Based on the thought of "preventive treatment of disease" to explore clinical study on new drugs of syndrome traditional Chinese medicine[J]. Pharmacology and Clinics of Chinese Materia Medica, 2017, 33(03):209-211.

[7] Wang Shaoqing, Gao Ying. Discussion on the Clinical Research Methods of New TCMs for Patterns from the Combination of TCM Syndromes and Diseases[J]. Global Traditional Chinese Medicine, 2014, 7(09):724-726.

[8] Lin Fangbing, Liu Qiang, Zhu Wenhao, et al. Discussion on the Research

and Development Strategy of the New Medicine of Syndrome TCM Based on Formulas and Patterns [J]. Global Traditional Chinese Medicine, 2015, 8(05):557-560.

[9] Shang Hongcai, Wang Baohe, Zhang Boli. Evaluation of Syndrome and Therapeutic Efficacy of New TCMs[J]. Traditional Chinese Drug Research and Clinical Pharmacology, 2004(05):365-368.

[10] An Yu, Wang Jie, Li Zhaoling. Study on the current situation and development in clinical efficacy evaluation of new traditional Chinese medicine[J]. China Journal of Traditional Chinese Medicine and Pharmacy, 2015, 30(01):9-11.

[11] Wang Shaoqing, Gao Ying, Wu Shengxian. Thoughts on the Clinical Evaluation Methodology of New Medicine of Syndrome TCM[J]. World Chinese Medicine, 2014, 9(08):1093-1095.

[12] Shen Chunti, Zhang Lei, Wang Zhong, et al. Discussion on the Standardization of the Collection of Information from the Four Diagnostic Methods in Clinical Trials of New TCMs for Patterns [J]. Journal of Traditional Chinese Medicine, 2013, 54(15):1265-1267.

[13] Wang Tianfang, Li Candong, Zhu Wenfeng, et al. Expert Consensus on Standardized Operations for the Four Diagnostic Methods in Traditional Chinese Medicine[J]. China Journal of Traditional Chinese Medicine and Pharmacy, 2018, 33(01):185-192.

证候类中药新药临床研究技术指导原则

　　证候（简称证）是对疾病（泛指非健康）发展到一定阶段的病因、病性、病位及病势等的高度概括，具体表现为一组有内在联系的症状和体征，是中医临床诊断和治疗的依据。为了更好地传承和发扬中医药特色和优势，国家药品监督管理局根据药品注册相关法规，特制定《证候类中药新药临床研究技术指导原则》（以下简称《指导原则》）。

　　证候类中药新药是指主治为证候的中药复方制剂新药。《指导原则》旨在为证候类中药新药临床试验的开展和有效性、安全性评价提供基础性指导，其正文内容中的每一个原则性要求都可以随着后续研究的不断深入，进一步丰富和发展为更详实具体的技术标准。

一、证候类中药新药的处方来源及基本要求

　　证候类中药新药的处方应来源于临床实践，符合中医药理论，体现理、法、方、药相一致的原则。证候类中药新药申请临床试验应有充分的人用历史证明性文献材料，包括处方来源、组方合理性、临床应用情况（包括提供临床实践完善处方的演变过程）、功能主治、用法用量等相关内容。如拟开发的证候类中药新药是来源于中医临床经验的积累，针对临床常见基本证候的，应提供相关证明；如是源于医案中对比分析研究所发现的相对成熟有效的处方，应提供典型医案和系列医案；如具有一定临床研究基础且有相应数据证明的成熟有效的处方，应提供相关临床研究总结报告，该总结报告应明确具体中医证候、疗效特点和安全性信息；如是源于国家科技立项的临床研究成果，应提供临床研究部分的总结资料及相关的成果鉴定材料。

　　证候类中药新药立项开发时，应注意评估与已上市同类药品的临床价值差异，以明确其是否具备临床开发价值。

二、证候类中药新药的临床定位

　　证候类中药新药临床应定位于消除、改善或控制具有内在关联性的一组疾病的主要临床症状、体征等，也可定位于通过证候改善达到疾病治疗等目的。

三、证候类中药新药的证候诊断

拟开发新药的中医证候确定应有与之相关的临床实践基础，并应遵循中医药理论。

中医证候诊断标准可以参照有关国家标准、行业标准或团体标准等进行制定，如无适用的诊断标准，可自行制定并经专家论证达成共识。证候诊断构成要素可采用定性或半定量方式，或主次症的方法，鼓励制定具有中医特色的证候诊断量表，并可根据具体研究内容辅以客观诊断指标。

四、证候类中药新药的基本研究思路及试验设计

（一）基本研究思路

证候类中药新药临床研究可有多种模式，如单纯中医证候研究模式、中医病证结合研究模式或中医证统西医病的研究模式，无论何种研究模式，证候类中药新药研究均应对所研究证候的动态变化规律及相关西医疾病所处特定阶段要有明确的界定。

1. 单纯中医证候研究

选择符合某个中医证候诊断标准的适应人群进行研究，观察药物对该中医证候所涉及的症状、体征以及相关指标的改善情况。

2. 中医病证研究

在符合某一中医疾病诊断标准的基础上，选取该病的某一证候进行研究，观察药物对该证候所涉及的症状、体征以及相关指标的改善情况。

3. 证病结合研究

在中医"异病同治""以证统病"诊治思维模式的指导下，基于不同疾病发生发展过程中的某个阶段出现有相同病机特点、相似证候要素的，可以在同一证候下选择至少 3 个不同西医疾病来进行研究，突出以证候为中心的设计理念，观察药物对中医证候疗效以及西医疾病的疗效。

（二）设计考虑

1. 纳入标准

纳入标准的制定，应考虑到临床试验目的以及实施过程，包括应符合相关诊断标准的规定，受试者在病情、病程等基线一致性方面的规定。建议纳入基础治疗和证候表现基本稳定的患者，对基础治疗处于动态调整阶段的患者不宜纳入。纳入西医疾病时应注意把握证候与西医治疗之间的关系。试验设计者可根据试验的需要制定合理的纳入标准。受试者应在充分知情同意的情况下自愿

参加临床试验。

2. 排除标准

应排除兼夹影响目标证候诊断或证候疗效判断的其他证候的人群。应基于受试者安全性的角度考虑排除标准，应排除通过改善症状可能导致掩盖病情进展的情形，排除服药后会发生严重后果或加速疾病进程的特定人群。

3. 试验设计

探索性研究可以根据试验目的采用多种试验设计。确证性研究应遵循随机、双盲、对照、重复的原则，并基于探索性研究的初步结果去估算样本量。

如采用加载设计，须事先规定好基础治疗，如基础治疗的用药指征、用药种类、用药剂量、用药方法、用药时间等。

4. 对照药

对照药宜首选安慰剂。如果已有用于该证候的中成药上市，可选择业内所公认的中成药进行阳性对照，但该药的有效性须经过安慰剂对照确证。

安慰剂应在剂型、外观、气味、口感、质感等特征上与试验药物尽量接近，确保临床研究者和受试者在盲态下开展研究。如采用阳性药对照且剂型不一致时，需通过双盲双模拟技术保证盲态实施。

临床研究如果涉及多个西医疾病，应结合所纳入的疾病情况，采用分层随机，以保证组间基线具有可比，以免影响药物的疗效评价。

五、疗程及随访

应根据药物特点和前期研究信息合理设置观测时点及疗程，并根据研究目的的不同，科学设计随访的方式、时点、内容等。

六、有效性评价

证候类中药新药应采用科学公认的中医证候疗效评价标准，根据研究目的确定好主要疗效指标和次要疗效指标，应重视证候疗效的临床价值评估。疗效指标选择如下：

1. 以改善目标症状或体征为目的者，应以目标症状或体征消失率/复常率，或临床控制率为疗效评价指标，但同时应注意观察目标症状或体征痊愈时间和/或起效时间的评价。

2. 建议引入患者报告结局指标，将患者"自评"与医生"他评"相结合。

3. 鼓励采用能够反映证候疗效的客观应答指标进行评价。证候疗效的客观指标，包括现代医学中的理化指标、生物标志物等。临床试验期间需观察评估中医证候疗效的起效时间、缓解时间或消失时间。

4. 基于生存质量或生活能力、适应能力改善等方面的考虑，推荐采用公认具有普适性或特异性的生存质量或生活能力、适应能力等量表进行疗效评价。也可采用基于科学原则所开发的中医证候疗效评价工具进行疗效评价。

5. 鼓励采用反映疾病的结局指标或替代指标进行疗效评价。

七、安全性评价

安全性评价可以结合受试者疾病相关检查去评估，如某些能够反映疾病病情进展的理化检查指标；安全性评价必须通过与安慰剂或阳性药的平行对照去反映试验药物的安全性。临床试验期间，研究者需关注中医证候的变化情况以及疾病进展情况，及时评估可能存在的用药风险。

八、试验质量控制与数据管理

（一）信息采集

中医四诊信息采集是现代中医证候研究的必需手段，中医数据的信息化采集有利于临床试验质量的控制。建议中医四诊信息采集应参照最新的"中医四诊操作规范（中华中医药学会中医诊断分会）"制定，研究者应据此制定"四诊信息采集标准操作规程（SOP）"并严格执行。临床试验前，应对各临床研究中心进行四诊信息采集规范化培训，并对各临床研究中心研究者的四诊信息采集进行一致性评价。

四诊信息采集应遵循客观化原则。其信息采集工具可以是纸质版采集表，或基于计算机软件的图文采集系统，乃至未来中医人工智能和云计算的应用。四诊信息采集表/系统，可以是普适性也可以是特异性，并以量化评定的形式呈现。鼓励引入经国家批准上市、较为成熟的四诊信息采集仪如舌诊仪、脉诊仪等配合使用，该仪器应具有实时显示、存储和复读功能，有利于临床试验数据可溯源。

（二）数据管理

申办方和研究者应加强数据管理工作，建议证候类中药新药临床研究项目须成立独立的数据监察委员会，鼓励研究者应通过电子数据采集系统采集数据以确保研究数据的真实性和可靠性。另外，临床研究项目应制定临床试验风险控制计划及措施、临床试验数据管理计划与报告、数据核查计划与报告、统计分析计划与报告等，以促进证候类中药新药临床试验整体质量控制水平的提升。

（三）研究人员

主要研究者必须是具备中医专业或中西医结合专业的正高级技术职称及其以上的人员。研究者必须是具备中医专业或中西医结合专业的副高级技术职称的人员。

九、说明书撰写原则

证候类中药新药的说明书【功能主治】项的内容应符合中医术语表述，【临床试验】项的内容会就支持该药上市的临床试验情况进行简要概述。说明书其余内容可参照《药品说明书和标签管理规定》和中药相关指导原则执行。

参考文献

［1］寇冠军，唐健元. 中医证候研究现状及证候中药研究关键［J］. 中药药理与临床，2017，33（04）：213-214.

［2］郭洁，董宇，唐健元. 中药复方新药立题依据的临床问题探讨［J］. 中国中药杂志，2017，42（05）：844-847.

［3］高颖，吴圣贤，王少卿，王忠，王永炎. 证候类中药新药临床试验的证候诊断路径思考［J］. 中西医结合心脑血管病杂志，2014，12（08）：1010-1012.

［4］李兵，王忠，张莹莹，等. 中医证候分类研究常用方法与应用概述［J］. 中国中医基础医学杂志，2014，20（01）：30-33+36.

［5］李兵，王忠，张莹莹，等. 基于文献的中医临床常见证型统计分析［J］. 中国中西医结合杂志，2014，34（08）：1013-1016.

［6］吴文斌，安娜，裴小静，等. 基于"治未病"探讨证候类中药新药的临床研究［J］. 中药药理与临床，2017，33（03）：209-211.

［7］王少卿，高颖. 从证病结合模式探讨证候类中药新药的临床研究方法［J］. 环球中医药，2014，7（09）：724-726.

［8］林芳冰，刘强，朱文浩，等. 浅谈基于方证的证候类中药新药研发策略［J］. 环球中医药，2015，8（05）：557-560.

［9］商洪才，王保和，张伯礼. 中药新药证候及疗效评价［J］. 中药新药与临床药理，2004（05）：365-368.

［10］安宇，王阶，李赵陵. 中药新药临床疗效评价的现状与发展［J］. 中华中医药杂志，2015，30（01）：9-11.

［11］王少卿，高颖，吴圣贤. 证候类中药新药临床评价方法的思考［J］.

世界中医药，2014，9（08）：1093–1095.

［12］申春悌，张磊，王忠，等. 试论证候类中药新药临床试验四诊信息采集规范［J］. 中医杂志，2013，54（15）：1265–1267.

［13］王天芳，李灿东，朱文锋. 中医四诊操作规范专家共识［J］. 中华中医药杂志，2018，33（01）：185–192.

Guideline for Writing of Reference Safety Information in Investigator's Brochures

I. Overview

Reference safety information (RSI) is usually a list of expected serious adverse reactions in Investigator's Brochures (IBs). The sponsor should assess the expectedness of all suspected serious adverse reactions occurring during the clinical trial based on the RSI.

These Guidelines are intended to guide the writing of RSI in IBs for approved drug clinical trials (including traditional Chinese medicines (TCMs), chemical drugs and biological products). In addition to these Guidelines, please also refer to the International Council for Harmonisation of Technical Requirements for Pharmaceuticals for Human Use (ICH) Guidelines, e.g., *E2A: Clinical Safety Data Management: Definitions and Standards for Expedited Reporting and E2F: Development Safety Update Report.*

These Guidelines only represent the current views and understandings of the drug regulatory authority, and are not legally binding. With the progress of scientific research, the relevant content in the Guidelines will be refined and updated. These Guidelines provide general considerations for writing RSI and may not be able to cover all situations. If any individual problems are not clarified herein, you may communicate with the Center for Drug Evaluation.

II. Contents of Reference Safety Information

(I) Expected serious adverse reactions

Expected serious adverse reactions (SARs) are serious adverse events (SAEs) that have occurred at least once in completed and ongoing drug clinical trials, for which there is reasonable evidence to establish a causal relationship with the investigational drug after a full and comprehensive assessment by the sponsor, such as by comparing the frequency of SAEs in clinical trials, or by making an adequate assessment of the causal relationship reported in individual cases. Adverse reactions (ARs) that are expected to occur based solely on pharmacological properties but have not been observed with the investigational drug are not considered expected ARs, which can also refer to other sections of the IB (e.g.,"Effects in the Humans" or "Summary of Data and Guidance for the Investigator").

In general, a suspected SAR that has occurred only once is not sufficient to be included in the RSI, unless based on the sponsor's medical judgment, there is strong evidence to prove that it has a clear causal relationship with the investigational drug, and relevant supporting evidence should be provided. Moreover, not all suspected SARs that have occurred more than once should be listed in the RSI as expected SARs. Instead, the sponsor needs to conduct a full and comprehensive assessment, and provides relevant supporting evidence while listing the expected SARs.

Given the fact that multiple causality assessment methods are currently available, it is allowed to use one or more methods to assess whether adverse events occurring in clinical trials are causally related to the investigational drug. According to the ICH E2A, an adverse drug reaction is one where there is at least a reasonable probability of correlation between the investigational drug and the AE, that is, a causal relationship cannot be ruled out. Therefore, an "unlikely related" causal relationship should be assessed with caution. If the investigator is unable to determine the correlation of an AE with the investigational drug (i.e., "unevaluable"), the sponsor should communicate with the investigator and encourage the investigator to assess the correlation rigorously. If the judgment result remains to be "unevaluable", the SAE should be considered to be related to the investigational drug and reported as a suspected unexpected serious adverse reaction (SUSAR). However, the inclusion of "unevaluable" SAEs as expected SARs in the RSI is not supported.

(II) Fatal and/or life-threatening serious adverse reactions

In general, the sponsor should not expect fatal and/or life-threatening SARs with the investigational drug. Therefore, even if a fatal and/or life-threatening SAR has occurred before, it is generally considered to be unexpected. However, fatal SARs that are stated in the package insert of marketed medicines can be regarded as expected SARs. Therefore, for investigational drugs that are not yet available on the market, fatal SARs should not be listed in the RSI.

If there are expected fatal and/or life-threatening SARs listed in the RSI section , the RSI should include the number and frequency of such SARs, these data should be provided in separate columns.If fatal and/or life-threatening expected SARs are included in the RSI, the number and frequency of such SARs should be listed separately. For other fatal and/or life-threatening suspected SARs that are considered to be unexpected, see the section of the IB "Effects in the Humans" or "Summary of Data and Guidance for the Investigator".

(III) Circumstances deemed as unexpected due to specificity and/or severity

A provision of severity grades using Common Terminology Criteria for Adverse Events (CTCAEs) grading system in the RSI is not required. However, if the specificity and/or severity of a suspected SAR in the individual case report is different from the expected SARs in the RSI, that is, the suspected SAR is more specific and/or of a higher severity grade than the expected SARs in the RSI, the suspected SAR is considered to be unexpected (refer to Table 1).

Table 1 Examples of SUSAR and reasons for reporting

Listed SARs in RSI	Suspected SARs in individual Case Reports	Unexpected due to specificity and/or severity
Acute renal failure	Interstitial nephritis	Specificity
Hepatitis	Fulminant hepatitis	Severity
Cerebral vascular accident	Cerebral thromboembolism	Specificity
Exfoliative dermatitis	Stevens-Johnson syndrome	Severity and specificity
Transient increase in liver function tests	Increased liver function tests persisting for several months	Severity

continued

Listed SARs in RSI	Suspected SARs in individual Case Reports	Unexpected due to specificity and/or severity
Hypertension	Hypertensive crisis	Severity
Herpes zoster	Multiple cutaneous herpes zoster	Severity
Sepsis	Septic shock	Severity
Supraventricular Cardiac Arrhythmia	Atrial fibrillation	Specificity

Note: The above examples are only circumstances that are more specific and/or of a higher severity grade, rather than the Preferred Terms (PTs) for expected SARs in the RSI.

A suspected SAR is considered to be unexpected if its frequency is higher than that of the expected SARs in the RSI.

It is recommended that a medical and scientific assessment of the specificity and/or severity of suspected SARs be performed by the sponsor's trained professionals.

(IV) Safety information not to be included in the reference safety information

The following safety information should not be included in the RSI, but should be presented in the "Effects in the Humans" or "Summary of Data and Guidance for the Investigator"section of the IB.

For example:

(1) Adverse events that were considered unrelated to the investigational drug by both the investigator and the sponsor, including SAEs and non-SAEs.

(2) Non-serious ARs.

(3) Unexpected SARs.

(4) SARs that have occurred only once, for which strong evidence based on medical judgment to prove that it has a clear causal relationship with the investigational drug cannot be provided.

(5) In the clinical trial protocol, death events and SAEs are often used as efficacy endpoints and considered disease-related, and not reported as SUSARs. However, if the investigational drug enhances the severity of AEs or increases the frequency of AEs, a careful assessment is required.

(6) SARs that are expected to occur based on pharmacological properties, have occurred with other similar medicines, but have not been observed with the investigational drug.

III. Form of Presentation of Reference Safety Information

(I) Location

The RSI is titled "Reference Safety Information", and located in the "Summary of Data and Guidance for the Investigator"chapter, or after the "Summary of Data and Guidance for the Investigator"chapter as a separate chapter.

The sponsor should clearly state that the RSI summarizes the current expected SARs of the investigational drug for reporting purposes to regulatory authorities, and that the RSI does not provide a comprehensive overview of the safety profile of the investigational drug.

(II) Form of presentation

The RSI should be presented in the form of a table, where the nature of the "expected SARs"must be listed by system organ class (SOC) and using preferred terms (PTs) as per the latest MedDRA version, in which previously observed suspected SARs are summarized and their frequencies are calculated. For the frequency categories, please refer to the classification of the frequency of adverse reactions in the package insert (such as Very Common, Common, and Uncommon, etc.). If there is an insufficient number of subjects exposed to the investigational drug, making classification impossible, or the number of expected SARs observed is small, the number of each"expected SAR"should be provided together with the number of subjects exposed (refer to Table 2).

The RSI may include SARs that have been observed in post-market experience, but the frequency should not be filled out as "unknown". Since the actual post-market frequency categories cannot be collected precisely, the number of reports for each SAR should be provided, or the frequency categories[1] can be provided according to the method in the *Guide for Spontaneous Reporting of Adverse Reactions* (refer to Table 2).

Table 2 Expected SARs of the investigational drug for
safety reporting purposes

SOC	SARs	Number of subjects exposed (N)=328		
		All SARs	Fatal SARs[1]	Life-threatening SARs[1]
		n (%)	n (%)	n (%)
Gastro-intestinal disorders	Intestinal perforation	9 (2.7)	3 (0.9)	6 (1.8)
Tests	Alanine aminotransferase increase	12 (3.6)	NA	NA
	Aspartate aminotransferase increase	9 (2.7)	NA	NA
Cardiac disorders	Myocarditis	33 (10.0)	NA	2 (0.6)
	Bradycardia	(Rare)[2]	NA	NA

Note: SOC: System Organ Class; SARs: Serious Adverse Reactions; n: Number of subjects who have experienced the SAR; NA: Not Applicable.

Note 1: Under special circumstances, if an investigational drug is considered to have the potential of causing fatal and/or life-threatening expected SARs, it should be clearly listed in the table. For other unexpected fatal and/or life-threatening SARs (lines), it is feasible to fill in "NA" and state in a footnote that "For unexpected fatal and/or life-threatening SARs, please refer to other sections of the IB". If the investigational drug is considered to be free of fatal and/or life-threatening expected SARs, it should be stated separately in the text of the RSI, and there is no need to list the corresponding column in the table.

Note 2: Bradycardia is derived from post-market safety information, and frequency categories are provided according to the methods in the *Guide for Spontaneous Reporting of Adverse Reactions*.

---

2 A Guideline on Summary of Product Characteristics (SmPC), September 2009, 2nd edition
https://ec.europa.eu/health/sites/default/files/files/eudralex/vol-2/c/smpc_guideline_rev2_en.pdf

While the sponsor is conducting clinical development of the investigational drug for different indications (e.g., tumor or non-tumor diseases) or different populations (e.g., adults or children), if the expected SARs are different, the RSI should be listed separately by indication or population.

(III) Terms for expected SARs

The use of medical concepts or unspecific terms in the RSI of an IB, e.g. "Rash", "Infections" or "Arrhythmia" is not acceptable. Only MedDRA preferred terms (PTs) e.g. exfoliative dermatitis, urticarial rash or hives, herpes zoster, pneumonia, sepsis, atrial fibrillation are allowed. If there are multiple lower level terms (LLTs) within a single PT they are all expected (for example if the PT hypophosphataemia is included in the RSI table, then the LLT hypophosphatemia is also considered expected). Immunosuppressive medicines may lead to infection, but not all types of infection can be considered as expected. An infection should be considered unexpected unless its PT is listed in the RSI.

Synonymous medical terms represent the same medical phenomenon, and if the RSI contains a term, its other synonymous medical terms are considered expected. However, for different forms of the same medical phenomenon, e.g. different forms of rash such as rash generalized, rash maculo-papular, rash papular, rash pustular, etc., specific PTs have to be used.

(IV) Reference safety information for expected SARs not found yet

In some cases, the investigational drug may not be expected to cause any SARs (such as early in the clinical development of an investigational drug when subject exposure is low), but a clearly defined section of the IB called RSI should still be present, followed by a brief text stating that no SARs are considered expected by the sponsor for the purpose of expedited reporting to regulatory authorities and identification of SUSARs in the "Cumulative Summary Tabulations of Serious Adverse Reactions" in the Development Safety Update Report (DSUR).

IV. Applicable Version of Reference Safety Information

The RSI in place at the time of occurrence of the suspected SAR should be used to assess expectedness. The same version of the RSI as the initial report should be used for follow-up reports, and SUSARs should not be downgraded on the basis that the RSI was updated.

V. Changes to Reference Safety Information

If there are changes to the RSI during the drug clinical trial, the sponsor should fully assess the impact on the safety of the subjects in accordance with the regulations. If the sponsor believes that it will not affect the safety of the subjects, the change can be directly implemented and reported in the DSUR.

It is recommended to update the RSI section of the IB once per year in accordance with the annual reporting cycle of DSUR. To identify SUSARs in the "Cumulative Summary Tabulations of Serious Adverse Reactions" in the DSUR, the sponsor should use the current version of the RSI at the beginning of the annual reporting cycle.

In some cases, the sponsor or regulatory authority may deem it necessary to make an emergency update to the safety information in the IB, and in this case, an emergency update can be made to the safety information in other sections of the IB (e.g., "Effects in the Humans" or "Summary of Data and Guidance of Investigator"). The sponsor may consider making changes to the RSI while preparing and writing the DSUR (after analysis and assessment of the SUSARs) rather than making multiple updates during the reporting period.

VI. Quality Management System for Reference Safety Information

The sponsor should clarify the RSI implementation and change management procedures (including but not limited to clear change management and traceability procedures, and the implementation time of RSI, etc.) and keep relevant documentation. In addition, the impact of MedDRA version updates on the RSI should be assessed.

VII. Circumstances Where Reference Can Be Made to the Adverse Reactions in the Package Inserts of Marketed Medicines for Reference Safety Information

For the RSI of clinical trials of medicines that have been marketed abroad but not marketed in China, if the indications are consistent with those approved overseas, reference can be made to SARs in the package inserts of marketed medicines. If the indications are different from those approved overseas or new indications are added to domestically marketed medicines, the sponsor should justify its use of the SARs in the approved indications as the RSI.

For generic medicines/biosimilar medicines, if there is evidence to prove that they are consistent with/biosimilar to the reference medicine, reference can be made to the RSI of the reference medicine.

VIII. Reference Safety Information for Combination Therapy

In clinical trials of combination therapy, the sponsor may formulate new RSI based on experience with combinations of the same active pharmaceutical ingredient in previous clinical trials, or refer to the RSI of each individual medicine.

IX. References

[1] EU. Clinical Trials Regulation (EU) NO 536/2014 Draft Questions & Answers Version 4.1. https://ec.europa.eu/health/sites/default/files/files/eudralex/vol-10/regulation5362014_qa_en.pdf.

[2] CTFG. Q&A document - Reference Safety Information. https://www.hma.eu/fileadmin/dateien/Human_Medicines/01-About_HMA/Working_Groups/CTFG/2017_11_CTFG_Question_and_Answer_on_Reference_Safety_

Information_2017.pdf.

[3] ICH. Clinical Safety Data Management: Definitions and Standards for Expedited Reporting E2A. https://database.ich.org/sites/default/files/E2A_Guideline.pdf.

[4] ICH. Development Safety Update Report E2F. https://database.ich.org/sites/default/files/E2F_Guideline.pdf.

[5] CDE. Notice on Issuing the Standard and Procedure for Expedited Reporting of Safety Data During Drug Clinical Trials https://www.cde.org.cn/main/news/viewInfoCommon/f86be6d655db5c711fe660bef22c3bf1.

[6] CDE. Notice on Issuing the Rules for the Management of Development Safety Update Report (Trial). https://www.cde.org.cn/main/news/viewInfoCommon/afced30f3c45431f04b47a7f3faee971.

[7] EC. A Guideline on Summary of Product Characteristics (SmPC). https://ec.europa.eu/health/sites/default/files/files/eudralex/vol-2/c/smpc_guideline_rev2_en.pdf.

X. Example

This example serves solely as a reference form of RSI. The sponsor may adjust the relevant content and format as appropriate on the basis of complying with these Guidelines.

Reference Safety Information

This chapter/section only provides an overview of expected SARs for the purpose of expedited reporting SUSARs to regulatory authorities and identifying SUSARs in the "Cumulative Summary Tabulations of Serious Adverse Reactions" of the DSUR, and does not provide a comprehensive overview of the safety profile of the investigational drug X. For more safety information, see Chapter X.

All fatal and life-threatening SARs of the investigational drug X are considered unexpected and will be submitted as SUSARs.

Table 1 Expected SARs of the investigational drug X for
safety reporting purposes

SOC	SARs	Frequency category[1]	Number of subjects exposed $(N)^2$=328
			All SARs
			n (%)
Gastro-intestinal disorders	Intestinal perforation	Common	9 (2.7)
Tests	Alanine aminotransferase increase	Common	12 (3.6)
	Aspartate aminotransferase increase	Common	9 (2.7)
Cardiac disorders	Myocarditis	Very common	33 (10.0)
	Bradycardia	Rare	(Rare)[3]

SOC: System Organ Class; SARs: Serious Adverse Reactions; n: Number of subjects who have experienced the SAR.

Notes: 1: Frequency category: Very common (≥ 1/10); common (≥ 1/100 to <1/10); uncommon (≥ 1/1000 to <1/100); rare (≥ 1/10000 to <1/1000); very rare (<1/10000).

2: Include Study 1, Study 2...

3: Bradycardia is derived from post-market safety information, and frequency categories are provided according to the methods in the *Guide for Spontaneous Reporting of Adverse Reactions*.

MedDRA Version 24.0, data lock date: May 1, 2021, based on Global Safety Database.

研究者手册中安全性参考信息撰写
技术指导原则

一、概述

安全性参考信息（Reference Safety Information，RSI）通常是研究者手册（Investigator's Brochure，IB）中的一个预期严重不良反应的列表。申办者应根据 RSI 评估临床试验期间发生的所有可疑严重不良反应的预期性。

本指导原则旨在指导获准开展药物（包括中药、化学药及生物制品）临床试验的 IB 中 RSI 的撰写。应用本指导原则时，请同时参考国际人用药品注册技术协调会（International Council for Harmonisation of Technical Requirements for Pharmaceuticals for Human Use，ICH）《E2A：临床安全性数据的管理：快速报告定义和标准》、《E2F：研发期间安全性更新报告》指导原则等。

本指导原则仅代表药品监管部门当前的观点和认识，不具有强制性的法律约束力。随着科学研究的进展，本指导原则中的相关内容将不断完善与更新。本指导原则为撰写安全性参考信息的一般考虑，尚不能涵盖所有情形。如有未能阐明的个性化问题，可与药审中心进行沟通。

二、安全性参考信息的内容

（一）预期严重不良反应

预期严重不良反应为已完成和正在进行的药物临床试验中观察到的至少发生一次的严重不良事件，经申办者充分和全面评估后，有合理证据证实其与试验药物存在因果关系，如通过比较临床试验中严重不良事件的发生频率，或对个例报告的因果关系进行充分的评估。仅基于药理学特性预期可能发生，但尚未在试验药物中观察到的不良反应不作为预期不良反应，可参见 IB 的其它章节（如"人体内作用"或"数据概要和研究者指南"）。

一般情况下，仅发生过一次的可疑严重不良反应不足以列入 RSI，除非基于申办者的医学判断，存在有力的证据证实其与试验药物存在明确的因果关系，且需提供相关支持证据。并且，不是所有发生超过一次的可疑严重不良反应均可作为预期严重不良反应列入 RSI，需由申办者进行充分和全面的评估，在增加预期严重不良反应的同时提供相关支持证据。

考虑目前存在多种因果关系评价方法，允许使用一种或多种方法评价临床试验中发生的不良事件与试验药物是否存在因果关系。根据 ICHE2A，药物不良反应是试验药物与不良事件至少存在合理的可能性，即因果关系无法排除。因此，应谨慎评估"可能无关"的因果关系。如果研究者无法判断不良事件与试验药物的相关性（即"无法评价"），申办者应与研究者沟通并鼓励其对相关性进行评估。如果判断结果仍然为"无法评价"，该严重不良事件应被认为与试验药物相关并报告为可疑且非预期严重不良反应（Suspected Unexpected Serious Adverse Reaction，SUSAR）。但是，不支持将"无法评价"的严重不良事件作为预期严重不良反应列入 RSI。

（二）致死和 / 或危及生命的严重不良反应

一般情况下，申办者不应预计试验药物会出现致死和 / 或危及生命的严重不良反应。因此，即使之前发生过致死和 / 或危及生命的严重不良反应，其通常被认为是非预期的。但已上市药品的说明书中载明致死的严重不良反应可作为预期严重不良反应。因此，对于尚未上市的试验药物，RSI 中不应包含致死的严重不良反应。

如果 RSI 中包含致死和 / 或危及生命的预期严重不良反应，应在列表中单独列出此类严重不良反应的数量和发生频率。其它被视为非预期的致死和 / 或危及生命的可疑严重不良反应可参见 IB 中"人体内作用"或"数据概要和研究者指南"章节。

（三）因特异性和 / 或严重程度视为非预期的情形

不强制要求在 RSI 中使用不良事件通用术语标准（Common Terminology Criteria for Adverse Events，CTCAE）进行严重程度分级。但是，如果个例报告中可疑严重不良反应的特异性和 / 或严重程度与 RSI 中预期严重不良反应不同，即可疑严重不良反应比 RSI 中预期严重不良反应更具特异性和 / 或严重程度更高时，该可疑严重不良反应被认为是非预期的（参见表 1）。

表 1　SUSAR 举例及其报告原因

RSI 中列出的严重 不良反应	个例报告中的可疑 严重不良反应	因特异性和 / 或严重 程度视为非预期
急性肾衰竭	间质性肾炎	特异性
肝炎	暴发性肝炎	严重程度
脑血管意外	脑血栓栓塞	特异性

续表

RSI 中列出的严重 不良反应	个例报告中的可疑 严重不良反应	因特异性和 / 或严重 程度视为非预期
剥脱性皮炎	史蒂文斯 – 约翰逊综合征	严重程度和特异性
肝脏功能检查值短暂升高	肝脏功能检查值升高持续数月	严重程度
高血压	高血压危象	严重程度
带状疱疹	多发性皮肤带状疱疹	严重程度
脓毒症	感染性休克	严重程度
室上性心律失常	房颤	特异性

注：上述举例仅阐述更具特异性和 / 或严重程度更高的情形，非 RSI 中预期严重不良反应的首选语（Preferred Term，PT）。

如果可疑严重不良反应的发生频率高于 RSI 中预期严重不良反应的发生频率，该可疑严重不良反应视为非预期。

建议由申办者经过培训的专业人员对可疑严重不良反应的特异性和 / 或严重程度进行医学和科学的评估。

（四）安全性参考信息中不应包含的安全性信息

以下安全性信息不应包含在 RSI 中，但可参见 IB 中"人体内作用"或"数据概要和研究者指南"章节。

例如：

（1）研究者和申办者均认为与试验药物无关的不良事件，包括严重不良事件和非严重不良事件；

（2）非严重的不良反应；

（3）非预期的严重不良反应；

（4）仅发生过一次的严重不良反应，且无法提供基于医学判断的有力证据证实其与试验药物存在明确的因果关系；

（5）试验方案中，死亡事件和严重不良事件常作为疗效终点，被认为与疾病相关，不作为 SUSAR 报告。但是，如果试验药物增强了不良事件的严重程度，或增加了不良事件的发生频率，应谨慎评估；

（6）基于药理学特性预期发生的、同类其它药物已经发生的，但尚未在本试验药物中观察到的严重不良反应。

三、安全性参考信息的呈现形式

（一）位置

RSI 的标题为"安全性参考信息"，位于"数据概要和研究者指南"章，或单独作为一章置于"数据概要和研究者指南"章之后。

申办者应明确指出 RSI 以向监管部门报告为目的，总结了试验药物当前的预期严重不良反应，且 RSI 并未全面概述试验药物的安全性特征。

（二）呈现形式

RSI 应以表格形式呈现，使用监管活动医学词典（Medical Dictionary for Regulatory Activities，MedDRA）最新版本的系统器官分类（System Organ Class，SOC）和 PT 来描述"预期严重不良反应"的性质。汇总先前观察到的可疑严重不良反应，计算其发生频率。发生频率类别可参考说明书中不良反应发生频率的分类（如十分常见、常见、偶见等）。当暴露于试验药物的受试者数量较少，无法进行分类或观察到的预期严重不良反应的数量较少时，应提供每个"预期严重不良反应"的数量以及暴露的受试者数量（参见表 2）。

表 2　以安全性报告为目的的试验药物的预期严重不良反应

SOC	SARs	暴露的受试者数量（N）=328		
		所有 SARs	致死 SARs[1]	危及生命 SARs[1]
		n（%）	n（%）	n（%）
胃肠系统疾病	肠穿孔	9（2.7）	3（0.9）	6（1.8）
各类检查	丙氨酸氨基转移酶升高	12（3.6）	NA	NA
	天门冬氨酸氨基转移酶升高	9（2.7）	NA	NA
心脏器官疾病	心肌炎	33（10.0）	NA	2（0.6）
	心动过缓	（罕见）[2]	NA	NA

注：SOC 系统器官分类；SARs 严重不良反应；n 发生 SAR 的受试者数量；NA 不适用

注 1：在特殊情况下，如果认为试验药物存在致死和 / 或危及生命的预期严重不良反应，应在表中明确列出。其它的非预期的致死和 / 或危及生命严重不良反应（行），可填写"不适用"，并在脚注中说明非预期的致死和 / 或危及生命的严重不良反应可参考 IB 的其它章节。如果认为试验药物无致死和 / 或危及生命的预期严重不良反应，则需在 RSI 的文字部分单独说明，表格中无需列出相应的列。

注 2：心动过缓来源于上市后安全性信息，根据自发报告不良反应指南中的方法提供发生频率类别。

RSI 中可包含上市后观察到的严重不良反应，但发生频率不应填写"未知"。由于上市后无法获知真实的发生频率类别，因此，应提供每个严重不良反应的报告数量，也可按照自发报告不良反应指南中的方法提供发生频率类别[1]（参见表 2）。

如果申办者正在针对试验药物进行不同适应症（如肿瘤、非肿瘤疾病）或不同人群（如成人、儿童）的临床开发，若其预期严重不良反应不同，应按适应症或人群单独列出 RSI。

（三）预期严重不良反应的术语

预期严重不良反应不应使用广义的医学术语或非特定的术语，如"皮疹"、"感染"或"心律失常"。应使用 MedDRA 的 PT，如剥脱性皮炎、荨麻疹、带状疱疹、感染性肺炎、脓毒症、房颤。如果 RSI 中的 PT 包含多个低位语（Lowest Level Term，LLT），则多个 LLT 均视为预期（如 RSI 包含 PT 低磷酸血症，则 LLT 血磷酸盐过少也视为预期）。已知免疫抑制的药物可能导致感染，但不能认为所有类型的感染都是预期的。除非 RSI 列出具体感染类型的 PT，否则均应被视为非预期。

同义医学术语表示同一医学现象，如果 RSI 包含一个术语，其它同义医学术语均视为预期。但对于同一种医学现象的不同类型，如不同类型的皮疹，即普通皮疹、斑丘疹、丘疹样皮疹、脓疱疹等，须使用特定的 PT。

（四）尚未发现预期严重不良反应的安全性参考信息

在某些情况下，试验药物预计可能不会导致任何严重不良反应（如在试验药物临床开发早期，暴露的受试者数量较少时），但 IB 中仍应有一个单独的 RSI 章节，其可以是一段简要的描述，说明为了向监管部门快速报告 SUSAR，并在研发期间安全性更新报告（Development Safety Update Report，DSUR）的"严重不良反应累计汇总表"中识别 SUSAR，截止到目前，申办者认为尚未发现预期严重不良反应。

四、安全性参考信息的适用版本

应使用可疑严重不良反应发生时的现行版 RSI 判断其预期性。随访报告使用与初始报告相同版本的 RSI，申办者不应以更新版 RSI 为依据降低 SUSAR 的等级。

2　产品特性概要（SmPC）指南，2009 年 9 月，第二版 https://ec.europa.eu/health/sites/default/files/files/eudralex/vol-2/c/smpc_guideline_rev2_en.pdf

五、安全性参考信息的变更

药物临床试验期间发生 RSI 的变更，申办者应当按照规定，充分评估对受试者安全的影响，认为不影响受试者安全的，可以直接实施并在 DSUR 中报告。

可根据 DSUR 的年度报告周期每年更新一次 IB 的 RSI。为了在 DSUR 的"严重不良反应累计汇总表"中识别 SUSAR，申办者应使用在年度报告周期开始时的现行版 RSI。

在某些情况下，申办者或监管部门可能认为需要紧急更新 IB 中的安全性信息，可在 IB 的其它章节（如"人体内作用"或"数据概要和研究者指南"）对安全性信息进行紧急更新。RSI 的变更可考虑在准备和撰写 DSUR 时（对 SUSAR 进行分析和评估后）进行，而非在报告周期内进行多次更新。

六、安全性参考信息的质量管理体系

申办者应明确 RSI 的实施及变更管理程序（包括但不限于清晰的变更管理及追溯流程，RSI 的实施时间等）并保留相关文件记录。此外，应评估 MedDRA 版本的更新对 RSI 产生的影响。

七、安全性参考信息参考已上市药品说明书中不良反应的情形

境外已上市境内未上市药物临床试验的 RSI，若适应症与境外已批准适应症一致，可参考已上市药品说明书中的严重不良反应。若适应症与境外已批准适应症不同或境内已上市药品增加新适应症的，如申办者仍使用已批准适应症说明书中的严重不良反应作为 RSI，应说明其合理性。

对于仿制药/生物类似药，若有证据证实其与参照药具有一致性/生物相似性，可参考参照药的 RSI。

八、联合用药的安全性参考信息

在联合用药临床试验中，申办者可以根据先前试验中相同活性药物联合用药的经验制订新的 RSI，或参考各单药的 RSI。

九、参考文献

［1］EU. Clinical Trials Regulation（EU）NO 536/2014 Draft Questions &

Answers Version 4.1.https://ec.europa.eu/health/sites/default/files/files/eudralex/vol-10/regulation5362014_qa_en.pdf.

［2］CTFG.Q&Adocument –Reference Safety Information. https://www.hma.eu/fileadmin/dateien/Human_Medicines/01–About_HMA/Working_Groups/CTFG/2017_11_CTFG_Question_and_Answer_on_Reference_Safety_Information_2017.pdf.

［3］ICH. Clinical Safety Data Management: Definitions and Standards for Expedited Reporting E2A. https://database.ich.org/sites/default/files/E2A_Guideline.pdf.

［4］ICH. Development Safety Update Report E2F. https://database.ich.org/sites/default/files/E2F_Guideline.pdf.

［5］CDE. 关于发布《药物临床试验期间安全性数据快速报告的标准和程序》的通知. https://www.cde.org.cn/main/news/viewInfoCommon/f86be6d655db5c711fe660bef22c3bf1.

［6］CDE. 关于发布《研发期间安全性更新报告管理规范（试行）》的通告. https://www.cde.org.cn/main/news/viewInfoCommon/afced30f3c45431f04b47a7f3faee971.

［7］EC. A Guideline on Summary of Product Characteristics（SmPC）. https://ec.europa.eu/health/sites/default/files/files/eudralex/vol–2/c/smpc_guideline_rev2_en.pdf.

示例：本示例仅是 RSI 的一种呈现形式，申办者可在符合指导原则的基础上酌情调整相关内容和格式。

安全性参考信息

本章 / 节仅概述了以向监管部门快速报告 SUSAR，并在 DSUR 的"严重不良反应累计汇总表"中识别 SUSAR 为目的的预期严重不良反应，并未全面概述试验药物 X 的安全性特征，更多安全性信息详见第 X 章。

试验药物 X 所有致死和危及生命的严重不良反应均视为非预期，将作为 SUSAR 递交。

表 1　以安全性报告为目的的试验药物 X 的预期严重不良反应

SOC	SARs	发生频率类别[1]	暴露的受试者数量（N）[2]=328
			所有 SARs
			n（%）
胃肠系统疾病	肠穿孔	常见	9（2.7）
各类检查	丙氨酸氨基转移酶升高	常见	12（3.6）
	天门冬氨酸氨基转移酶升高	常见	9（2.7）
心脏器官疾病	心肌炎	十分常见	33（10.0）
	心动过缓	罕见	（罕见）[3]

SOC 系统器官分类；SARs 严重不良反应；n 发生 SAR 的受试者数量

注 1：发生频率类别：十分常见（≥ 1/10）；常见（≥ 1/100 至＜ 1/10）；偶见（≥ 1/1000 至＜ 1/100）；罕见（≥ 1/10000 至＜ 1/1000）；十分罕见（＜ 1/10000）。

2：包含研究 1、研究 2……。

3：心动过缓来源于上市后安全性信息，根据自发报告不良反应指南中的方法提供发生频率类别。

MedDRA 版本 24.0，数据锁定日期 2021 年 5 月 1 日，基于全球安全性数据库。

Guideline for Naming of Generic Names of Chinese Proprietary Medicines

I. Overview

This guideline is hereby formulated for the purpose of strengthening registration management, standardizing naming of Chinese Proprietary Medicines (CPMs), embodying characteristics of traditional Chinese medicine (TCM), showing respect for culture, and inheriting the tradition.

This Guideline is based on previous technical requirements and principles for naming of generic names of traditional Chinese medicines (TCMs), under the current situation of naming of CPMs, and also in combination with new progress in studies on the naming of CPMs in recent years.

II. Basic Principles

(I) Scientific, concise and avoiding duplication

1. Generic names of CPMs should be scientific, clear, short, and unambiguous, avoiding the use of obscure terms. The names should generally consist of not more than 8 characters (except for ethno-medicine, which may adopt the conventional translated name in Chinese).

2. Vulgar or superstitious language should not be used.

3. The names should clearly indicate the dosage form which should be placed at the end of the names.

4. The name of a CPM, except for its dosage form, should not duplicate the existing generic names to avoid the occurrence of different formulas with identical name or identical formula with different names.

(II) Normative naming and avoiding exaggeration of efficacy

1. Generally, names of people, places, enterprises, or endangered animals

and plants should not be used.

2. Names that use code names or homophonic words with specific inherent meanings should not be adopted, such as X0X and homophonic words of celebrities' names, etc.

3. The names should not be derived from terms related to modern medicine, pharmacology, anatomy, physiology, pathology or therapeutics, such as cancer, anti-inflammation, glucose-lowering, anti-hypertensive, and lipid-lowering, etc.

4. The names should not be exaggerated, self-praising and unrealistic terms, such as strong, quick-acting, made by the emperor's order, secretly-made, as well as "Ling" (miracle), "Bao" (treasure) and "Jing" (essence), etc. (except for names containing full name of TCM crude drugs and TCM terms).

(III) Embodying characteristics of traditional culture

Incorporating traditional cultural characteristics into the naming of TCM formulas is one of the TCM cultural characteristics. Therefore, the naming of CPMs can draw on the advantages of ancient formula naming combined with aesthetic concepts, making the names of CPMs both scientific and standardized, and reflective of traditional Chinese cultural heritage. However, the culturally characteristic terms used in the names should have clear literature basis or recognized cultural origins, and should avoid exaggerating the efficacy.

III. Naming of Single-ingredient Preparation

1. Generally, the names should consist of TCM crude drugs, prepared slices/decoction pieces, active components, and medicinal parts, plus the dosage forms, such as Huaruishi Powder, Danshen Oral Liquid, and Bajitian Guatang Capsule, etc.

2. The names could consist of active components, medicinal parts and their functions plus the dosage forms.

3. The names of artificially manufactured products of TCM crude drugs should differ from those natural ones, and generally should not be named as "Artificial XX" plus the dosage form.

IV. Naming of Compound Preparation

Compound preparations of CPMs could be named as the following:

1. The names should be formed by using abbreviations of the main TCM crude drugs in the formula plus the dosage form. The abbreviations should not be combined to form meanings that violate other naming requirements. Examples include Xianglian Pills, formulated by Muxiang (*Aucklandiae Radix*) and Huanglian (*Coptidis Rhizoma*); Guifu Dihuang Pills, formulated by Rougui (*Cinnamomi Cortex*), Fuzi (*Aconiti Lateralis*), Shudihuang (*Rehmanniae Radix Praeparata*), Shanyao (*Dioscoreae Rhizoma*), Shanzhuyu (*Corni Fructus*), Fuling (*Poria*), Danpi (*Moutan Cotex*), and Zexie (*Alismatis Rhizoma*); and Gegen Qinlian Tablets, formulated by Gegen (*Puerariae Lobatae Racis*), Huangqin (*Scutellariae Radix*), Huanglian (*Cortidis Rhizoma*), and Gancao (*Glycyrrhizae Radix Et Rhizoma*).

2. The names can be formed by the primary functions (using only TCM terminology to describe the functions, the same below) plus the dosage form. In this type of naming, the functions can be used directly for naming. Examples include Buzhong Yiqi Mixture (invigorating spleen-stomach and replenishing qi), Chutan Zhisou Pills (dispelling phlegm and relieving cough), Buxin Pills (tonifying heart), and Dingzhi Pills (settling mind), etc.; formula functions can also be conveyed through various rhetorical devices such as metaphor, pun, metonymy and antithesis, etc., such as Jiaotai Pills, Yunu Brew, Yuehua Pills, and Yupingfeng Powder, etc. Examples are as follows:

(1) Naming with metaphor. Based on the similarity between things, using concrete, simple and familiar things to explain abstract, profound and unfamiliar things, such as Yupingfeng Powder and Yuehua Pills, etc.

Yupingfeng Powder: "pingfeng"(screen) symbolizes guarding the skin surface and defend against exogenous evil (wind). The name "Yupingfeng" uses "pingfeng" to represent the screen of human body's defense against external factors, reflecting traditional cultural depth and embodies the characteristics of image thinking in the TCM.

Yuehua Pills: "Yuehua" (moonlight) refers to the moon or its halo. This formula nourishes yin and moisturizes the lungs, treating the consumption-related diseases. Since the lung is associated with yin and serves as the canopy of the five internal organs, similar to the shining moon, the formula is named "Yuehua Pills".

(2) Naming with pun. In a certain linguistic context, puns take advantage of the polysemy or homophone of the words to deliberately give sentences a double meaning, with the intention of conveying one meaning while alluding to another, such as Didang Decoction, etc.

Didang Decoction consists of *Hirudo, Tabanus, Persicae Semen* and *Rhei Radix Et Rhizoma*. It is used to treat symptoms caused by blood stasis in the lower Jiao, such as abdominal fullness and pain, spontaneous urination, yellow body such as jaundice, mania and others by purgating blood stasis. "Didang" might be alias for the main ingredient, *Hirudo*, but more often it means "washing away", indicating that this formula can wash away and purge blood stasis.

(3) Naming with metonymy. Use one thing to substitute another, such as Gengyi Pills, etc.

Gengyi Pills contain *Cinnabaris* and *Aloe*, and should be taken orally with yellow rice wine. It plays the function of purging intense heat and relaxing the bowels, and is used to treat dryness in intestines and stomach, constipation, restlessness and irritability, and disturbed sleep. "Gengyi" is the euphemism for urination and defection in ancient times; therefore, use "Gengyi" to substitute "go to the toilet" is not only elegant but also clarifies the meaning of the formula.

(4) Naming with antithesis. Use two phrases or sentences with the same structure, equal number of characters, and symmetric meaning to express opposite, similar or relevant meanings, such as Xiexin Daochi Powder, etc.

Xiexin Daochi Powder acts to alleviate excessive heat within the heart and spleen. This formula is commonly employed to address oral ulcers stemming from excessive heat in these organs. The terms "Xiexin" (indicating heat-purging within the heart) and "Daochi" (signifying heat-draining) are skillfully combined, creating a concept of "positive antithesis". This linguistic pairing suggests that these terms share akin or comparable meanings that synergistically enhance one another.

3. Naming with the number of drug ingredients plus the dosage form, such as Siwu Decoction, etc.

Siwu Decoction is a representative formula of blood tonic made up of four ingredients, namely *Angelica Sinensis Radix*, *Chuanxiong Rhizoma*, *Paeoniae Radix Alba* and *Rehmanniae Radix Praeparata*.

4. Naming with dosage (dosage in the formula, dosage ratio of TCM crude drugs in the formula, single dose) plus the dosage form, such as Qili Powder and Liuyi Powder, etc.

Qili Powder acts to disperse blood stasis and reduce swelling, alleviate pain and stopping bleeding. Overdose of this formula is prone to consume and damage healthy qi of the body, thus it cannot be taken at a great dose for a long time. Therefore, it is named after the dose per time which is only "qili" (seven "li", "li" is a traditional Chinese unit of weight).

Liuyi Powder is made of *Talci Pulvis* and *Glycyrrhizae Radix Et Rhizoma* at the ratio of 6:1. "Liuyi" literally means "six to one", hence the name.

5. Naming with the color of the TCM crude drugs plus the dosage form. Formulas named after colors are mostly due to the distinctive color of the finished products, leaving a deep impression on people. Therefore, these formulas are named accordingly to facilitate promotion and application, such as Taohua Decoction, etc.

Taohua Decoction consists of one catty of *Halloysitum Rubrum*, one liang (a traditional Chinese unit of weight) of *Zingiberis Rhizoma* and one catty of polished round-grained rice. Due to the red and white color, *Halloysitum Rubrum* is also known as Taohua stone (peach blossom stone). After being boiled, the decoction is light red, resembling fresh peach blossoms, hence the name Taohua Decoction (peach blossom decoction).

6. Naming after the time of administration plus the dosage form, such as Jiming Powder, etc.

Jiming Powder: "Jiming" refers to the time when rooster crows. This formula must be taken on an empty stomach in the early morning, hence the name "Jiming Powder".

7. Naming with sovereign or primary TCM crude drugs plus functions and the dosage form, such as Longdanxiegan Pills and Danggui Buxue Decoction, etc.

Longdan Xiegan Pills acts to purge liver and gallbladder fire and remove lower-Jiao damp heat. The sovereign crude drug in the formula, Longdan (*Gentianae Radix et Rhizoma*), plays a key role in purging liver and gallbladder fire.

Danggui Buxue Decoction plays the role of tonifying qi and nourishing blood. The primary TCM crude drug in the formula, Danggui (*Angelicae Sinensis Radix*), plays the role of benefiting blood and nutrition.

8. Naming with the number of ingredients and names of primary TCM crude drugs, or naming with the number of ingredients and functions or usage plus the dosage form, such as Wuling Powder and Sansheng Decoction, etc.

Wuling Powder consists of five TCM crude drugs, namely *Polyporus, Alismatis Rhizoma, Atractylodis Macrocephalae Rhizoma, Poria* and *Cinnamomni Ramulus*, and it gets its name since it contains two "Ling", namely "Zhuling" (*Polyporus*) and "Fuling (*Poria*)".

The formula of Sansheng Decoction consists of *Aconiti Kusnezoffii Radix, Magnoliae Officinalis Cortex*, and *Glycyrrhizae Radix et Rhizoma*, all of which are used in a no processing or simple processing state ("sheng"). *Glycyrrhizae Radix Et Rhizoma* is mostly used in the state of "sheng", but *Aconiti Kusnezoffii Radix* is mostly processed before use. Different from other formulas, this formula is unique in its emphasis on using all TCM crude drugs in the state of "sheng".

9. Naming with the source of formula (excluding the dynasty), and functions or TCM crude drugs, plus the dosage form, such as Zhimi Fuling Pills, etc.

Many formulas contain "Fuling Pills" in their names. Zhimi Fuling Pills refer to the Fuling Pills coming from *Quansheng Zhimi Formulas*. The term

"Zhimi" distinguishes this particular formula based on its source, among other similar formulas.

10. Naming with functions and action sites of the medicine (TCM term) plus the dosage form, such as Wendan Decoction, Yangyin Qingfei Pills (nourishing yin and clearing lung-heat), Qingre Xiepi Powder (clearing heat and purging spleen-fire), Qingwei Powder (clearing stomach), Shaofu Zhuyu Decoction (expelling lower abdomen stasis), and Huazhi Rougan Capsules (dissolving stasis and nourishing liver) etc.

11. Naming with the primary TCM crude drugs and guiding medicine plus the dosage form, such as Chuanxiong Chatiao Powder, which gets its name since it is taken together with cha (tea).

12. Naming of pediatric drugs may contain clinical department name of the drugs, such as Xiao'er Xiaoshi Tablets (children's indigestion) etc.

13. The names can also include the usage of the medicine, such as Xiao'er Fuqi Zhixie Power (compressing children's navel and anti-diarrheal), Hanhua Shangqing Pills (for buccal administration), and Waiyong Zijin Troches (for external use), etc.

14. While adhering to naming principles, formula names can reflect concepts such as yin-yang, the five elements, ancient academic school thoughts, and names of ancient items, etc., to highlight characteristics of traditional Chinese culture, such as Zuojin Pills and Yuquan Pills, etc.

Zuojin Pills have the effects of clearing and purifying liver fire and descending the adverse qi to stopping vomiting. The heart pertains to fire, liver to wood, and the lungs to metal. The liver is located on the right side of the body, but has the qi running on the left. When liver wood is restrained by lung metal, normal process of growth and transformation are maintained. By clearing the heart fire and assisting the lung metal (jin), the liver on the left (zuo) is regulated, hence the name "Zuojin Pills".

Yuquan Pills have the effects of tonifying qi and nourishing yin, and clearing heat and generating fluids. "Yuquan" is a beautiful name for spring water and also refers to the fluids from the acupoint Lian Quan (RN23) under the tongue. This formula consists of several ingredients that nourish yin, moisten dryness, supplement qi and generate fluids. Upon administration, the yin fluids become replenished, and the fluids return naturally, keeping the mouth constantly moist, much like an inexhaustible source of spring water, hence the name "Yuquan Pills".

中成药通用名称命名技术指导原则

一、概述

为加强注册管理，规范中成药的命名，体现中医药特色，尊重文化，继承传统，特制定本指导原则。

本指导原则是在既往中药通用名命名的技术要求、原则的基础上，根据中成药命名现状，结合近年来有关中成药命名的研究新进展而制定。

二、基本原则

（一）"科学简明，避免重名"原则

1. 中成药通用名称应科学、明确、简短、不易产生歧义和误导，避免使用生涩用语。一般字数不超过 8 个字（民族药除外，可采用约定俗成的汉译名）。

2. 不应采用低俗、迷信用语。

3. 名称中应明确剂型，且剂型应放在名称最后。

4. 名称中除剂型外，不应与已有中成药通用名重复，避免同名异方、同方异名的产生。

（二）"规范命名，避免夸大疗效"原则

1. 一般不应采用人名、地名、企业名称或濒危受保护动、植物名称命名。

2. 不应采用代号、固有特定含义名词的谐音命名。如：X0X、名人名字的谐音等。

3. 不应采用现代医学药理学、解剖学、生理学、病理学或治疗学的相关用语命名。如：癌、消炎、降糖、降压、降脂等。

4. 不应采用夸大、自诩、不切实际的用语。如：强力、速效、御制、秘制以及灵、宝、精等（名称中含药材名全称及中医术语的除外）。

（三）"体现传统文化特色"原则

将传统文化特色赋予中药方剂命名是中医药的文化特色之一，因此，中成药命名可借鉴古方命名充分结合美学观念的优点，使中成药的名称既科学规范，又体现一定的中华传统文化底蕴。但是，名称中所采用的具有文化特色的用语应当具有明确的文献依据或公认的文化渊源，并避免夸大疗效。

三、单味制剂命名

1.一般应采用中药材、中药饮片、中药有效成份、中药有效部位加剂型命名。如：花蕊石散、丹参口服液、巴戟天寡糖胶囊等。

2.可采用中药有效成份、中药有效部位与功能结合剂型命名。

3.中药材人工制成品的名称应与天然品的名称有所区别，一般不应以"人工XX"加剂型命名。

四、复方制剂命名

中成药复方制剂根据处方组成的不同情况可酌情采用下列方法命名。

1.采用处方主要药材名称的缩写加剂型命名，但其缩写不能组合成违反其他命名要求的含义。如：香连丸，由木香、黄连组成；桂附地黄丸由肉桂、附子、熟地黄、山药、山茱萸、茯苓、丹皮、泽泻组成；葛根芩连片由葛根、黄芩、黄连、甘草组成。

2.采用主要功能（只能采用中医术语表述功能，下同）加剂型命名。该类型命名中，可直接以功能命名，如：补中益气合剂、除痰止嗽丸、补心丹、定志丸等；也可采用比喻、双关、借代、对偶等各种修辞手法来表示方剂功能，如：交泰丸、玉女煎、月华丸、玉屏风散等。示例如下：

（1）采用比喻修辞命名，即根据事物的相似点，用具体的、浅显的、熟知的事物来说明抽象的、深奥的、生疏的事物的修辞手法。如：玉屏风散、月华丸等。

玉屏风散："屏风"二字，取其固卫肌表，抵御外邪（风）之义。"玉屏风"之名，以屏风指代人体抵御外界的屏障，具浓郁的传统文化气息，体现了中医形象思维的特质。

月华丸："月华"，古人指月亮或月亮周围的光环。本方能滋阴润肺，治疗肺痨之病。因肺属阴，为五藏之华盖，犹如月亮之光彩华美，故名"月华丸"。

（2）采用双关修辞命名，即在一定的语言环境中，利用词的多义或同音的条件，有意使语句具有双重意义，言在此而意在彼。如：抵当汤等。

抵当汤，由水蛭、虻虫、桃仁、大黄组成。用于下焦蓄血所致之少腹满痛，小便自利，身黄如疸，精神发狂等症。有攻逐蓄血之功。"抵当"可能是主药水蛭之别名，但更多意义上是通"涤荡"，意指此方具有涤荡攻逐瘀血之力。

（3）采用借代修辞命名，即借一物来代替另一物出现，如：更衣丸等。

更衣丸，由朱砂、芦荟组成，取酒和丸，用黄酒冲服，有泻火通便之功，用于治疗肠胃燥结，大便不通，心烦易怒，睡眠不安诸证。"更衣"，古时称大、小便之婉辞，方名更衣。以更衣代如厕，既不失文雅，又明了方义。

（4）采用对偶修辞，即用两个结构相同、字数相等、意义对称的词组或句子来表达相反、相似或相关意思的一种修辞方式。如：泻心导赤散等。

泻心导赤散，功能泻心脾积热，临床常用于治疗心脾积热的口舌生疮。"泻心"与"导赤"是属于对偶中的"正对偶"，前后表达的意思同类或相近，互为补充。

3.采用药物味数加剂型命名。如：四物汤等。

四物汤，由当归、川芎、白芍、熟地组成，为补血剂的代表方。

4.采用剂量（入药剂量、方中药物剂量比例、单次剂量）加剂型命名。如：七厘散、六一散等。

七厘散，具有散瘀消肿，定痛止血的功能。本方过服易耗伤正气，不宜大量久服，一般每次只服"七厘"，即以每次用量来命名。

六一散，则由滑石粉、甘草组成，两药剂量比例为6∶1，故名。

5.以药物颜色加剂型命名。以颜色来命名的方剂大多因成品颜色有一定的特征性，给人留下深刻的印象，故据此命名，便于推广与应用，如：桃花汤等。

桃花汤，方中药物组成为赤石脂一斤，干姜一两，粳米一斤，因赤石脂色赤白相间，别名桃花石，煎煮成汤后，其色淡红，鲜艳犹若桃花，故称桃花汤。

6.以服用时间加剂型命名。如：鸡鸣散等。

鸡鸣散，所谓"鸡鸣"，是指鸡鸣时分，此方须在清晨空腹时服下，故名"鸡鸣散"。

7.可采用君药或主要药材名称加功能及剂型命名。如：龙胆泻肝丸、当归补血汤等。

龙胆泻肝丸，具有泻肝胆经实火，除下焦湿热之功效。方中君药龙胆草，有泻肝胆实火作用。

当归补血汤，具有补气生血之功效。方中主药当归，有益血和营作用。

8.可采用药味数与主要药材名称，或者药味数与功能或用法加剂型命名。如：五苓散、三生饮等。

五苓散，方中有猪苓、泽泻、白术、茯苓、桂枝，同时含两个"苓"，故名。

三生饮，方中草乌、厚朴、甘草均生用，不需炮制，甘草生用较为常见，但草乌多炮制后入药，有别于其他方，强调诸药生用，是其特征。

9. 可采用处方来源（不包括朝代）与功能或药名加剂型命名。如：指迷茯苓丸等。

名称中含"茯苓丸"的方剂数量较多。指迷茯苓丸，是指来自于《全生指迷方》的茯苓丸，缀以"指迷"，意在从方剂来源区分之。

10. 可采用功能与药物作用的病位（中医术语）加剂型命名。如：温胆汤、养阴清肺丸、清热泻脾散、清胃散、少腹逐瘀汤、化滞柔肝胶囊等。

11. 可采用主要药材和药引结合并加剂型命名。如：川芎茶调散，以茶水调服，故名。

12. 儿科用药可加该药临床所用的科名，如：小儿消食片等。

13. 可在命名中加该药的用法，如：小儿敷脐止泻散、含化上清片、外用紫金锭等。

14. 在遵照命名原则条件下，命名可体现阴阳五行、古代学术派别思想、古代物品的名称等，以突出中国传统文化特色，如：左金丸、玉泉丸等。

左金丸，有清泻肝火，降逆止呕之功。心属火，肝属木，肺属金，肝位于右而行气于左，肝木得肺金所制则生化正常。清心火以佐肺金而制肝于左，所以名曰"左金丸"。

玉泉丸，有益气养阴，清热生津之效。"玉泉"为泉水之美称，亦指口中舌下两脉之津液。用数味滋阴润燥、益气生津之品组方，服之可使阴津得充，津液自回，口中津津常润，犹如玉泉之水，源源不断，故名"玉泉丸"。